P9-APB-933

HUMAN PARASITOLOGY

SECOND EDITION

HUMAN PARASITOLOGY

SECOND EDITION

Burton J. Bogitsh
Vanderbilt University
Nashville, Tennessee

Thomas C. Cheng
Marine Research Institute
Charleston, South Carolina

ACADEMIC PRESS
San Diego London Boston New York Sydney Tokyo Toronto

Cover photo credit: SEM of an intestinal villus. Courtesy of Dr. Robert L. Owen. ©1979 University of Chicago Press. For more details please see Figure 5-2c in the chapter "Visceral Protozoa II: Flagellates." For complete source reference, please see page 467.

This book is printed on acid-free paper. ♾

Academic Press
A Harcourt Science and Technology Company
525 B Street, Suite 1900, San Diego, California 92101-4495, USA
http://www.academicpress.com

Academic Press
Harcourt Place, 32 Jamestown Road, London NW17BY, UK
http://www.academicpress.com

Library of Congress Catalog Card Number: 98-84421

International Standard Book Number: 0-12-110870-8

PRINTED IN THE UNITED STATES OF AMERICA
03 QW 9 8 7 6 5 4

To Glenn and Libby,
who left us too soon.

Contents

PART ONE

THE PROTOZOA

Chapter Three

GENERAL CHARACTERISTICS OF THE PROTOZOA

Chapter Four

VISCERAL PROTOZOA I: AMOEBAE AND CILIATES

Chapter Five

VISCERAL PROTOZOA II: FLAGELLATES

Chapter Six

BLOOD AND TISSUE PROTOZOA I: HEMOFLAGELLATES

Chapter Seven
BLOOD AND TISSUE PROTOZOA II: HUMAN MALARIA

Chapter Eight
BLOOD AND TISSUE PROTOZOA III: OTHER APICOMPLEXANS

PART TWO
THE TREMATODA

Chapter Nine
GENERAL CHARACTERISTICS OF THE TREMATODA

Chapter Ten
VISCERAL FLUKES

Chapter Eleven
BLOOD FLUKES

PART THREE
THE CESTOIDEA

Chapter Twelve
GENERAL CHARACTERISTICS OF THE CESTOIDEA

Chapter Thirteen
INTESTINAL TAPEWORMS

Chapter Fourteen

EXTRAINTESTINAL TAPEWORMS

PART FOUR

THE NEMATODA

Chapter Fifteen

GENERAL CHARACTERISTICS OF THE NEMATODA

Chapter Sixteen

INTESTINAL NEMATODES

Chapter Seventeen

BLOOD AND TISSUE NEMATODES

PART FIVE

ARTHROPODA

Chapter Eighteen

ARTHROPODS AS VECTORS

Preface to the Second Edition

Several years ago, we recognized the need for a textbook of human parasitology designed specifically for premedical, medical technology, and biology students who required basic knowledge of the biology of parasitism, and we began to consider collaborating on such a text. As the idea germinated, we decided that, while emphasizing the medical aspects of the topic, the book should incorporate sufficient functional morphology, physiology, biochemistry, and immunology to enhance appreciation of the diverse implications of parasitism. It would also explore the potential of certain parasites for producing morbidity and mortality and would present available data regarding the *modus operandi* of certain modern chemotherapeutic agents. Through considerable discussion and several revisions of the manuscript, the first edition of *Human Parasitology* evolved. One of the goals for *Human Parasitology* was that it would also serve as a bridge between classical clinical parasitology texts and more traditional encyclopedic, advanced treatises that include in-depth consideration of biochemistry and immunology as well as more exotic parasites, such as strigeids of fishes and birds.

In this era of expanded use of radiation therapy and immunosuppressive drugs to treat cancer, tissue rejection in organ transplants, and AIDS, all of which serve to reduce immunocompetence in the human host, a number of parasites, some of which were formerly considered inconsequential, have become life-threatening. Although this aspect of parasitology was discussed throughout the first edition of *Human Parasitology,* its significance has expanded to such an extent that a new section titled "Opportunistic Parasites" was deemed essential for the second edition. The marked increase in world travel and immigration has made it imperative that students preparing for careers in the allied health sciences, medicine, and public health, as well as those interested in various aspects of environmental studies, acquire a working knowledge of parasitic diseases and how they affect their human hosts. To that end, we include expanded coverage of such topics as water-borne parasitic diseases and food-borne zoonoses.

So as not to diminish the importance of the biological aspects of parasites, the opening chapter of the segment devoted to each major group of parasites is titled "General Characteristics." These introductory chapters deal with the evolution and biology of each group and include ample light and electron micrographs to illustrate the various points of the text. An abridged classification of parasites covering the major nomenclature of only those forms discussed in the text has been placed at the end of each "General Characteristics" chapter. Updated references recommended as ancillary reading are found at the end of each chapter.

The field of chemotherapy is advancing at such a rapid pace that new drugs become available continually. Consequently, sections of the book dealing with information about current drugs of choice will become obsolete more rapidly than other sections of the book. Nevertheless, in the individual sections and at the end of the book, specific, currently prescribed chemotherapeutic regimens are included and may prove useful to prospective medical students.

Newly discovered organisms that parasitize humans, as well as adaptations among normally nonpathogenic parasites, continue to be documented. For instance, during the past few years a number of essentially unheralded protozoans such as *Cryptosporidium parvum* and *Cyclospora cayentanensis* have become public health problems. We have not attempted to identify and discuss all parasites that have been reported from humans, concentrating instead on only those considered to be of major significance.

Because the second edition, like the first, is designed for a one-semester or one-quarter course, the material is somewhat condensed, particularly in the areas of physiology and biochemistry. We believe this edition will appeal particularly to those students interested not only in the medical aspects of parasitology but also to those who require a solid foundation in the biology of parasites in order to further their studies in a graduate school of their choice.

Preface to the First Edition

Several years ago, the authors began to consider writing a textbook of human parasitology designed for premedical, medical technology, and biology students in need of basic knowledge of the biology of parasitism. While emphasizing the medical aspects, the book would include sufficient functional morphology, physiology, biochemistry, and immunology to foster greater apppreciation of the diverse implications of parasitism. In addition, it would explore the means by which certain parasites cause morbidity and mortality and would present, where known, the modes of action of certain modern chemotherapeutic agents. Through considerable discussion and several revisions of the manuscript, this volume evolved. The authors believe that *Human Parasitology* serves as an intermediate between textbooks devoted almost exclusively to the "classical" clinical parasitology approach and more advanced treatises that provide in-depth treatments of parasite taxonomy, physiology, biochemistry, and immunology.

In this age of radiation therapy, immunosuppressive drugs, and AIDS (Acquired Immune Deficiency Syndrome)–all of which serve to reduce immunocompetence in the human host–the importance of parasites once considered inconsequential has mushroomed. Toxoplasmosis, pneumocystosis, and other parasitic infections have become diseases of major consequence. For this reason and others, including marked increases in world travel and immigration, it has become imperative that students preparing for careers in the allied health sciences, medicine, and public health acquire some knowledge of parasitic diseases of humans. This book has been written with such students in mind.

Classification of parasites is an integral part of the discipline. This book has been organized by placing the classification schemes most widely favored in current usage at the end of the first chapter in each part. This leaves the level of emphasis to the discretion of the instructor. References that are recommended as ancillary reading are also included at the end of each chapter.

It must be recognized that the field of chemotherapy is advancing at such a rapid pace that new drugs become available constantly. Consequently, current information about drugs of choice will become obsolete more rapidly than will information presented in other sections of the book. Nevertheless, at the end of the book is an appendix listing the specific, currently prescribed chemotherapeutic regimens that may prove useful to prospective medical students.

Newly discovered organisms that can and do parasitize humans, as well as adaptations among normally nonpathogenic parasites, continue to be documented. For instance, during the past three decades there have been fascinating discoveries that free-living amoebae such as *Naegleria fowleri* and Acanthamoeba species can become highly lethal pathogens as a result of facultative parasitism. Furthermore, it has been established that a number of essentially benign protozoans can become highly pathogenic in immunologically compromised hosts. The authors have not attempted to identify and discuss all parasites that have been reported from humans but only those considered to be of major significance.

This volume is designed for a one-semester or one-quarter course and, as such, presents the material in a less detailed format.

ACKNOWLEDGMENTS

Numerous friends and associates have been kind enough to review and criticize several versions of this book during manuscript preparation. Among these we want to thank especially Dr. Frank J. Etges of the University of Cincinnati; Dr. Grover C. Miller of

North Carolina State University; Dr. Stuart A. Krassner of the University of California, Irvine; and Dr. John Mackiewicz of the State University of New York, Albany. We also thank Dr. Laverne Buldhaupt, University of Wisconsin–La Crosse; Dr. Albert Canaris, University of Texas at El Paso; Dr. Gerald Coles, University of Massachusetts at Amherst; Dr. Paul Nollen, Western Illinois University; Dr. Leslie Uhazy, University of Missouri at Columbia; Dr. Steven Zam, University of Florida; Dr. William Chobotar, Andrews University; Dr. Brent Nickol, University of Nebraska at Lincoln; and Dr. Peter Castro, California Polytechnic State Univeristy at Pomona.

Chapter One

SYMBIOSIS AND PARASITISM

Parasitology, the study of parasites and their relationships to their hosts, is one of the most fascinating areas of biology. The study of parasitism is interdisciplinary, encompassing aspects of systematics and phylogeny, ecology, morphology, embryology, physiology, biochemistry, immunology, pharmacology, and nutrition, among others. Newly developed techniques in biochemistry and cellular and molecular biology have also opened significant new avenues for research on parasites.

Not only does parasitology touch upon many disciplines, but the varied nature of parasites renders their study multifaceted. While it is entirely proper to classify many bacteria and fungi and all viruses as parasites, parasitology has traditionally been limited to parasitic protozoa, helminths, and arthropods, as well as those species of arthropods that serve as vectors for parasites. It follows, then, that parasitology encompasses elements of protozoology, helminthology, entomology, and acarology. The World Health Organization has proclaimed that, of the six major unconquered human tropical diseases, five—schistosomiasis, malaria, filariasis, African trypanosomiasis, and leishmaniasis—are parasitic in the traditional sense. Leprosy, the sixth major disease, is caused by a bacterium.

DEFINITIONS

The complexity of the host–parasite relationship has often led to misunderstandings of the precise nature of parasitism. In order to avoid such misperceptions, researchers have devised the following concepts to distinguish among the several types of associations involving heterospecific organisms.

Any organism that spends a portion or all of its life intimately associated with another living organism of a different species is known as a **symbiont** (or symbiote), and the relationship is designated as **symbiosis.** The term *symbiosis*, as used here, does not imply mutual or unilateral physiologic dependency; rather, it is used in its original sense (living together) without any reference to "benefit" or "damage" to the symbionts.

Although the lines of demarcation between them are indistinct, at least four categories of symbiosis are commonly recognized: commensalism, phoresis, parasitism, and mutualism. The scope of this text is limited to relationships of medical importance, and, since parasitism is the major type of symbiosis meeting this criterion, definitions of the other forms are included for clarification only.

COMMENSALISM

Commensalism does not involve physiologic interaction or dependency between the two partners, the **host** and the **commensal.** Literally, the term means "eating at the same table." In other words, commensalism is a type of symbiosis in which spatial proximity allows the commensal to feed on substances captured or ingested by the host. The two partners can survive independently. Although at times certain nonpathogenic organisms (e.g., protozoa) are referred to as commensals, this interpretation is incorrect because they are physiologically dependent on the host and are, therefore, parasites. An example of commensalism is the association between hermit crabs and the sea anemones they carry on their borrowed shells.

PHORESIS

The term *phoresis* is derived from the Greek word meaning "to carry." In this type of symbiotic relationship, the **phoront,** usually the smaller organism, is mechanically carried by the host, which is usually a larger organism. Unlike commensalism, there is no dependency in the procurement of food by either partner, and no physiologic interaction is involved. Both commensalism and phoresis can be considered spatial rather than physiologic relationships. Examples of phoresis are the relationships in which numerous sedentary protozoans, algae, and fungi are attached to the bodies of aquatic animals such as arthropods and turtles.

PARASITISM

Parasitism is another type of symbiotic relationship between two organisms: a **parasite,** usually the smaller of the two, and a **host**, upon which the parasite is physiologically dependent. The relationship may be permanent, as in the case of tapeworms found in the vertebrate intestine, or temporary, as with female mosquitoes, some leeches, and ticks, which feed intermittently on host blood. **Obligatory parasites** are physiologically dependent upon their hosts and usually cannot survive if kept isolated from them. **Facultative parasites**, on the other hand, are essentially free-living organisms that are capable of becoming parasitic if placed in a situation conducive to such a mode. An example of a facultative parasite is the amoeba *Naegleria.*

The physiologic requirements of most parasites are only partially known and understood, but there is sufficient information to indicate certain categories of dependence, such as nutritional. Unlike commensals, parasites derive essential nutrients directly from the host, usually from such nutritive substances as blood, lymph, cytoplasm, tissue fluids, and host-digested food.

The intimate relationship between parasite and host generally exposes the host to antigens produced by the parasite. These antigens may be molecules that make up the surface of the parasite (**somatic antigens**), or substances secreted or excreted by the parasite (**metabolic antigens**). In either case, the host typically responds to the presence of such antigens by synthesizing antibodies. Thus, unlike phoresis and commensalism, parasitism usually involves immunological responses by the host. The effect upon the host is usually the result of the host's reaction to the presence of the parasite. The reaction may be localized at the site of attachment or deposition or may be more generalized, perhaps throughout the entire host body. One of the more important consequences of such reactions is the limitation of parasite populations. It is axiomatic in helminthology that all species of worms are harmful when present in massive numbers (Fig. 1-1); therefore, internal defense responses by the host help to reduce pathological effects of the parasite.

While there are numerous systems for classifying host–parasite relationships, the one used here distinguishes between two major types of parasites—endoparasites and ectoparasites—according to location. Endoparasites live within the body of the host at sites such as the alimentary tract, liver, lungs, and urinary

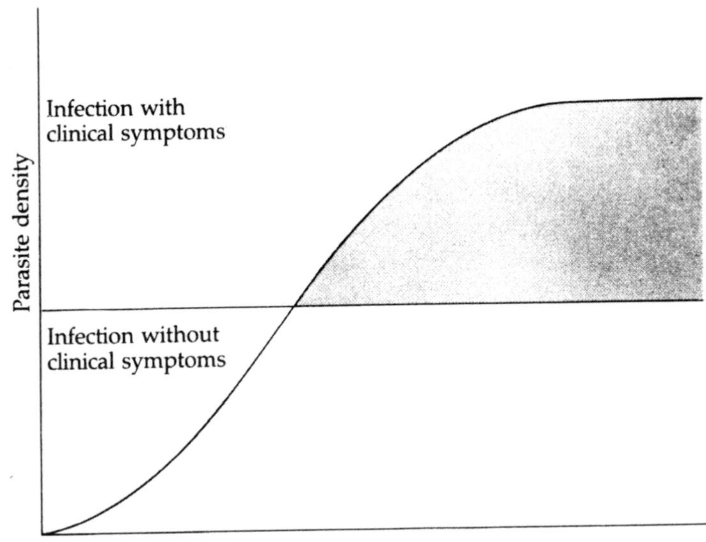

FIGURE 1-1
Correlation between diseases with clinical symptoms and parasite density.

bladder; ectoparasites are attached to the outer surface of the host or are superficially embedded in the body surface.

A host may be classified as (1) a **definitive host,** if the parasite attains sexual maturity therein; (2) an **intermediate host,** if the host serves as a temporary but essential environment for the development or metamorphosis of the parasite short of sexual maturity; or (3) a transfer or **paratenic host,** if the host is not necessary for the completion of the parasite's life cycle but is utilized as a temporary refuge and vehicle for reaching an obligatory host, usually the definitive host.

Generally, an arthropod or some other invertebrate that serves as a host as well as a carrier for a parasite is referred to as a **vector.** Unlike a transfer host, a vector is essential for completion of the life cycle. In this text, the term *vector* is used to designate an organism, usually an arthropod, that transmits a parasite to a human or other vertebrate host; for example, various species of anopheline mosquitoes serve as vectors for the malaria-producing protozoan *Plasmodium*, which they transmit to humans. Some intermediate hosts or vectors may have evolved from definitive hosts or paratenic hosts.

Infected animals that serve as sources of infective organisms for humans are known as **reservoir hosts.** A wild animal in this role is called a **sylvatic reservoir host,** while a domestic animal is called a **domestic reservoir host.** For example, one type of human filariasis is caused by a filarial worm, *Brugia malayi*, which is transmitted to humans by a mosquito. Although the parasite is usually transmitted from one person to another via the mosquito, it can also be transmitted to humans from cats (domestic reservoirs) or monkeys (sylvatic reservoirs). Thus, the reservoir host, by definition, shares the same stage of the parasite with humans. Often, the reservoir host tolerates the parasitic infection better than the human host does.

The term **zoonosis** can be used in various contexts; it is used here to denote a disease of humans that is caused by a pathogenic parasite normally found in wild or domestic vertebrate animals. Person-to-person transmission does not normally occur in zoonosis. An example of a zoonotic disease of significant medical importance is trichinellosis, caused by the nematode *Trichinella spiralis*. The worm is found in a variety of sylvatic and domestic reservoirs, notably pigs, bears, and rodents. Humans become infected by consuming raw or undercooked meat from infected animals.

MUTUALISM

The fourth category of symbiosis, mutualism, is an association in which the **mutualist** and the host depend on each other physiologically. A classic example of this type of relationship occurs between certain species of flagellated protozoans and the termites in whose gut they live. The protozoan, which depends almost entirely on a carbohydrate diet, acquires nutrients from wood chips ingested by the host termite. In return, the protozoan synthesizes and secretes cellulases, enzymes that catabolize cellulose into compounds the termite can utilize. Incapable of synthesizing its own cellulases, the termite is dependent on the mutualist and, in turn, provides developmental stimuli to the mutualist and a hospitable environment for reproduction. If the termite is defaunated, it will die; conversely, the flagellate cannot survive outside the termite.

It has been suggested that there may be a complete and progressive gradation among the various types of symbiosis. Furthermore, it is important to note that the definitions of symbiosis and its subcategories are often arbitrary and subject to considerable overlap. Figure 1-2 illustrates, for example, that

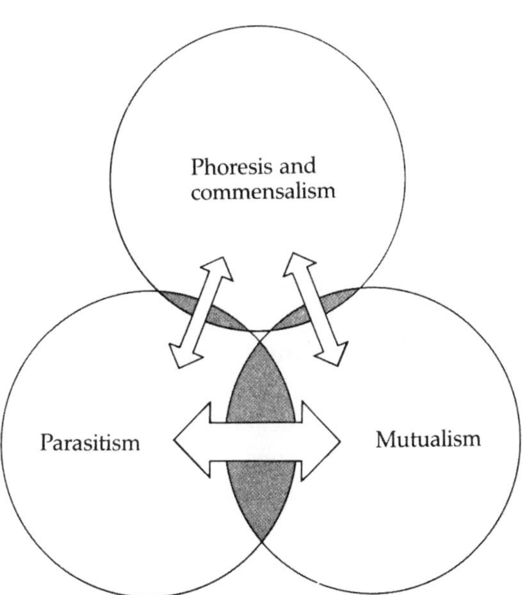

FIGURE 1-2
Overlap between the major categories of symbiosis. Note that there is less overlap between phoresis/commensalism and parasitism or between phoresis/commensalism and mutualism than between parasitism and mutualism.

some associations qualify as both phoresis and commensalism or as both commensalism and parasitism. Such overlapping relationships may be transitional stages that reflect evolutionary shifts from one category to another. In the shift from parasitism to mutualism, for example, a parasite initially may give off some nonessential metabolic by-product that can be utilized by the host; eventually, the host becomes physiologically dependent not only on this by-product but on other factors as well, and the relationship evolves into a mutualistic one.

ECOLOGY OF PARASITISM

Conceptually, the body of a host constitutes the environment on or in which the parasite spends some or all of its life. Further, the host's environment, whether tropical jungle or freshwater pond, also affects the parasite via the host. Some parasite ecologists have proposed the use of techniques employed in quantitative life-history studies of free-living populations (i.e., r- and K-selection analysis) for determining certain quantitative aspects of the population biology of parasites. By definition, **r-selection** occurs when selective forces upon organisms (**r-strategists**) are unstable and environmental conditions are variable. **K-selection**, on the other hand, prevails when forces influencing the organisms (**K-strategists**) remain relatively stable over a period of time. Most r-strategists are characterized by high fecundity, high, density-independent mortality rates, short life spans, effective dispersal mechanisms, and population sizes that vary over time and are usually below the carrying capacity of the environment. K-strategists are generally characterized by relatively low fecundity, low, density-dependent mortality rates, longer life spans, and relatively stable population sizes. It can be seen, then, that the mechanisms that regulate populations of r-strategists are independent of population density, whereas those that regulate populations of K-strategists are density-dependent. As an example, digenetic trematodes are considered r-strategists, since both their biotic potential and their mortality rates are high as a result of selective pressures in their environments, which is unstable because it differs at practically every phase of the life cycle. It should be emphasized that r- and K-strategy designations are relative. Species B, for example, may be an r-strategist when compared to species C, but a K-strategist when compared to species A.

A number of influences, such as the presence or absence of certain biological, chemical, and physical factors, dictate the geographic distribution of a parasite. For instance, the ability of a particular species of parasite to survive depends upon the availability of all hosts needed to complete its life cycle; therefore, factors governing the survival of hosts indirectly govern the presence of parasites. Another feature affecting the distribution of a parasite is **host specificity**, or the adaptability of a species of parasite to a certain host or group of hosts. The degree of specificity varies from species to species. Host specificity is determined by genetic, immunological, physiological, and/or ecological factors.

Many of these ecological aspects play important roles in defining the **epidemiology** of a disease-producing parasite. Epidemiology is the study of factors responsible for the transmission and distribution of disease. The distribution and characteristics of various hosts (including vectors), host specificity, cultural patterns of human hosts (such as diet, which is often influenced by religion, economic status, and other factors), and the density of host and parasite populations all influence the epidemiology of pathogenic parasites.

MEDICAL IMPLICATIONS

The area of human pathology attributable to parasitic diseases is known as **tropical** or **geographic medicine**, because many of these diseases occur most commonly or exclusively in the tropical regions of the world. The conditions that make these regions suitable for such diseases will be discussed later in this section.

The causative agents of parasitic diseases of humans include organisms commonly known as protozoans (one-celled eukaryotes, p. 38), flatworms (trematodes and tapeworms, pp. 117–307), roundworms (nematodes, pp. 311–337), and certain arthropods (insects, ticks, and mites, pp. 405–442). Parasitic diseases differ from viral, bacterial, and fungal diseases in several ways. First, viruses, bacteria, and fungi generally multiply rapidly, producing large numbers of progeny within the human host, whereas parasites generally reproduce more slowly and produce fewer offspring. Also, viral and bacterial infections are usually more acute and are often highly virulent and potentially lethal; parasitic diseases, in contrast, are usually chronic, and if they do cause death, it commonly comes after a lengthy period of debilitation. Finally, except for certain viral infections, parasitic diseases are generally more difficult to control than other infectious diseases. Reasons for the difficulty in controlling parasitic diseases lie in the epidemiology of these diseases, as described below.

CONTROL IMPEDIMENTS

Intermediate Hosts

The life cycles of certain parasites depend upon the presence of at least one intermediate host. Trematodes that parasitize humans, for example, require specific snail intermediate hosts and conditions that ensure host–parasite contact. Specific chemical qualities of the water, physical characteristics of the aquatic environment, the type and quantity of aquatic vegetation, and other factors are also essential to the successful completion of the life cycle. Many of the intermediate hosts are so specialized that they can protect themselves from a number of control measures. For example, the snail intermediate host of *Schistosoma mansoni*, one of the causative agents of human schistosomiasis, can burrow into the mud, shielding itself from adverse conditions such as drought as well as from molluscicides. Also, while alteration of one or more characteristics of the aquatic environment for the purpose of disease control could disrupt the cycle and subvert the transmission of schistosomiasis, such alterations might also disrupt the biology of cohabitant plants and animals and upset the entire ecological balance of the immediate environment.

Vectors

Plasmodium falciparum is the causative agent of one type of malaria known as malignant tertian malaria (pp. 139–140), in which the vector is a female mosquito of the genus *Anopheles*. These mosquitoes breed by the millions in small, isolated bodies of fresh water. Because of the inaccessibility of many of these breeding sites, the use of insecticides for eradication of the mosquito population is of limited value; therefore, combatting the spread of malaria by this method is never completely effective. In addition, the use of insecticides often leads to the emergence of strains of mosquitoes that are resistant to insecticides. Another danger inherent in the widespread use of insecticides is their potential to destroy or contaminate beneficial life forms along with the vectors.

Leishmania braziliensis, the protozoan parasite that causes mucocutaneous leishmaniasis (pp. 109–112), is transmitted by sandflies of the genus *Lutzomyia*. Essential to the development of these sandflies is an environment of low light intensity, high humidity, and organic debris upon which the larvae feed. Breeding sites are commonly located under logs and decaying leaves, inside hollow trees, and in animal burrows. As with the mosquito vector of *P. falciparum*, the inaccessibility of breeding sites limits the effectiveness of insecticides in eliminating the vectors. Hence, only partial eradication of the disease has been achieved by targeting the vector.

Several genera of mosquitoes serve as vectors for a form of human Bancroftian filariasis caused by the nematode *Wuchereria bancrofti*. The incidence of periodic filariasis, common in areas of dense population and poor sanitation, parallels the distribution of the principal vector, *Culex fatigans*, which breeds in sewage-contaminated water. In economically depressed areas of the world, contaminated water is common and, as previously noted, the widespread use of insecticides to control mosquitoes is not totally reliable. In recent years, the combined use of screens, insect repellents, and insecticides, augmented by mass treatment of patients with chemotherapeutic drugs, has proven effective in combatting this type of filariasis in the U.S. Virgin Islands, Puerto Rico, and Tahiti. Nevertheless, failure to find an effective means of eliminating the vector essential to its transmission has complicated the control of Bancroftian filariasis.

Resistance and Resurgence

During the past decade, there have been spectacular resurgences of several parasitic diseases that had been considered under control or eradicated, the most dramatic of which has been malaria. The upsurge in malaria is due primarily to the emergence of drug-resistant strains of the malaria-causing parasite as well as insecticide-resistant mosquito vectors. In addition, the crowded conditions resulting from resettlement of refugees from war and famine expedite transmission of the disease.

Diagnosis

Diagnosis of human parasitic diseases is often complicated. Emphasis on medical parasitology in North American medical curricula has traditionally been woefully lacking and continues to be increasingly neglected. Consequently, the actual and potential impact of these diseases is not being addressed, and younger clinicians have little appreciation for the hazard they represent. This lack of awareness results in few, if any, diagnostic tests being ordered. This, in turn, produces a cyclical effect wherein there is a corresponding reduction in the medical technology curricula dealing with diagnostic laboratory tests designed to identify parasitic diseases. The cycle continues in a failure by physicians to recognize the need for diagnostic tests, resulting in misdiagnosis of parasitic diseases. This indictment applies to almost all North American medical schools and hospitals. In contrast, instruction in the diagnosis of such diseases in Central and South American medical schools is commendable. The greatest deficiency, however, remains in the field clinics in tropical and subtropical Africa and parts of southeast Asia. Inadequacies in funding, supplies, and trained staff thwart courageous efforts to achieve significant progress in the struggle against these insidious diseases.

FACTORS INFLUENCING PREVALENCE

A variety of conditions contribute to the prevalence of parasitic diseases in the tropics and subtropics, among them unsanitary living conditions, inadequate funding for disease control and treatment, poor nutrition, lack of health education (although this is improving), regional and ethnic customs conducive to infection by parasites, climatic conditions, and compromised immune systems.

Unsanitary Living Conditions

In most tropical and subtropical countries, construction of modern sewage systems is still in the planning or preliminary stages. Consequently, raw sewage contaminating open trenches and streams remains very common. In rural Southeast Asia, for example, shacks built on stilts overhang streams polluted with human and animal excreta, and vegetation growing in these streams is often gathered for human consumption. Such scenarios create an ideal environment for the transmission of parasitic and other diseases.

Disease Control and Treatment

Third world nations, including most tropical countries, invariably have limited funds in their national budgets for public health, and the research and other programs essential to improving conditions are costly. The control of snails that transmit schistosomiasis, for example, is an expensive undertaking involving vehicles, pumps and other machinery, and chemicals. Consequently, in spite of aid from such international agencies as the World Health Organization, funding for disease control is vastly inadequate.

Parasitic diseases most commonly afflict the poor, and, unfortunately, pharmaceutical companies are reluctant to invest large sums in research and development of new drugs that victims are unlikely to be able to afford. Where significant progress has been made over the past two decades in developing new drugs, limited production has kept the price high, beyond the means of most of the afflicted population.

Poor Nutrition

Immunological defense mechanisms in all animals, including humans, are influenced by several physiological processes, including nutrition. In most parts of the world where parasitic diseases abound, malnutrition plays an important role in susceptibility to disease and the manifestation of clinical symptoms. Undernourished persons, especially children suffering from protein deficiency, are particularly vulnerable to infection, and physical and physiological deviations from the norm are also markedly more pronounced, especially among the young. For example, hookworm infection (pp. 356–363) exacerbated by malnutrition commonly results in anemia, significant loss of body weight, abdominal distension, and mental malaise.

Health Education

Education of the population in endemic areas concerning methods of reducing or eliminating parasitic infections is probably the most economical approach to disease control. Educational programs usually involve teams that present illustrated lectures to school children in rural areas. Longstanding practices and attitudes often produce stubborn resistance to change. However, while such efforts alone have limited effect, they can be useful when incorporated into more comprehensive programs involving the media and other advertising ploys such as road signs. Indeed, recent growth in such programs has been helpful in reducing diseases such as schistosomiasis in rural Egypt.

Regional and Ethnic Customs

Epidemiologists have long recognized that certain regional and ethnic customs practiced by inhabitants of third world countries in the tropics and subtropics contribute significantly to the spread of parasitic diseases. In Moslem countries, for example, ablution is a common practice. The use of communal pools for this ritual bathing of previously unwashed body parts leads to contamination of the water and facilitates the spread of diseases such as schistosomiasis (pp. 229–248).

In many parts of the Orient, raw and lightly pickled crabs and other crustaceans are considered delicacies. These hosts harbor one of the larval stages of the Oriental lung fluke, *Paragonimus westermani* (pp. 223–228). The encysted larva, known as a metacercaria, is ingested in crustacean meat and, upon excystation, penetrates the human gut and enters the peritoneal cavity, eventually reaching the lungs.

In Egypt, especially in parts of the lower Nile Valley, there is a high incidence of *Heterophyes heterophyes*, an intestinal fluke of humans. This parasite also occurs in Greece, Israel, Korea, and Taiwan, and it has been reported in Hawaii among persons of Philippine origin. Human infections are contracted through consumption of raw or poorly cooked fish. The mullet, a favored delicacy when served raw, is most often responsible for heterophyidiasis as well as some other parasitic diseases.

Climatic Conditions

The climate in tropical and subtropical lands favors the transmission of several parasitic diseases, especially those transmitted by arthropods. Exposed bare skin and perspiration invite insect bites, and, because various insects serve as vectors of protozoan and nematode pathogens, there is a higher incidence of insect-transmitted parasitic diseases in warm and hot climates. Going barefoot facilitates invasion of the skin by parasites such as hookworm (pp. 356–365), whose infective stage lives in warm soil and penetrates the bare skin of the victim. In addition, the abundance of bodies of stagnant water, in conjunction with the prolonged elevated temperatures of the tropics and subtropics, provides ideal, essentially year-round breeding environments that enhance the survival of intermediate hosts and arthropod vectors. The favorable habitat for intermediate hosts and the uninterrupted life cycles of vectors help to establish and perpetuate parasitic diseases in these areas, further impeding eradication efforts.

Opportunistic Parasitism

Any organism or agent that weakens the immune system increases a person's vulnerability to "opportunistic" parasites (pp. 27–33) and other disease-causing organisms. For example, the human immunodeficiency virus (HIV), the virus responsible for the current world-wide AIDS epidemic, so compromises the immune system of its victims that they are left virtually defenseless. Even relatively benign parasites that cause only mild symptoms, if any, in a healthy person can be quite devastating to a patient suffering from AIDS.

EVOLUTION OF PARASITISM

When and how did parasites arise? Although there is no definitive answer, it is agreed that parasites have evolved among very diverse groups of free-living progenitors. One of these earlier organisms probably formed an initially casual association with another organism, and one member of the pair, perhaps due to **preadaptation**, developed a gradually increasing dependency on the other. In the context of parasitism, the term *preadaptation* denotes the potential in a free-living organism for adaptation to a parasitic (symbiotic) lifestyle. This potential may never be realized as long as the organism remains free-living; however, if the organism becomes associated with a suitable host, its potential for parasitism becomes critically important for survival should hostile environmental conditions develop. Preadaptations can be structural, developmental, and/or physiological.

Parasites of the alimentary tract probably became such after having been swallowed, either accidentally or intentionally, by the host. If they were preadapted to withstand the environment or were capable of subsequent adaptation to it, they might have become progressively more dependent upon the new environment or might even have migrated to other more hospitable areas, such as the lungs or the liver. Parasites requiring two or more hosts very likely developed their multi-host life cycles sequentially. For instance, blood-inhabiting flagellates first parasitized the alimentary tracts of insects and, when introduced into vertebrate blood while the insect was feeding, adapted to that environment secondarily. Thus, present intermediate hosts once may have been definitive hosts. Recent studies suggest, however, that the advancement to parasitism is best represented by a bell-shaped curve (Fig. 1-3), in which an increasing number of intermediate

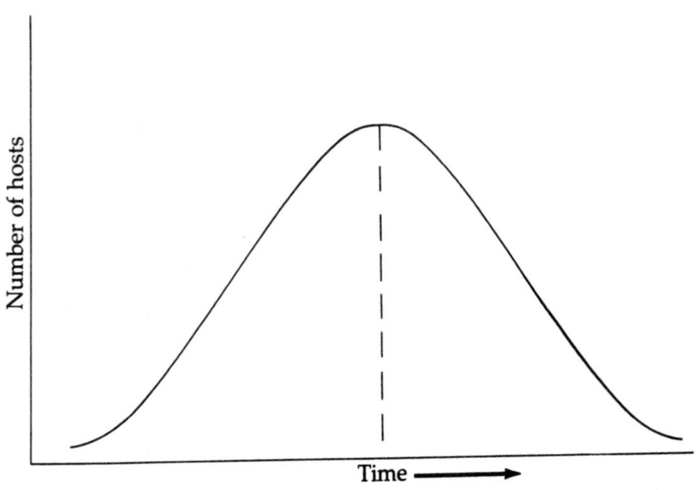

FIGURE 1-3
Hypothetical scheme showing an increase in the number of obligatory hosts in the evolution of parasites. As time increases, the number of obligatory hosts decreases.

hosts signifies higher adaptability only up to a point. Past that point, elimination of certain hosts represents a more successful state, because simplification of the life cycle may enhance the parasite's chance of reaching the definitive host.

SELECTED READINGS

Anderson, R. M., and May, R. M. 1982. Coevolution of hosts and parasites. *Parasitology* **85**, 411–426.

Blair, D., Campos, A., Cummings, M. P., and Laclette, J. P. 1996. Evolutionary biology of parasitic helminths: The role of molecular phylogenetics. *Parasitology Today* **12**, 66–71.

Brooks, D. R., and McLellan, D. 1991. *Phylogeny, Ecology, and Behavior: A Research Program in Comparative Biology*. Univ. of Chicago, IL.

Ebert, D., and Herre, E. A. 1996. The evolution of parasitic diseases. *Parasitology Today* **12**, 96–101.

Force, D. C. 1974. Succession of r and k strategists in parasitoids. In *Evolutionary Strategies of Parasitic Insects and Mites* (P. W. Price, Ed.), pp. 112–129. Plenum, New York.

Poulin, R. 1996. The evolution of life history strategies in parasitic animals. *Advances in Parasitology* **37**, 107–134.

Read, C. P. 1970. *Parasitism and Symbiosis*. Ronald Press, New York.

Chapter Two

PARASITE–HOST INTERACTIONS

An integral part of modern parasitology is the study of host–parasite relationships. A knowledge of how a parasite survives in its host often serves as the basis for the eventual control of the parasite. For instance, new chemotherapeutic agents may be synthesized on the basis of biochemical differences between the parasite and its host, or the elaboration of vaccines may be possible if the immunological responses of the host to the parasite and the parasite's evasion of these responses are known. Other avenues involving genetic engineering may open as additional knowledge is gained.

EFFECTS OF PARASITES ON HOSTS

Parasites trigger varying degrees of change within their hosts. Although not inevitably, disease often results. As previously noted, parasitic diseases are usually functions of parasite density, especially when caused by metazoan parasites. Two factors commonly influence the onset of recognizable disease symptoms: the number and species (or strains) of parasites and the physiological condition of the host. Small numbers of parasites often elicit no clinical symptoms. Several of the conditions that most often develop in parasitic diseases are discussed in the following sections.

TISSUE DAMAGE

Beyond the erosion caused by ingestion or by mechanical disruption of cells by the parasite, three major types of histopathological cell damage occur in parasite-injured tissues.

Parenchymatous or Albuminous Degeneration

This type of damage is characterized by swollen cells packed with albuminous or fatty granules, indistinct nuclei, and pale cytoplasm. It is often seen in infected liver, cardiac muscle, and kidney cells.

Fatty Degeneration

This type of degeneration results in the deposition of abnormal amounts of fat in cells, imparting a yellowish color to the cells. It is common among parasite-laden liver cells.

Necrosis

Persistent cell degeneration of any type causes death of cells or tissues. The dead cells give tissues an opaque appearance. Encystment and calcification of *Trichinella spiralis* larvae in mammalian skeletal muscle cells cause necrosis of surrounding tissue.

TISSUE CHANGES

Cell and tissue parasites sometimes evoke changes in the growth pattern of the affected tissue. Some of these changes are very deleterious; others are merely structural with no serious systemic consequences to the host organism. Tissue changes of parasitic origin are of four major types.

Hyperplasia

Elevation of the metabolic rate of cells causes cell proliferation by accelerating cell division. This condition, when associated with parasitism, is precipitated by the marked increase in host body repair activity that commonly follows inflammation. For example, inflammation caused by the liver fluke *Fasciola hepatica* stimulates excessive division of epithelial cells lining the bile duct, with a resultant thickening of the duct wall.

Hypertrophy

An increase in cell or organ size in victims of parasitic diseases is usually due to engorgement by intracellular parasites. For example, during the erythrocytic phase in the life cycle of the malaria-producing organism *Plasmodium vivax*, the parasitized red blood cells and the spleen commonly become enlarged.

Metaplasia

One type of tissue may be converted into another without the intervention of embryonic tissue. In patients infected with the lung fluke *Paragonimus westermani*, the parasite is surrounded by a host capsule consisting of fibrocytes that have been transformed from other types of cells.

Neoplasia

Abnormal cell growth may occur in a tissue, producing an entirely new entity, such as a tumor. The neoplastic tumor is not inflammatory, is not required for the repair of organs, and does not conform to the normal growth pattern. Neoplasms may be **benign**, remaining localized with no invasion of adjacent tissues; alternatively, they may be **malignant**, invading adjacent tissues or spreading (metastasizing) to other parts of the body through the blood or lymph. Cancers are malignant neoplasms. The human blood fluke *Schistosoma haematobium* is sometimes associated with malignant neoplasia of the urinary bladder.

BIOLOGICAL ADAPTATIONS OF PARASITISM

The intimacy of parasite–host associations invariably involves physiological, biochemical, morphological, and immunological adaptations. In this section, aspects of physiology, biochemistry, and immunology will be addressed briefly; morphological adaptations will be considered in subsequent chapters.

PHYSIOLOGY AND BIOCHEMISTRY OF PARASITISM

The study of parasitism deals with a number of basic questions: How are parasites physiologically dependent upon their hosts? How do parasites affect their hosts? How do hosts affect the parasites? Since the antigenicity of parasites has somatic as well as physiological origins, increasing attention is also being focused upon the chemical composition of parasite bodies and metabolites. Therefore, it is important for anyone interested in parasitism and parasites to understand the enzymatic activities, pathways associated with energy production, protective mechanisms, secretions and excretions, respiration, and general metabolism of parasites. From a practical viewpoint, the prime requisite in modern chemotherapeutic research as it relates to parasitic diseases is the identification of an essential metabolic process in the pathogenic parasite that does not occur in the host or that can be chemically impaired or halted in the parasite with no adverse effect upon the host. After such identification, potential therapeutic agents can be developed to inhibit the process, killing the pathogen without harming the host. The discussion of chemotherapy in subsequent sections includes the information available about targets within the parasite toward which such agents are directed. Chemotherapy must be upgraded continuously as parasites evolve resistance to a particular drug or family of drugs and as research suggests new, more effective targets for drug action.

IMMUNOLOGY

The following discussion is aimed at providing a basic overview of some of the principles of immunology as they relate to the parasite–host relationship. For more detailed information, the reader is directed to the Selected Readings at the end of this chapter.

The guiding principle in immunology is the recognition by animals of *self* and *nonself*. Immunoparasitological implications of this principle are manifested in several ways. For instance, either the host recognizes the parasite as foreign (nonself) and reacts against it, or the parasite manages to evade immune recognition by the host. In one highly successful type of evasion, known as **molecular mimicry**, the parasite produces hostlike molecules on its body surface or its surface becomes covered with host molecules and, as a result, the host is duped into accepting the parasite as self.

A parasite, whether protozoan or metazoan, is a mosaic of various molecules that, when recognized by the host as nonself, are known as **immunogens** or **antigens.** For the purpose of this discussion, the terms *immunogen* and *antigen* will be considered synonyms. An antigen is any substance that is capable, under appropriate conditions, of inducing the synthesis of **antibodies.** The two substances interact to form an antigen–antibody complex. Antibodies are proteins synthesized in response to an antigen and may react, in varying degrees, to molecules whose structure is similar to that of the antigen. A parasite or any portion thereof

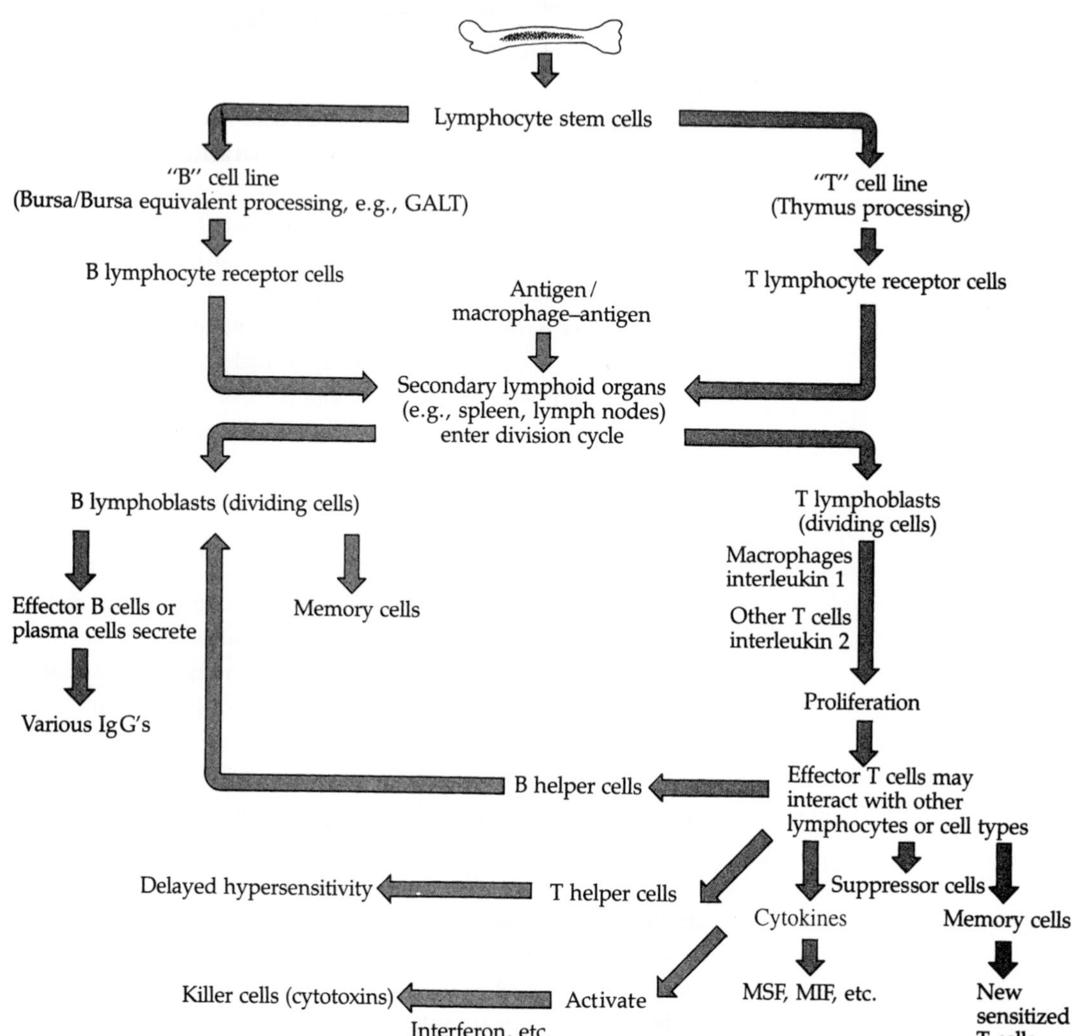

FIGURE 2-1
Generalized scheme showing the basic patterns of lymphocyte development and differentiation to become immunocompetent.

recognized by the host as antigenic generally elicits **cellular** (or **cell-mediated**) and **humoral reactions.** In a cellular reaction, specialized cells are mobilized to arrest and eventually destroy the parasite; in a humoral reaction, specialized molecules in the circulatory system interact with the parasite, seeking to immobilize or destroy it. Humoral antibodies may also react with excretory–secretory products (ESPs) of the parasite, forming immune complexes that may precipitate, which may cause host organ dysfunction.

When a host is immunologically challenged, it signals a functionally specialized type of lymphocyte, a **receptor cell,** to produce a specific antibody (Fig. 2-1). This signal originates from the direct binding of the antigen to a receptor cell and/or the processing and presentation of the antigen by an antigen-presenting cell (such as a macrophage) to specific receptors on a receptor cell's surface. Each receptor cell carries only one type of specific receptor and will, therefore, respond to only a few closely related antigenic determinants. Under appropriate conditions, the binding of the antigen to the receptor site stimulates the receptor cell to proliferate, forming a clone of cells. Each cell in the clone displays surface receptors with the same specificity as the originally stimulated cell. Receptor cells originate from bone marrow and are of two types: **B cells (B lymphocytes)** and **T cells (T lymphocytes).** B cells are so designated because they were originally recognized by their dependence upon processing through the bursa of Fabricius, an avian lymphoid tissue attached to the intestine near the cloaca. In mammals, however, processing of B cells is believed to occur in primary lymph tissue such as spleen, lymph nodes, and gut-associated lymphoid tissue (GALT). T cells, on the other hand, are so designated because they must be processed through the thymus. B cells produce humoral, or circulating, antibodies, while T cells may elicit cell-mediated reactions usually independent of circulating antibodies. In certain situations, however, humoral antibodies also participate in cell-mediated reactions, as in the case of antibody-dependent, cell-mediated cytotoxicity, described in the following sections.

The introduction of parasite antigens into a vertebrate sometimes triggers a series of events involving T cells. After the antigen is endocytosed by antigen-presenting cells (e.g., macrophages), the surfaces of these cells present specific antigenic determinants. T cells that are equipped with complementary surface receptors enter lymph tissues, such as spleen and lymph nodes, and come in contact with antigen-presenting cells. Upon recognition of the antigen, the T cells proliferate and differentiate into **effector T cells.** On entering the general circulation, these specialized T cells function in several ways. For example, one type, called **memory cells,** reverts to a "resting state" and serves as a source of new, antigen-specific T cells whenever the same antigen reenters the body. Most T cells, however, are involved with the synthesis and release of various chemical mediators called **cytokines.** Cytokines react with a wide variety of cells essential to the inflammatory process. For instance, **macrophage stimulating factor** (**MSF**) and **macrophage inhibitory factor** (**MIF**) regulate the activity of macrophages, **chemotactic factor** attracts other types of cells to the inflamed site, and **cytostatic factor** delays or blocks cell proliferation.

Two other types of effector T cells are **helper T cells,** which facilitate B and T cell differentiation and proliferation, and **cytotoxic** or **killer T cells,** which eliminate foreign cells either directly or through various cytokines.

An example of T cell action against a specific parasite is seen in the mammalian host reaction in schistosomiasis (see pp. 229–248). Much of the pathology in this disease results from granuloma formation, an immunological response to parasite eggs trapped in host tissues. Antigens released through the porous shells of trapped eggs stimulate T cells, which in turn release cytokines. The cytokines attract white blood cells to the eggs and stimulate phagocytosis. Cellular participants in this reaction include eosinophils, neutrophils, and fibroblasts, which accumulate at the site of antigen production. Finally, intercellular collagenous fibers are deposited to form a granuloma, sealing off the eggs from surrounding tissue. Reaction to the parasite's antigens also elicits **delayed hypersensitivity,** an increased reactivity to specific antigens mediated by cells rather than antibodies. It is termed *delayed* because of its slow onset; it requires 24 hours or longer to reach maximum intensity.

The B cell follows basically the same pattern of stimulation described for T cells, i.e., processing in lymph tissues, differentiation, and proliferation into **plasma cells** (Fig. 2-2) and **memory cells.** The plasma cell, which has a half-life of only a few days, secretes into the circulation large numbers of antibodies of the same idiotype and antigen-recognition specificity as its cell surface receptors. These antibodies occur in five classes and are known collectively as **immunoglobulins** (**Igs**) (Table 2-1). The first Ig secreted is **IgM** (mu), but with the aid of helper T cells, the B cell can shift to production of any of the other four classes: **IgG** (gamma), **IgE** (epsilon), **IgA** (alpha), or **IgD** (delta). All classes of Igs are found in blood and tissue fluids to some extent. IgA is also the primary Ig in the intestinal lumen. IgE levels are often elevated in helminthic infections and can bind via their Fc regions to

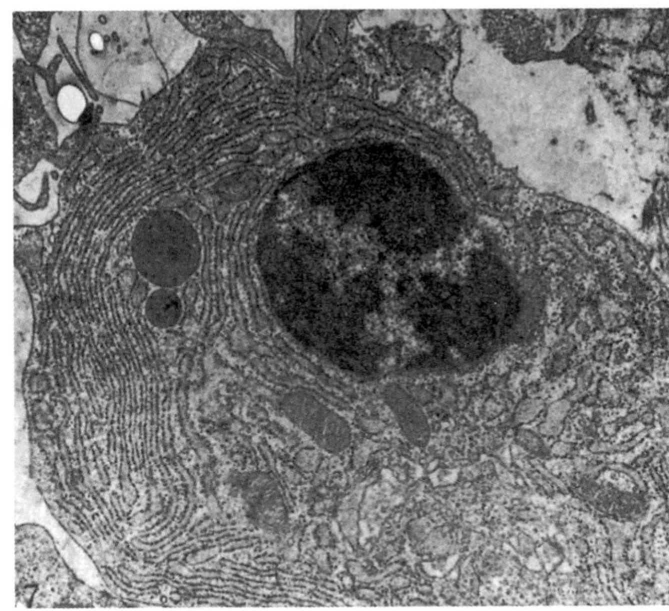

FIGURE 2-2
Electron micrograph of plasma cell from rat trachea. Note the extensive rough endoplasmic reticulum and the finely granular contents in the cisternae.

the surfaces of mast cells and basophils, sensitizing these cells to release histamines and other vasoactive substances, which increase capillary permeability.

The currently accepted concept of B cell selection with specific idiotypes is known as the **clonal selection hypothesis.** Briefly,

TABLE 2-1
Classes of Immunoglobulins

Class	Molecular weight	Biological function
IgG	150,000	Fix complement Bind to amine-containing cells (e.g., mast cells and basophils) Bind to macrophages and granulocytes Cross placenta
IgA	170,000	Secreted across mucus surface
IgM	890,000	Fix complement Secreted across mucus surface
IgD	150,000	?
IgE	196,000	Bind to amine-containing cells (e.g., mast cells and basophils)

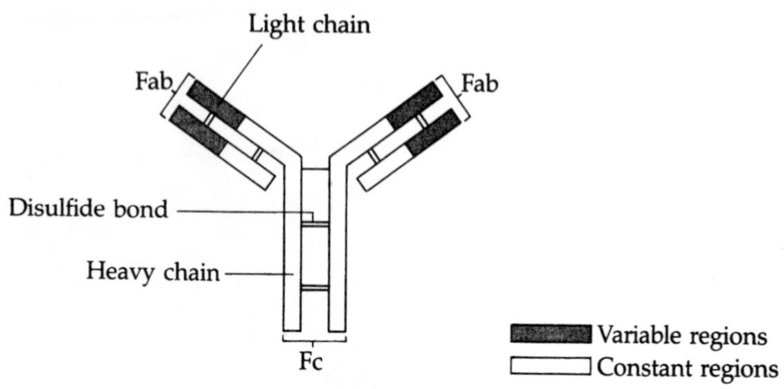

FIGURE 2-3
IgG molecule.

this hypothesis states that B lymphocytes are committed to the production of a specific B cell receptor (immunoglobulin). There is a huge population of B lymphocytes, each bearing a surface receptor of different antigenic specificity. When an antigen of appropriate structure is introduced to the B cell surface and combines with the specific receptor, the combination stimulates the B cell to differentiate and proliferate into a clone of plasma cells, each of which synthesizes Igs that have the same specificity as the parent cell. The cells of one portion of the clone remain small, serving as memory cells.

The IgG molecule (Fig. 2-3) illustrates the basic molecular structure of immunoglobulins. The molecule is composed of two identical light chains and two identical heavy chains held together by disulfide bonds. Antigenic specificity lies in regions of the chains susceptible to variation in amino acid sequences (**Fab portions**). Regions where the amino acid sequences remain constant (**Fc portions**) determine the biological properties of the particular class of immunoglobulin.

An example of an antigen–antibody reaction to a parasitic helminth is the **antibody-dependent cell-mediated cytotoxicity** reaction, referred to earlier. This interaction usually involves membrane-bound antigens associated with parasite surfaces. As shown in Fig. 2-4, one class of immunoglobulin, IgE, recognizes and attaches to the parasite surface antigens by means of its Fab portions, exposing its Fc portions to the environment. White blood cells, such as eosinophils with surface IgE-Fc receptor sites, attach to the parasite surface and destroy the parasite by releasing lysosomal hydrolases or other cytotoxic factors.

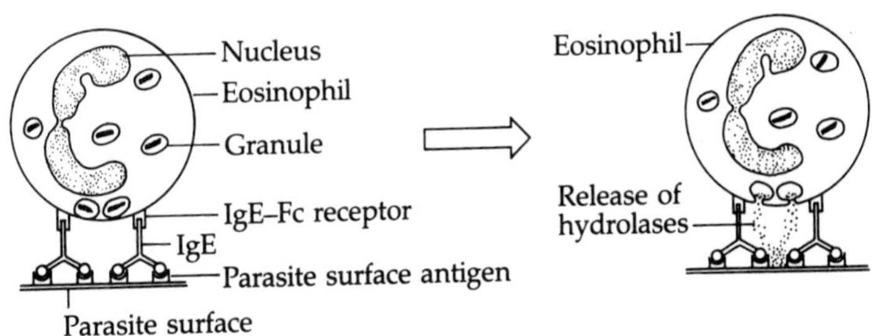

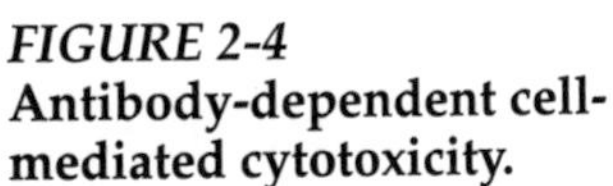
FIGURE 2-4
Antibody-dependent cell-mediated cytotoxicity.

OPPORTUNISTIC PARASITES

Immunosuppression in humans is sometimes brought on by therapy following successful grafts or used in the treatment of certain types of cancer; it can also be produced by several infectious diseases, including AIDS and measles. A number of parasites, some of which were formerly considered inconsequential, have become life-threatening to individuals thus compromised.

One of the major roles in the human immune system affected by immunosuppression is that of the **CD4$^+$ T cell** (Fig. 2-5). There are two subsets of CD4$^+$ T cells: (1) **Th1 cells** are responsible for the primary inflammatory response through the cytokines (see pp. 22, 24), **interleukin-2** (**IL-2**), and **gamma interferon** (**IFN-γ**). IL-2 targets the growth and cytokine production of B cells, other T cell subpopulations (including cytotoxic lymphocytes, which participate in the killing of infected cells), and **natural killer** (**NK**) cells; **IFN-γ** activates NK cells and macrophages and inhibits the activity of Th2 CD4$^+$ T cells. (2) **Th2 cells,** which constitute the primary helper cell subset, secrete a number of cytokines, including IL-3, IL-4, and IL-5. **IL-3** promotes proliferation of mast cells and the release of **granulocyte-macrophage colony stimulating factor** (**GM-CSF**); **IL-4** and **IL-5** stimulate B cell differentiation into antibody-producing cells, eosinophil growth and development, TH2 cell growth, and IgE and IgG synthesis, and they inhibit Th1 cells.

Macrophage activation is a major force by which the body rids itself of infectious organisms. INF-γ stimulates monocytes to become activated macrophages which, in turn, produce short-range effectors such as toxic oxygen radical intermediates, **tumor necrosis factor** (**TNF**), and lysosomal enzymes that act in concert to kill intracellular parasites. In many instances, intracellular par-

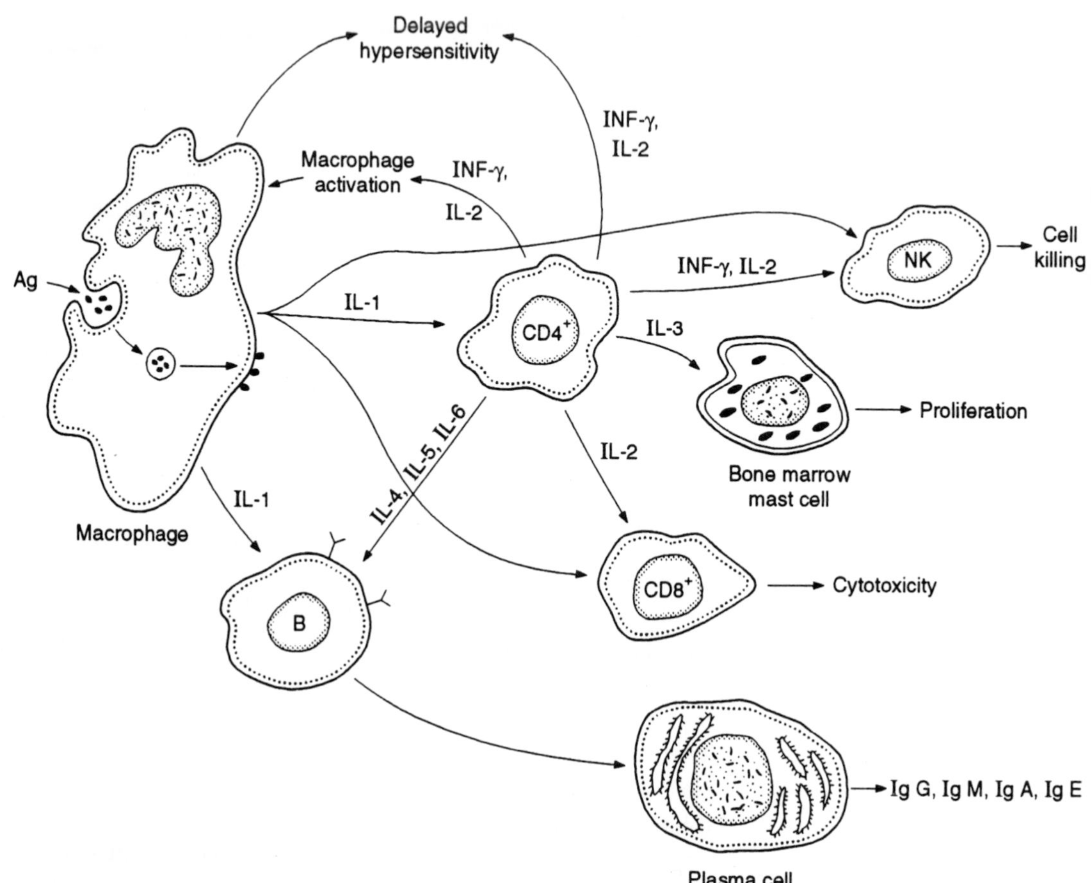

FIGURE 2-5
Role of CD4+ T cell in the immune response.

asites are not totally eliminated, but their numbers are kept in check by such macrophage activity.

Worldwide, parasitic infections account for a higher incidence of morbidity and mortality than diseases produced by any other group of organisms. This is especially true in developing countries where the effects of parasitic infections are exacerbated by poor nutrition. Perhaps the most insidious disease that compromises the immune system in the greatest number of people throughout the world is AIDS. AIDS victims concomitantly infected with certain parasites are the individuals most severely impacted by immunosuppression.

The human immunodeficiency virus (HIV) attacks $CD4^+$ T cells. A brief review of the mechanisms used by the virus to infect these cells follows. The virus possesses two important **chemo-**

kines associated with its outer surface, GP120 and GP41. GP120 binds to the **chemokine receptor** CD4 on the surfaces of T cells and mononuclear phagocytes, permitting one end of the GP41 molecule to penetrate the plasma membrane of the host cell, initiating fusion of the virus with the membrane. HIV's genetic material passes between the two cells, ultimately causing death of the infected cell subsequent to replication and release of the virus. HIV infection results in a 10-fold reduction in the number of $CD4^+$ and helper T cells in the patient. Of the many effects attributed to a depletion of $CD4^+$ T cells, three are of particular significance in patients with concomitant parasitic infections: (1) killer function of macrophages is impaired, (2) Th1 cell cytokine synthesis decreases and Th2 cell cytokine synthesis increases, and (3) differentiation of B cells and **cytolytic T lymphocytes** (**CTLs** or **$CD8^+$ cells**) is inhibited. In the discussion that follows, parasites are considered in decreasing order of their adaptability to opportunism.

PNEUMOCYSTIS CARINII

Pneumocystis carinii (see pp. 162–167) is an extracellular parasite of indeterminate taxonomic status that parasitizes the interstitial tissues of the lungs and alveoli. Most people probably harbor latent infections of *P. carinii*. Such infections are asymptomatic, since the normal immune system enables activated alveolar macrophages to phagocytose and thus control the organisms. The absence of sufficient numbers of $CD4^+$ T cells undoubtedly impairs this ability, allowing the organism to flourish in the lungs and cause ***Pneumocystis carinii* pneumonia** (**PCP**), one of the leading causes of death among AIDS patients. PCP affects an estimated 60% of AIDS patients. PCP is also common in children and premature infants who are malnourished or debilitated or who suffer from primary immune deficiency disorders, and it occurs in cancer and transplant patients who are being treated with immunosuppressive drugs.

TOXOPLASMA GONDII

Toxoplasma gondii (see pp. 156–162) is an intracellular parasite that infects a wide variety of cells. As is the case with *P. carinii*, large segments of the world's population are likely to have been exposed to *T. gondii*. This observation is based on serological surveys showing that prevalence of antibodies against *T. gondii* in humans increases with age. One response of a normal immune system to *T. gondii* infection is the formation of pseudocysts containing bradyzoites (see p. 160). Cerebral toxoplasmosis is the most common manifestation of neural involvement of a parasite in immunosuppressed patients. Bradyzoites, released from ruptured pseudocysts, invade neighboring cells of the central nervous system. Normally, cysts in the central nervous system are prevented from rupturing either by the protection afforded by immune mechanisms or, some believe, by the intraneural environment. However, if pseudocyst-infected nerve cells bearing CD4 receptors are invaded by HIV, bradyzoites are freed to infect new nerve cells, causing toxoplasma encephalitis. The absence of a T cell helper response allows bradyzoites to spread unimpeded.

CRYPTOSPORIDIUM PARVUM

Cryptosporidium parvum (see pp. 167–171) infects the microvilli of the small intestine of humans and other animals. HIV patients infected with *C. parvum* develop cholera-like symptoms. Experimental evidence indicates that, in individuals with normal immune systems, the infection is controlled by IFN-γ which, in turn, activates the intracellular defense mechanisms described previously.

LEISHMANIA SPP.

The amastigotes of *Leishmania* spp. (see pp. 102–104), the cystlike stages of this polymorphic protozoan, reside exclusively in macrophages. Normally, the infection is regulated by the infected macrophages themselves, which induce cell-mediated immunity by stimulating Th1 T cells to produce macrophage-activating factors such as IFN-γ. Infected individuals that have Th1 T cell deficiency, on the other hand, will experience macrophage dysfunction allowing the infection to exacerbate. Macrophages infected with both *Leishmania* and HIV display an intensification of both infections. The infection with *Leishmania* stimulates the release of **tumor necrosis factor (TNF-α)** which, in turn, induces

HIV replication in the macrophage. Not only does HIV suppress cell-mediated immunity due to T cell inhibition, but infection by *Leishmania* promotes HIV infection of the macrophages resulting in the worst of both worlds.

TRYPANOSOMA CRUZI

Trypanosoma cruzi (see pp. 120–122) amastigotes also infect macrophages of humans. As in leishmaniasis, activated macrophages regulate the disease, especially the acute phase, by controlling the number of intracellular parasites. Any breakdown in T cell function serves to upgrade the infection. However, *T. cruzi* does not appear to exacerbate the effects of dual infections with HIV as *Leishmania* does.

PLASMODIUM SPP.

Plasmodium, the causative agent of human malaria (see pp. 129–151), displays two life cycle phases in its human host, an extraerythrocytic phase initiated when sporozoites infect hepatocytes, and an erythocytic phase involving the infection of red blood cells by merozoites. Suppression of $CD4^+$ T helper cell functions inhibits CD8 cytotoxic cell differentiation and release of IFN-γ. Both of these processes are important in the immunology of human malaria, especially for the extraerythrocytic stages. Inhibition of cytotoxic cell functions prevents the lysis of sporozoite-infected hepatocytes, while suppression of IFN-γ prevents the activation of macrophages and results in the release of uncontrolled numbers of merozoites during the extraerythrocytic phase.

GIARDIA LAMBLIA

The flagellate *Giardia lamblia* (see pp. 82–86) is an extracellular parasite of the small intestine. While *Giardia* infections are ostensibly controlled by IgA and IgM secretions of the host, there is evidence that depletion of $CD4^+$ T cells results in a marked decrease in the clearance of the motile trophozoites.

ENTEROCYTOZOON BIENEUSI

Enterocytozoon bieneusi (see pp. 76–77) is a protist of the phylum Microspora, which consists of obligate intracellular parasites that infect a wide variety of invertebrates and vertebrates, including mammals. Human infection by microsporidia is rare. However, with the advent of AIDS, there has been a dramatic rise in the number of human cases. *E. bieneusi* is one of the primary causes of chronic diarrhea in such individuals. In human microsporidiosis there is a decrease in the number of $CD4^+$ T cells, notably Th1 cells, in the patient. The microbiostatic activity of IFN-γ-activated macrophages has been shown experimentally in mice to be essential for the control of microsporidia. In HIV-infected patients, depletion of Th1 cells reduces the ability of macrophages to control the organisms, allowing the disease to flourish.

SCHISTOSOMA SPP.

In most helminth infections, Th2 cells, the primary helper cell subset, predominate. However, of the helminths that infect humans, only the blood flukes of the genus *Schistosoma* (see pp. 229–245) appear to be affected by Th2 cell inhibition.

Because the primary pathology of human schistosomiasis is the granulomatous response to eggs in the urinary tract, liver, spleen, and gastrointestinal tract (see pp. 244–245), depletion of the factors responsible for this inflammatory reaction might be considered beneficial to persons infected with schistosomes. The granulomatous response is normally triggered when $CD4^+$ T cells are stimulated by trapped eggs; the stimulated $CD4^+$ T cells activate macrophages, which, in turn, induce **delayed hypersensitivity reactions.** The granuloma serves to isolate the eggs in the tissue. Concurrently, the fibrous granulomas may disrupt blood and lymph flow and destroy neighboring cells; accompanying side effects may include enlargement of organs and cirrhosis (see p. 243–244). In immunosuppressed patients, there is a reduced response to the eggs, which leads to a reduction in the cell-mediated response and, consequently, a reduction in the granulomatous response. Concomitantly, fewer eggs reach the environment, suggesting that a certain level of inflammatory response is requisite for the propulsion of eggs through the intestinal and bladder walls. In addition to a reduction in the chronic inflammatory response, reduced T helper cell activity diminishes the level of concomitant immunity (see below).

RESISTANCE

Defined as the ability of a host to withstand infection by a parasite, **resistance** may develop in several ways. (1) It may result from the presence of some physical or chemical barrier that prevents the parasite from penetrating or migrating in the host. Such a barrier is thought to prevent the larval form of avian blood flukes from entering the circulatory system of abnormal hosts, such as humans. (2) Resistance may also be due to **natural** or **innate immunity.** An example of this type of immunity is conferred when certain proteins naturally present within an organism display structural properties of antibodies to specific antigens even though the organism (i.e., the potential host) has had no previous exposure to those antigens. Natural immunity may also be influenced by such factors as the host's genetic makeup, age, nutritional status, receptor molecules on cells, and gender. (3) **Acquired immunity** is conferred by a host's immune response to previous parasitic infection. This type of resistance, like natural immunity, is attracting a great deal of attention in the development of vaccines. **Premunition,** a form of acquired immunity, is resistance to reinfection dependent upon retention of the infectious agent. This type of resistance is seen in regions where malaria is endemic and low parasitemia is maintained in the victim when the disease is left untreated. **Concomitant immunity**, another form of acquired immunity, is the survival of some cells or organisms with the immune destruction of other cells or organisms of the same line. This type of resistance is typical of schistosomiasis. Hosts infected with adult schistosomes are able to destroy a challenge infection, but are unable to clear themselves of the original infection.

SELECTED READINGS

Bloom, B. R. 1979. Games parasites play: How parasites evade immune surveillance. *Nature* **279,** 21–26.

Campbell, W. C. 1986. The chemotherapy of parasitic infections. *Journal of Parasitology* **72**, 45–61.

Coffman, R. L., Varkila, K., Scott, P., and Chatelain, R. 1991. Role of cytokines in the differentiation of $CD4^+$ T-cell subsets *in vivo*. *Immunological Reviews* **123**, 189–207.

Damian, R. 1964. Molecular mimicry: Antigen sharing by parasite and host and its consequences. *American Naturalist* **98**, 129–149.

Hall, R. 1994. Molecular mimicry. *Advances in Parasitology* **34**, 81–132.

Leder, P. 1982. The genetics of antibody diversity. *Scientific American* **246**, 102–115.

Liew, F. Y., and O'Donnell, C. A. 1993. Immunology of leishmaniasis. *Advances in Parasitology* **32**, 162–259.

Pham, T. S., Mansfield, L. S., and Turiansky, G. W. 1997. Zoonoses in HIV-infected patients: Risk factors and prevention. *The AIDS Reader* **7**, 41–52.

Trager, W. 1986. *Living Together.* Plenum, New York.

PART ONE

THE PROTOZOA

Chapter Three

GENERAL CHARACTERISTICS OF THE PROTOZOA

Despite immense diversity, organisms of the kingdom Protista share a number of characteristics. Perhaps the most distinctive of these characteristics are: (1) the organisms are all single-celled or colonial and (2) they are eukaryotic. Beyond these broad criteria, however, sufficient diversity exists, even within the subkingdom Protozoa, to cause frequent confusion in taxonomy. In the taxonomic scheme adopted for this text, protozoans parasitic to humans are assigned to three phyla—Sarcomastigophora, Apicomplexa, and Ciliophora—with their mode of locomotion being one criterion for identification. In the phylum Sarcomastigophora, for example, the amoebae (subphylum Sarcodina) move by means of pseudopodia, and the flagellates (subphylum Mastigophora) use flagella as their primary locomotor apparatus. The ciliates (phylum Ciliophora) propel themselves by cilia. Members of the phylum Apicomplexa, primarily intracellular parasites, require no locomotor organelles except at some stages of their life cycles (e.g., flagellated gametes in some species). In some species limited movement is accomplished by contraction of intracellular microfilaments.

Light microscopy studies have given rise to a terminology unique to the protozoans in many ways. Increased use of electron microscopy, however, has shown that many of the structures typical of protozoans are ubiquitous among eukaryotic cells. To avoid confusion arising from the use of two sets of terms, those used in cell biology will be employed in this text with attempts to correlate them to their older counterparts.

Structurally, protozoa are unicellular organisms, each cell a self-sufficient unit capable of carrying out all of the metabolic functions of which multicellular organisms are capable. Each protozoan is surrounded by a unit membrane chemically similar to the plasma membrane common to all eukaryotic cells (i.e., a bilipid layer associated with a variety of proteins). Among the sarcodinans, this tends to be a very thin, flexible layer often called the **plasmalemma.** On the other hand, a more rigid body wall, usually supported by microtubules and characteristic of some flagellates and most ciliates, is termed a **pellicle.** It results in a more constant and uniform shape than that of the more amorphic amoebae.

The cytoplasm is usually divided into two areas: the cortical **ectoplasm** and the medullary **endoplasm.** The consistency, extent, and appearance of these two zones differ among species. Typically, the ectoplasm is a **gel** containing the basal bodies of cilia or flagella, microfilaments, and, in some protozoa, microtubules for rigidity and/or contractility. The endoplasm, or **sol,** is more fluid than ectoplasm and contains such organelles as nuclei, mitochondria, and various types of vacuoles and vesicles.

LOCOMOTOR ORGANELLES

FLAGELLA

Mastigophorans, commonly known as flagellates, include all protozoans usually exhibiting in their **trophozoite** (motile) stage one or more flagella (Fig. 3-1). The ability to swim has facilitated the flagellates' adaptation to a variety of habitats in their hosts. Unlike amoebae, which require a substrate on which to move, flagellates thrive in a liquid medium and, thus, are well suited for survival in the blood, lymph, and cerebrospinal fluid of the host. Their elongate, torpedo-shaped form enables them to swim in the host's body fluids with little resistance, a further adaptation for life in a liquid medium.

While flagella occur in the developmental stages of some amoebae and in the microgametes of some members of the phylum Apicomplexa, they are always present in the trophozoite stage of flagellates. The number of flagella per organism varies widely according to species.

The single flagellum is a filamentous cytoplasmic projection. Electron microscopy reveals this projection to be a sheath consisting of a cytoplasmic matrix enclosed by a plasma membrane within which is embedded an axial filament or **axoneme** (Fig. 3-2). The axoneme, extending the length of the flagellum, is comprised of a series of regularly oriented microtubules arranged in a specific pattern consisting of two central microtubules surrounded by an outer circle of nine pairs of microtubules or doublets (Fig. 3-3). Each flagellum is anchored in the cytoplasm by a

FIGURE 3-1
A typical flagellate as viewed with a light microscope, showing the flagellum, nucleus, basal body, and undulating membrane.

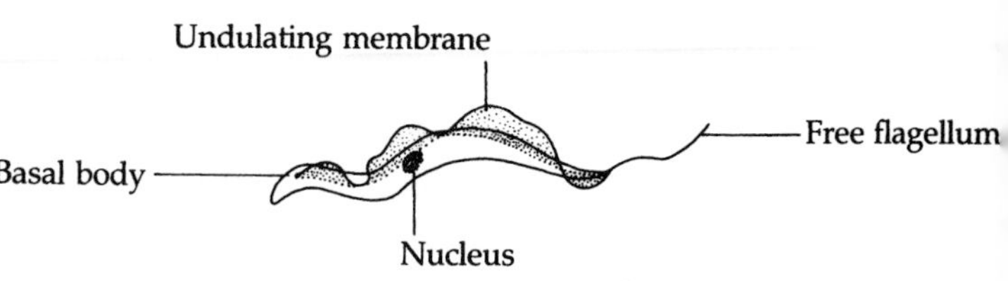

basal body (also called a **blepharoplast** or **kinetosome**) (Fig. 3-4a). Ultrastructural studies demonstrate that the basal body is morphologically identical to the centriole of the cell, and it is from the former organelle that the flagellum (or cilium) arises. The centriole and basal body consist of microtubules arranged in a circle of nine triplets, with two members of each triplet probably giving rise to and extending distally as one of the peripheral doublets of the flagellum (Fig. 3-4b).

In most flagellated cells, the flagellum extends from the basal body to the exterior; in some, however, one or more flagella may loop back in a complete reversal of their original direction. A flagellum of this type is known as a **recurrent flagellum.** A recurrent flagellum may extend into a cytostome, where it aids in the procurement of food. Or it may be attached to the plasma membrane

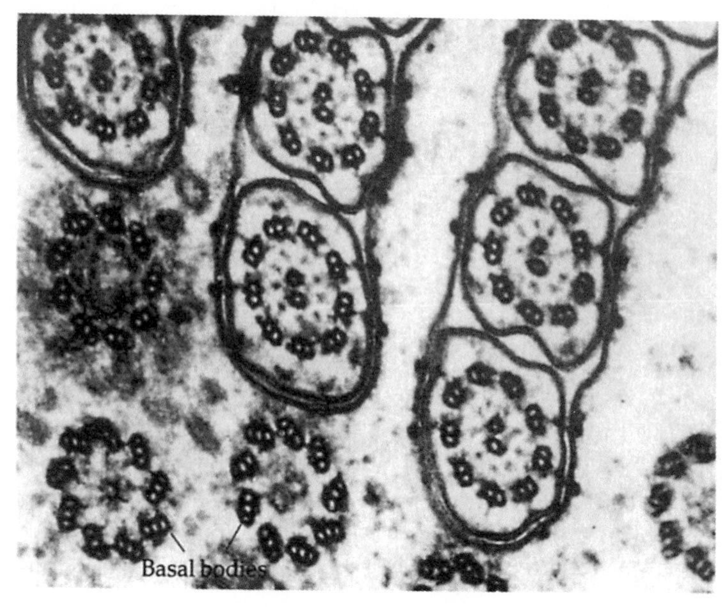

FIGURE 3-2
Transmission electron micrograph of cross sections of flagella of *Pseudotrichonympha* from the gut of a termite.
Note that the two median microtubules are single and the marginal ones are double. Sections through basal bodies are seen below the flagella.

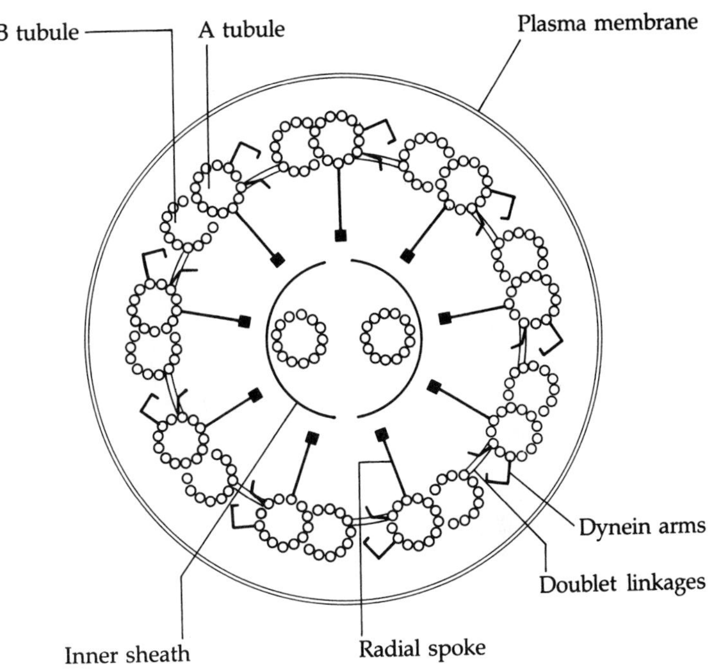

FIGURE 3-3
Schematic representation of flagellar organization.

by a series of desmosomes, in which case, during the beating process, it pulls the plasma membrane and a portion of the cytoplasm away from the body of the cell, producing an **undulating membrane** (Figs. 3-1, 3-5).

It is seen, then, that flagellar movement propels and directs the organism and at times assists in procuring food. The movement may also promote tactility and secretion of mating substances.

The so-called "beat" of a flagellum (or cilium) is actually the propagation of a series of wavelike bends along the length of the organelle. These bends are associated with the connections between outer microtubules and the inner sheath containing the two central microtubules. Energy to fuel this movement comes from the ATPase activity of the **dynein** arms associated with one member of each of the outer doublets (Fig. 3-3). This energy allows the doublet microtubules to slide past each other; however, because the sliding is restricted by chemical cross-links between the two microtubules, a bending occurs, which becomes a wave as the cross-links are broken and reformed along the axoneme (Fig. 3-6). When this phenomenon occurs sequentially, a regular beat pattern emerges, resulting in directional movement of the cell.

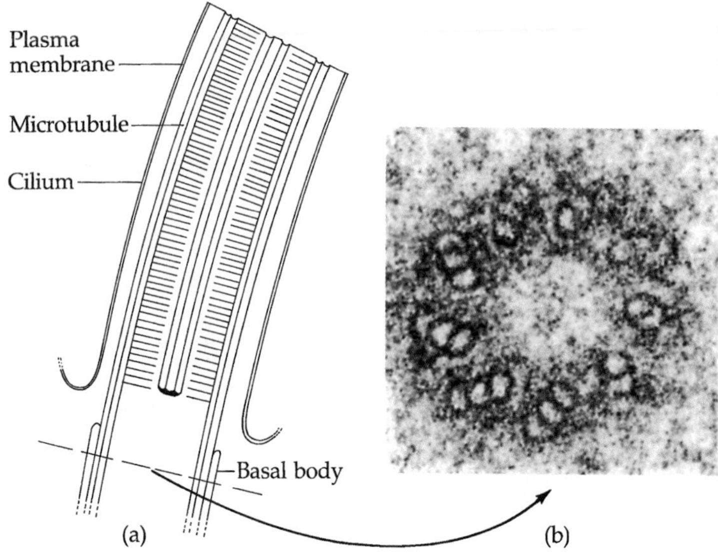

FIGURE 3-4
General structure of a cilium or flagellum.
(a) Longitudinal aspect of the cilium and basal body. (b) Transmission electron micrograph of a cross section through the basal body.

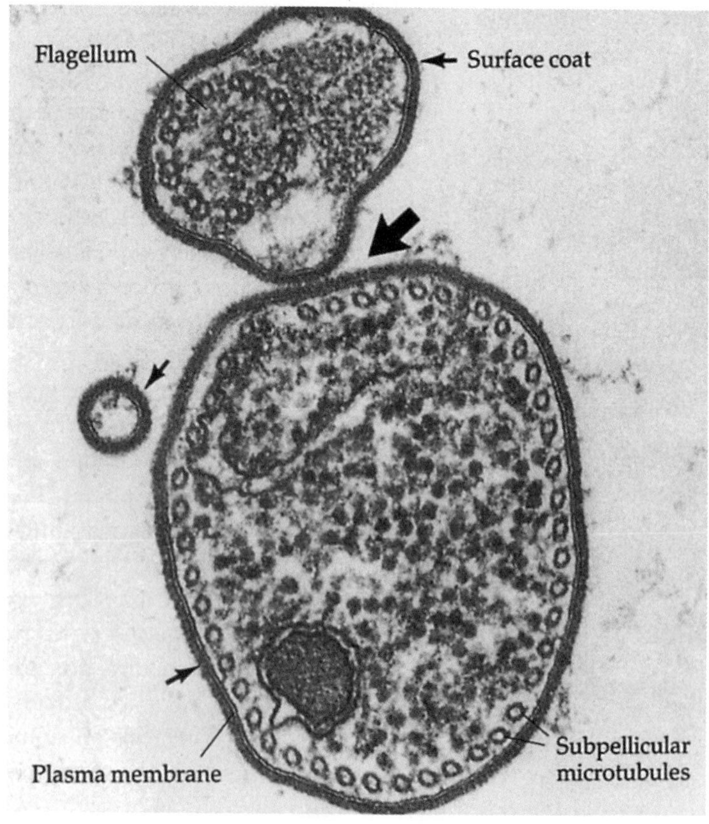

FIGURE 3-5
Transmission electron micrograph of *Trypanosoma brucei rhodesiense* (slender form) in transverse section.
The surface coat (small arrows) is seen as a dense layer covering the plasma membrane of both the body (below) and the flagellum (above). Large arrowhead points to the desmosome-like attachment of the flagellar membrane to the surface membrane. On the left, also in transverse section, is one of the streamerlike extensions that may represent a mechanism for shedding the variable antigen coat.

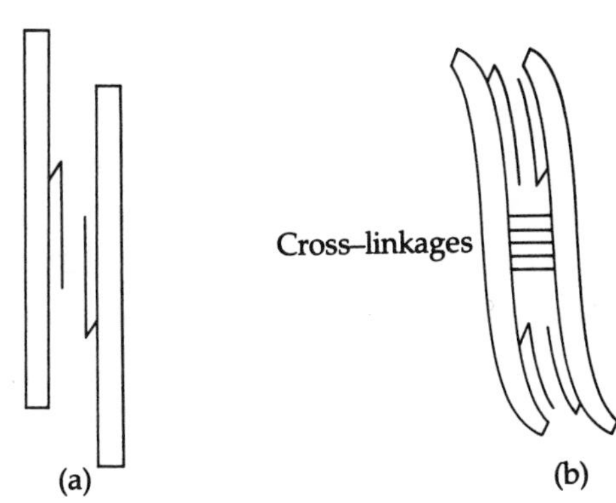

FIGURE 3-6
Sliding-filament mechanism of ciliary and flagellar bending.
(a) With no resistance to sliding, the doublets slide past one another. (b) Cross-links cause a resistance to sliding at one region. Displacement of doublets in the nonlinked regions is accommodated by bending.

CILIA

The fine structure of the axoneme of flagella and cilia is identical. Cilia may, therefore, be considered miniature flagella. In addition to noticeable differences in length, however, there are other fundamental differences between these two types of organelles, the most obvious of which is their number. Flagella usually number no more than ten on a given cell surface, while there may be literally thousands of cilia on a surface. An exception is found in the flagellate order Hypermastigida, whose members possess large numbers of flagella. In ciliates, the numerous basal bodies are interconnected by a series of subpellicular **microfilaments** or **neurofibrils,** forming an **infraciliature** believed to be responsible for either coordinating or providing support for the ciliary beat of the cell. The precise mechanics of this coordination are not presently understood.

PSEUDOPODIA

Amoebae are usually capable of producing **pseudopodia,** which are used as locomotor and food-acquiring organelles. These transitory body extensions depend for their function on the association between actin and myosin. These two molecules function in amoebae much as they function in the contraction of vertebrate muscle. Activated by ATP-derived energy and certain cations, such as calcium and magnesium, actin and myosin become intimately associated at the tip of the forming pseudopodium. This association produces a localized contractile response in the cytoplasm, whereupon the cytoplasm everts at the plasma

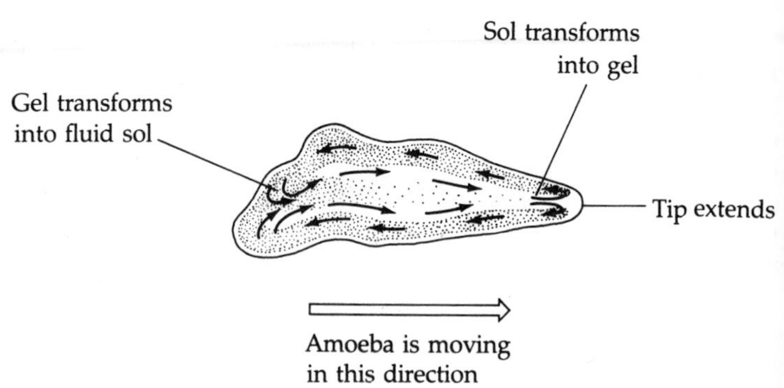

FIGURE 3-7
One type of amoeboid motion.
The extension of a pseudopodium by an amoeba is accompanied by the constant flowing of cytoplasm in the direction of the extension. There appears to be a continual transformation of gelated ectoplasm to fluid endoplasm at the trailing end and a reverse transformation at the leading end.

membrane and moves posteriad in the cell, forming an outer zone of cytoplasm known as the ectoplasm. At the rear of the cell, actin and myosin become dissociated; the ectoplasm reverts to the relaxed state, becoming more fluid, and moves inward to form endoplasm. When the endoplasm streams forward under the pressure of the contractile ectoplasm, actin again becomes associated with myosin, producing anew the contractile state. The overall effect, then, is a recurrent outward and posteriad flow of ectoplasm away from the direction of movement and a concomitant movement of the endoplasm from the rear of the cell in the direction of the forming pseudopod (Fig. 3-7).

Morphologically, pseudopodia can be assigned to one of four types: **filopodia, lobopodia, rhizopodia,** and **axopodia.** Lobopodia (Fig. 3-8), the most common form among parasitic amoebae, are blunt and may be composed of both ectoplasm and endoplasm or of ectoplasm only. In most species, lobopodia form slowly. Observation of living specimens clearly shows the gradual flow of granular endoplasm, when present, into the broad projection. *Entamoeba histolytica*, an important parasite of the human intestine, is exceptional in that the lobopodia are produced abruptly and withdrawn almost as quickly. Another exception is observed among certain amoebae that appear to move on a substratum with no obvious cytoplasmic protrusions. Such amoebae are termed **limax forms** after the slug, *Limax* spp., whose movement they appear to mimic.

Although the formation of pseudopodia by trophozoites is usually considered a distinguishing characteristic of amoebae, some flagellates are also capable of pseudopodial movement at some stage during their life and, conversely, some amoebae (*Naegleria*, for example) possess flagella during their developmental stages. As a general rule, however, among flagellates the princi-

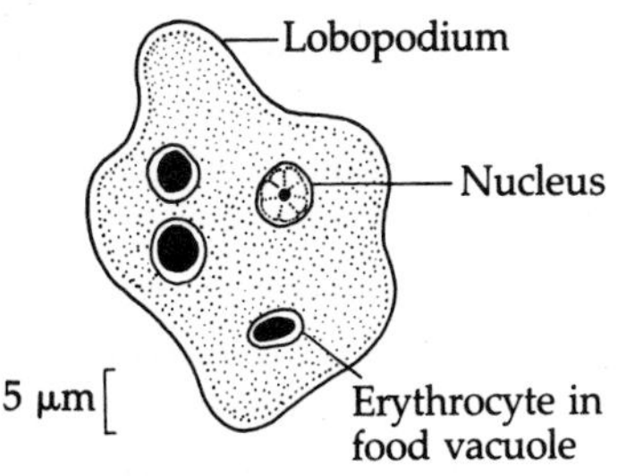

FIGURE 3-8
Lobopodial type of pseudopodium in an *Entamoeba histolytica* trophozoite.

pal means of locomotion is flagellar, while among amoebae it is pseudopodial.

Most amoebae cannot swim; pseudopodial locomotion requires a substrate on which these organisms can glide. Parasitic species, therefore, are commonly found in the alimentary tract of their hosts, intimately associated with the epithelial lining.

OTHER ORGANELLES

NUCLEUS

Well-defined nuclei bounded by nuclear envelopes are characteristic of all protozoa. Some protozoa have a single nucleus; others have two or more essentially identical nuclei; still others, such as the ciliophorans, have two different types of nuclei: a **macronucleus** and one or more **micronuclei.** As the name indicates, the macronucleus is larger than the micronuclei, and it is involved with trophic activities of the cell. Micronuclei are involved in reproductive functions, both asexual and sexual.

In addition to size classification as macro- or micronuclei, nuclei may be defined morphologically as either **vesicular** or **compact.** This distinction is often used in identification of species infecting humans, since nuclei of such species are commonly vesicular.

Vesicular Nucleus

The nuclear envelope of a vesicular nucleus, although delicate in appearance, is visible by light microscopy. The term *vesicular* denotes numerous clear areas resulting from the irregular distribution of chromatin, creating the impression of many small sacs or vesicles. The chromatin areas may be concentrated peripherally or internally. The nucleoplasm contains one or more **endosomes** or **karyosomes,** which are DNA-negative and probably analogous to metazoan nucleoli; unlike nucleoli, however, they do not disappear during mitosis.

Compact Nucleus

A compact nucleus contains a larger amount of more densely packed chromatin than does a vesicular nucleus. It is also generally larger than a vesicular nucleus and may vary in shape from round to ovate. Compact nuclei are found in the ciliophorans, where they are involved in the sexual process called **conjugation.** During this process, two cells join (or conjugate), one micronucleus of each cell undergoes meiosis, and some of the resulting haploid micronuclei are exchanged between the two individuals. The micronuclei then fuse, resulting in a genetically new set of micronuclei for each partner cell. During the meiotic division, exchange, and fusion of micronuclei, the macronuclei disappear and subsequently reform. They seem to serve as directors of the phenotypic expression of the cells. Following conjugation, the two cells separate and then usually divide mitotically.

MITOCHONDRIA

Double-unit, membrane-bound mitochondria provide sites for intracellular aerobic metabolism and are similar in ultrastructure to those of most eukaryotes. A feature peculiar to protistan mitochondria is the tubular shape of the cristae. Similar cristae are observed in mitochondria of multicellular eukaryotes (Fig. 3-9) but less consistently than in those of protists. The significance of this structural variation is presently unexplained. It should be noted that a number of parasitic protozoans (such as *Entamoe-*

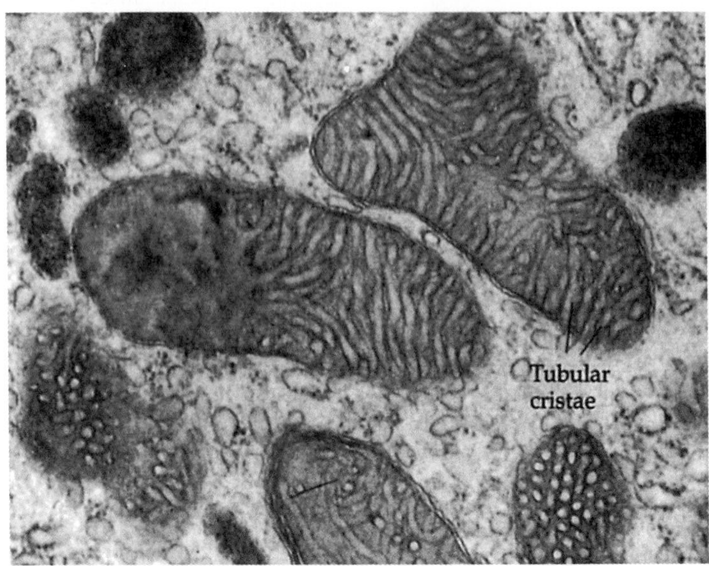

FIGURE 3-9
Several mitochondria showing profiles of tubular cristae, from hamster suprarenal cortex.

ba histolytica) possess no mitochondria, a deficiency associated with anaerobic metabolism.

GOLGI COMPLEX

The Golgi complex is a cytoplasmic organelle whose specific function in protozoans is essentially identical to that in other eukaryotes. The Golgi complex is the seat of glycosylation of a number of secretory products of the cell. It is in the cisternae of the Golgi complex, for instance, that the final carbohydrate moieties are added to the glycocalyx associated with the plasma membrane. The arrangement and number of Golgi complexes vary during the life cycle of many protozoans. Thus, cyst-forming protozoans may lose their Golgi complexes during encystation, only to resynthesize them when they excyst. The so-called **parabasal body** of protozoans is homologous to the Golgi complex of other eukaryotic cells but has several morphological differences, the most notable of which is the frequent presence of a fibril, the **parabasal filament,** running from the cisternae of the Golgi complex to one or more basal bodies.

LYSOSOMES

The lysosome (Fig. 3-10), an organelle ubiquitous among eukaryotes, is bounded by a single-unit membrane enclosing various hydrolytic enzymes whose optimum activities occur in the acid pH range. Such enzymes, therefore, are designated **acid hydrolases.** Lysosomes, with their battery of acid hydrolases, function in autophagy as well as in intracellular digestion of exogenous foodstuffs. In certain parasitic amoebae, for instance, **food vacuoles** are formed by the engulfment of exogenous food, including host cells. The food vacuoles then fuse with lysosomes, forming a **digestive vacuole,** and the lysosomal enzymes mix with and degrade the ingested material. Among a number of protozoans, ingestion occurs at a specialized site on the plasma membrane called the **cytostome** (Fig. 3-11). After digestion, undigested residues are egested through the plasma membrane. Among amoebae, such egestion may occur anywhere on the plasmalemma, while in ciliates there is a permanent pellicular site, the **cytopyge,** through which undigested residues are emitted.

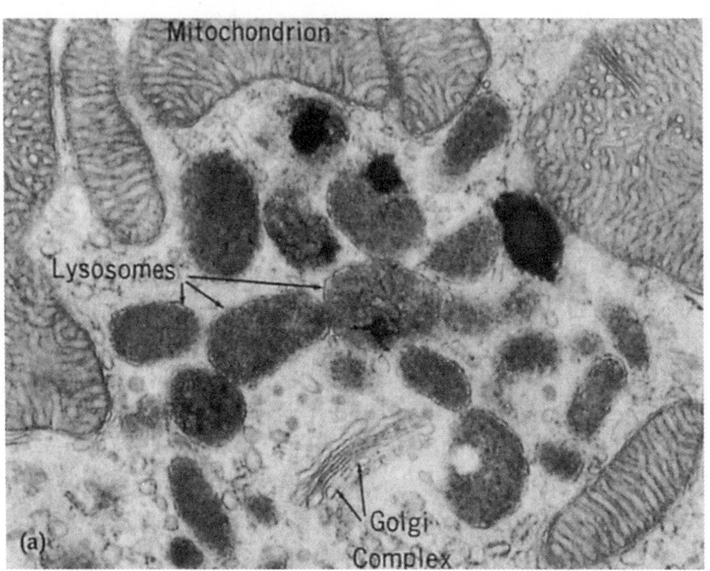

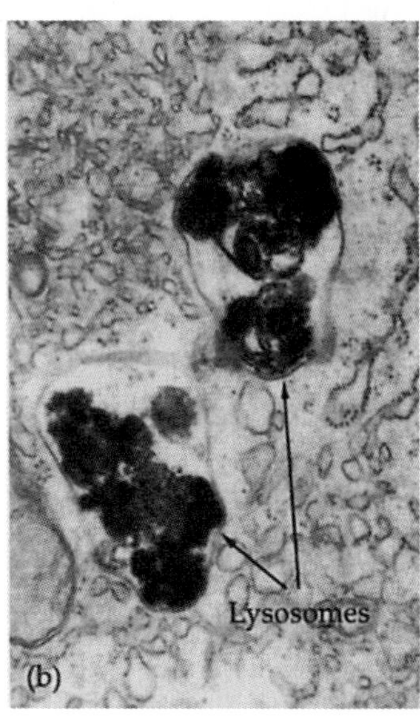

FIGURE 3-10
Transmission electron micrographs of lysosomes.
(a) A cluster of lysosomes. (b) Two secondary lysosomes enclosing dense inclusions.

CYTOPLASMIC FOOD STORAGE

Reserve food inclusions are seen in various species of parasitic protozoa. The nature and amount of stored nutrients vary with the environment and the species involved. For example, glycogen and/or amylopectin are sometimes found in cysts of amoebae that inhabit the human intestine. This stored food, accumulated shortly before encystation and used during the nonfeeding stage, is usually completely exhausted by the time of excystation. In addition to these polysaccharides, lipid droplets and nucleic acid reserves may be present in both trophozoites and cysts.

RIBOSOMES

These organelles, the sites of cellular protein synthesis, are part of the organelle population of all eukaryotes and are abundant in those cells that actively synthesize protein for either secretion or internal use. They occur in association with the endoplasmic reticulum or free in the cytoplasm, either singly or in clusters

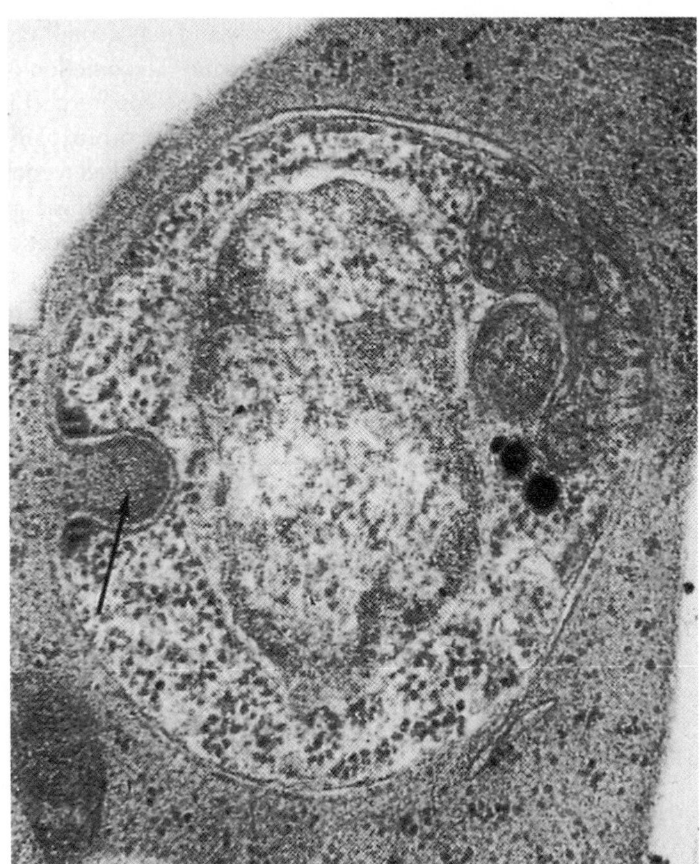

FIGURE 3-11
A uninucleate trophozoite of *Plasmodium cathemerium* ingesting host cell cytoplasm through a cytostome (arrow).

known as **polyribosomes.** During encystation, much of the ribosomal constituency of the cell is exhausted.

COSTA, AXOSTYLE, AND VACUOLES

Associated with the basal bodies of many flagellates is a prominent, striated rod, the **costa.** This structure usually courses from one of the basal bodies along the base of the undulating membrane. It can best be described as a modified, **striated rootlet.** Rootlets are found at the bases of many cilia and flagella in other eukaryotes, penetrating deep into the cytoplasm where they are believed to serve as anchors. In addition to the costa, a sheath of microtubules in the shape of a tube, the **axostyle,** is observed in many flagellates. This structure extends posteriorly from the basal body and may actually appear to protrude through the plasma membrane. The function of the axostyle is unknown, and the organelle has no counterpart in other eukaryotic cells.

Some parasitic protozoans, such as the ciliate *Balantidium coli*, possess fluid-filled vesicles called **contractile vacuoles.** In protozoans generally, these are considered osmoregulatory organelles, ridding the cell of excess water as well as some dissolved metabolic wastes. However, since most parasitic protozoa, like their marine counterparts, are isosmotic to their environment, they do not commonly contain contractile vacuoles.

ENCYSTATION

Many parasitic protozoa are capable of encystation, during which the rounded cytoplasmic mass is surrounded by a rigid or semirigid cyst wall secreted by the organism. The cyst wall may be single- or multi-layered. Cysts of parasitic protozoa serve three primary functions: (1) protection against unfavorable external environmental conditions, (2) morphogenesis and nuclear division, and (3) transmission from one host to another.

Examples of the first function are seen in the human pathogens *Entamoeba histolytica*, an amoeba, and *Giardia lamblia*, a flagellate, which form cysts in the intestinal tract that are expelled in fecal material. Such cysts may remain viable for many weeks under normal conditions and for days at higher and lower temperatures and during periods of dessication. Further, the cyst wall protects the ingested organism as it passes through the host's hostile gastric fluids.

Cysts of many parasitic protozoa also serve as sites for nuclear and cytoplasmic reorganization and division. Shortly after the trophozoite encysts, cytoplasmic reorganization occurs, sometimes followed by nuclear divisions, after which the mature cyst may enclose from one (in the absence of nuclear division) to eight vesicular nuclei. In *E. histolytica*, for instance, two consecutive mitotic divisions result in four vesicular nuclei (see Fig. 4-2, p. 63). If mature cysts are reintroduced into a suitable host, excystation occurs, and each escaping motile trophozoite usually divides once more, resulting in eight small trophozoites produced from the single, tetranucleated mass of cytoplasm encased within the cyst wall. After excystation, the newly excysted trophozoites begin a period of active feeding, followed by rapid growth and binary fission.

Finally, intestinal protozoa are transmitted to a new host (or become reestablished in the same host) when that host swallows the cysts. Thus, the cysts serve as a vehicle for transmission.

The precise environmental conditions that trigger encystation are not totally defined. In many species, the process often occurs in response to a deficiency in the host of nutrients essential to the parasite. In addition, increased osmotic pressure, temperature changes, low pH, accumulation of waste products in the medium, and crowding all appear to stimulate encystation.

REPRODUCTION

Parasitic protozoa most commonly reproduce by means of an asexual process called **fission,** a type of mitosis whereby each parent gives rise to two progeny. The plane of division is random among amoebae, usually longitudinal in flagellates, and transverse in ciliates. The sequence of division in a typical protozoan is as follows: organelles, nucleus, and finally cytoplasm.

In apicomplexans, two types of **multiple fission** occur: **schizogony** (**merogony**) and **endopolyogeny.** Both are characterized by rapid organelle and nuclear divisions, followed by multiple cytokinesis. In schizogony, the multinucleated cell is called the **schizont** or **segmenter.** After cytoplasmic division, the nuclei, with their attendant cytoplasm, form separate organisms, **merozoites**, at the periphery of the mother cell, which usually break away from the aggregate to infect new host cells. Once a merozoite enters a new host cell, it may either enter another schizogonic cycle or become a macro- or microgametocyte. **Syngamy,** the union of gametes derived from the gametocytes, initiates the sexual cycle. The resulting zygote undergoes **sporogony**, which produces **sporozoites.** The organisms that cause malaria are apicomplexans capable of both schizogonic (asexual) and sporogonic (sexual) reproduction. In fact, many apicomplexans are considered unique among protists in exhibiting alternation of generations, a characteristic more commonly associated with plants and some invertebrate animals, such as cnidarians. The other type of asexual reproduction, endopolyogeny, is sometimes considered a form of internal budding. It differs from schizogony only in the location of the daughter cells relative to the mother cell. In endopolyogeny, the daughter cells form in the center of the mother cell rather than at the periphery. The form of endopolyogeny in which the mother cell produces only two daughter cells is termed **endodyogeny.**

Conjugation, the specialized sexual mechanism in the ciliates, has already been discussed; it is distinguishable from syngamy in that conjugation involves nuclear exchange and union, whereas syngamy involves the union of entire cells (i.e., gametes).

SELECTED READINGS

Bailey, G. B., Day, D. B., and McCoomer, N. E. 1992. *Entamoeba* motility: Dynamics of cytoplasmic streaming, locomotion and translocation of surface-bound particles, and organization of the actin cytoskeleton in *Entamoeba invadens*. *Journal of Protozoology* **39**, 267–272.

Corliss, J. O. 1991. Introduction to the protozoa. In *Microscopic Anatomy of Invertebrates* (Harrison, F. W., and Corliss, J. O., Eds.), Vol. 1, pp. 1–12. Wiley-Liss, New York.

Lee, J. J., Hutner, S. H., and Bovee, E. C. 1986. *An Illustrated Guide to the Protozoa*. Society of Protozoologists, Lawrence, Kansas.

Pitelka, D. R. 1963. *Electron-microscopic Structure of Protozoa*. Pergamon, Elmsford, NY.

Satir, P. 1974. How cilia move. *Scientific American* **231**, 45–52.

Stossel, T. P. 1994. The machinery of cell crawling. *Scientific American* **71**, 54–63.

CLASSIFICATION OF THE PROTOZOA*

PHYLUM SARCOMASTIGOPHORA

Single type of nucleus; sexuality, when present, essentially syngamy; with flagella, pseudopodia, or both types of locomotor organelles.

*Only those taxa that include parasitic species discussed in this text are defined.

Subphylum Mastigophora

One or more flagella typically present in trophozoites; asexual reproduction basically by intrakinetal (symmetrogenic) binary fission; sexual reproduction known in some groups.

CLASS ZOOMASTIGOPHOREA

Chloroplasts absent; one to many flagella; amoeboid forms, with or without flagella, in some groups; sexuality known in a few groups; a polyphyletic class.

ORDER KINETOPLASTIDA

One or two flagella arising from a depression; flagella typically equipped with paraxial rod in addition to axoneme; single mitochondrion (nonfunctional in some forms) extending length of body as a single tube, hoop, or network of branching tubes, usually containing conspicuous Feulgen-positive (DNA-containing) kinetoplast located near flagellar kinetosomes; Golgi complex typically in region of flagellar depression, not connected to kinetosomes and flagella; parasitic (majority of species) and free-living.

Suborder Trypanosomatina

Single flagellum either free or attached to body by undulating membrane; kinetoplast relatively small and compact; parasitic. (Genera mentioned in text: *Leishmania, Trypanosoma*)

ORDER RETORTAMONADIDA

Two to four flagella, one directed posteriorly and associated with ventrally located cytostomal area bordered by fibril; mitochondria and Golgi apparatus absent; cysts present; parasitic. (Genera mentioned in text: *Chilomastix, Retortamonas*)

ORDER DIPLOMONADIDA

One or two karyomastigonts; genera with two karyomastigonts exhibit twofold rotational symmetry or, in one genus, primarily mirror symmetry; individual mastigonts with one to four flagella, typically one recurrent and associated with cytostome, or, in more advanced genera, with organelles forming cell axis; mitochondria and Golgi apparatus absent; intranuclear division spindle; cysts present; free-living or parasitic.

Suborder Diplomonadina

Two karyomastigonts; body with twofold rotational symmetry or, in one genus, bilateral symmetry; with four flagella, one recurrent; with a variety of microtubular bands; cysts present; free-living or parasitic. (Genus mentioned in text: *Giardia*)

ORDER TRICHOMONADIDA

Typically, karyomastigonts with four to six flagella, but one genus exhibiting only a single flagellum and another none; karyomastigonts and akaryomastigonts in one family with permanent polymonad organization; in mastigonts of typical genera, one flagellum recurrent, free, or with proximal or entire length adherent to body surface; undulating membrane, if present, associated with adherent segment of recurrent flagellum; pelta and noncontractile axostyle in each mastigont, except in one genus; hydrogenosomes present; true cysts known in very few species; all or nearly all parasitic. (Genera mentioned in text: *Dientamoeba, Trichomonas, Pentatrichomonas*)

Subphylum Sarcodina

Pseudopodia, or locomotive protoplasmic flow without discrete pseudopodia; flagella, when present, usually restricted to developmental or other temporary stages; body naked or with external or internal test or skeleton; asexual reproduction by fission; sexuality, if present, associated with flagellate or, more rarely, amoeboid gametes; most species free-living.

SUPERCLASS RHIZOPODA

Locomotion by lobopodia, filopodia, or reticulopodia, or by protoplasmic flow without production of discrete pseudopodia.

CLASS LOBOSEA

Pseudopodia lobose or more or less filiform but produced from broader hyaline lobe; usually uninucleate.

ORDER AMOEBIDA

Typically uninucleate; mitochondria typically present; no flagellate stage.

Suborder Tubulina

Body a branched or unbranched cylinder; no bidirectional flow of cytoplasm; nuclear division mesomitotic. (Genera mentioned in text: *Hartmannella, Entamoeba, Endolimax, Iodamoeba*)

Suborder Acanthopodina

More or less finely tipped, sometimes filiform, often furcate hyaline pseudopodia produced from a broad hyaline lobe; not regularly discoid; cysts usually formed; nuclear division mesomitotic or metamitotic. (Genus mentioned in text: *Acanthamoeba*)

ORDER SCHIZOPYRENIDA

Body with shape of monopodial cylinder; movement usually accomplished by means of more or less eruptive, hyaline, hemispheric bulges; typically uninucleate; nuclear division promitotic; temporary flagellated stages in most species. (Genus mentioned in text: *Naegleria*)

PHYLUM APICOMPLEXA

Apical complex (visible with electron microscope), generally consisting of one or more polar rings, rhoptries, micronemes, conoid, and subpellicular microtubules present at some stage; one or more micropores generally present at some stage; cilia absent; sexuality by syngamy; all species parasitic.

CLASS SPOROZOASIDA

Conoid, if present, forming complete cone; reproduction generally both sexual and asexual; oocysts generally containing infective sporozoites resulting from sporogony; locomotion of mature organisms by body flexion, gliding, or undulation of longitudinal ridges; flagella present only in microgametes of some groups; pseudopods ordinarily absent, but if present, used for feeding rather than locomotion; homoxenous or heteroxenous.

Subclass Coccidiasina

Gamonts ordinarily present; mature gamonts typically intracellular, without mucron or epimerite; syzygy generally absent, but if present, involves markedly anisogamous gametes; life cycle characteristically consists of schizogony (merogony), gametogony, and sporogony; most species in vertebrates.

ORDER EUCOCCIDIORIDA

Merogony present; in vertebrates and/or invertebrates.

Suborder Eimeriorina

Macrogamete and microgamont developing independently; no syzygy; microgamont typically producing many microgametes; zygote nonmotile; sporozoites typically enclosed in sporocyst within oocyst; homoxenous or heteroxenous. (Genera mentioned in text: *Toxoplasma, Isospora*)

Suborder Haemosporina

Macrogamete and microgamete developing independently; conoid usually absent; microgamont producing eight flagellated microgametes; zygote motile (ookinete); sporozoites naked, with three-membraned wall; heteroxenous, with schizogony (merogony) in vertebrates and sporogony in invertebrates; transmitted by blood-sucking insects. (Genus mentioned in text: *Plasmodium*)

Subclass Piroplasmasina

Piriform, round, rod-shaped, or amoeboid; conoid absent; no oocysts, spores, or pseudocysts; flagella absent; usually without subpellicular microtubules; with polar ring and rhoptries; asexual and probably sexual reproduction; parasitic in erythrocytes and sometimes also in other circulating and fixed cells; heteroxenous, with merogony in vertebrates and sporogony in invertebrates; sporozoites with single-membraned wall; vectors are usually ticks. (Genus mentioned in text: *Babesia*)

PHYLUM MICROSPORA

Unicellular spores, each with imperforate wall, containing one uninucleate or dinucleate sporoplasm and simple or complex extrusion apparatus always with polar tube and polar cap; without mitochondria; often dimorphic in sporulation sequence; obligatory intracellular parasites in nearly all major animal groups. (Genus mentioned in text: *Enterocytozoon*)

PHYLUM CILIOPHORA

Simple cilia or compound ciliary organelles typical in at least one stage of life cycle; with subpellicular infraciliature present even when cilia absent; two types of nuclei, with rare exceptions; binary fission transverse, but budding and multiple fission also occur; sexuality involving conjugation, autogamy, and cytogamy; contractile vacuole typically present; most species free-living, but many commensal, some parasitic, and a large number found as phoronts on a variety of hosts.

CLASS LITOSTOMATEA

Body monokinetids with tangential transverse ribbon and non-overlapping, laterally directed kinetodesmal fibrils; simple oral cilia usually not as polykinetids.

ORDER VESTIBULIFERIDA

Apical or near apical densely ciliated vestibulum commonly present; no polykinetids; free-living or parasitic, especially in digestive tracts of vertebrates and invertebrates. (Genus mentioned in text: *Balantidium*)

Chapter Four

VISCERAL PROTOZOA I: AMOEBAE AND CILIATES

Amoebae

Entamoeba histolytica

Entamoeba dispar

Entamoeba hartmanni

Entamoeba coli

Entamoeba polecki

Entamoeba gingivalis

Iodamoeba butschlii

Endolimax nana

Pathogenic Free-Living Amoebae

Naegleria fowleri

Acanthamoeba

Microsporidians

Ciliates

Balantidium coli

Selected Readings

AMOEBAE

This category of parasites consists of members of the subphylum Sarcodina. All species in this subphylum that are parasitic in humans belong to the order Amoebida and, with few exceptions, are nonpathogenic or produce only minor diseases; however, they require special emphasis in order to distinguish them from the potentially highly pathogenic *Entamoeba histolytica* (Table 4-1). Such attention is amply justified, since *E. histolytica* can produce extreme illness and even death. Furthermore, because side effects from chemotherapy may be pronounced, it is of great importance that diagnosis of the condition be precise and accurate in order to assure treatment only when absolutely necessary, not merely to eliminate a protozoan that resembles *E. histolytica.*

At least eight species of amoebae belonging to three genera are known to parasitize humans. These are *Entamoeba histolytica*, *E. hartmanni*, *E. dispar*, *E. coli*, *E. polecki*, *E. gingivalis*, *Endolimax nana*, and *Iodamoeba butschlii*. All inhabit the large intestine except *E. gingivalis*, which is found in the mouth. In addition, amoebae belonging to at least three genera, *Naegleria*, *Acanthamoeba*, and *Hartmannella*, normally free-living, have been shown on occasion to parasitize humans by accident.

ENTAMOEBA HISTOLYTICA

Undoubtedly, the best-known species of amoebae parasitizing humans is *E. histolytica* (Fig. 4-1), the causative agent of amoebic dysentery or amoebiasis. First discovered in Russia by Losch in 1875, it is global in distribution, although its prevalence varies markedly from one area to another. For example, it has been reported to infect 85% of the population of Merida, Yucatan, Mexico, but no more than an average of 13.6% (range, 0.8–38%) of several populations surveyed in the United States. It is, nevertheless, important to remember that amoebiasis is not restricted to

TABLE 4-1
Some Important Enteric Amoebae of Humans

	Entamoeba histolytica	***Entamoeba coli***	***Endolimax nana***	***Iodamoeba butschlii***	***Entamoeba gingivalis***	***Dientamoeba fragilis****
Trophozoite						
Size (range)	25 μm (15–60)	25 μm (15–40)	9 μm (5–14)	10 μm (6–25)	15 μm (5–35)	10 μm (6–25)
Motility	active, directional, progressive	sluggish, nondirectional, nonprogressive	similar to *E. coli*	similar to *E. coli*	moderately active, progressive	active, progressive
Pseudopodia	fingerlike, explosive	short, blunt, broad, slow	similar to *E. coli*	similar to *E. coli*	blunt, rapidly formed	thin, leaflike, multiple, rapidly formed
Nucleus (stained)	delicate envelope & chromatin; central endosome	coarse envelope & chromatin, eccentric endosome	large endosome; no peripheral chromatin	large endosome surrounded by granules	similar ro *E. histolytica*	similar to *E. histolytica;* endosome divided into 4–6 granules
Cyst						
Size (range)	12 μm (10–20)	17 μm (10–33)	9 μm (5–14)	10 μm (5–18)	none	none
Inclusions						
Glycogen	diffuse	ill defined	absent	large mass		
Chromatoidal bars	in young cysts; rounded ends	in young cysts; splintered ends	occasionally as granules	usually absent		
Number of nuclei	1–4	1–8	1–4	1		

*Mastigophora

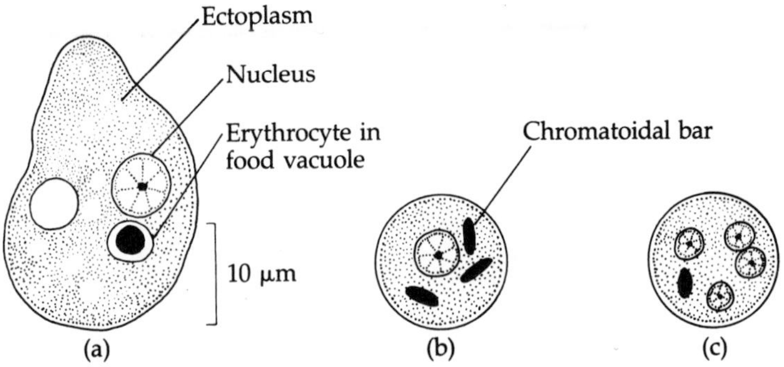

Ectoplasm
Nucleus
Erythrocyte in food vacuole
10 μm
Chromatoidal bar
(a) (b) (c)

FIGURE 4-1
Entamoeba histolytica.
(a) Trophozoite. (b) Early cyst with chromatoidal bars. (c) Later cyst.

the tropics and subtropics; it also occurs in temperate and even in arctic and antarctic zones. The usual mode of infection—ingestion of cysts from contaminated hands, food, or water—causes the incidence to increase considerably in densely populated areas, where contact with infected individuals is more likely. Children's homes and mental health institutions often produce conditions favorable to transmission of amoebiasis.

Life Cycle

The uninucleate trophozoite of *E. histolytica* inhabits the colon, rectum and, at times, the lower end of the small intestine of humans and other primates (Fig. 4-2). The motile trophozoite averages 25 μm in diameter (range, 15–60 μm) and is typically monopodial, producing one large, fingerlike pseudopodium at a time (Fig. 4-1a). The single pseudopodium erupts and is withdrawn so rapidly that, in prepared slides, trophozoites with pseudopodia extended are rarely seen. The cytoplasm is differentiated into two zones: a clear, refractile ectoplasm and a finely granular endoplasm in which food vacuoles occur. Such vacuoles may contain host erythrocytes, leukocytes, and epithelial cells, as well as bacteria and other intestinal material. Trophozoites proliferate mitotically (binary fission) within the host's gut.

The nucleus is of special importance in differentiating *E. histolytica* from most of the other intestinal amoebae. In saline preparations, the nucleus has a barely discernible nuclear envelope. In stained preparations, however, the vesicular nucleus is clearly visible. Ideally, it has a well-defined envelope, lined on the inner surface with fine peripheral chromatin granules and a minute, centrally located endosome. This nuclear morphology is

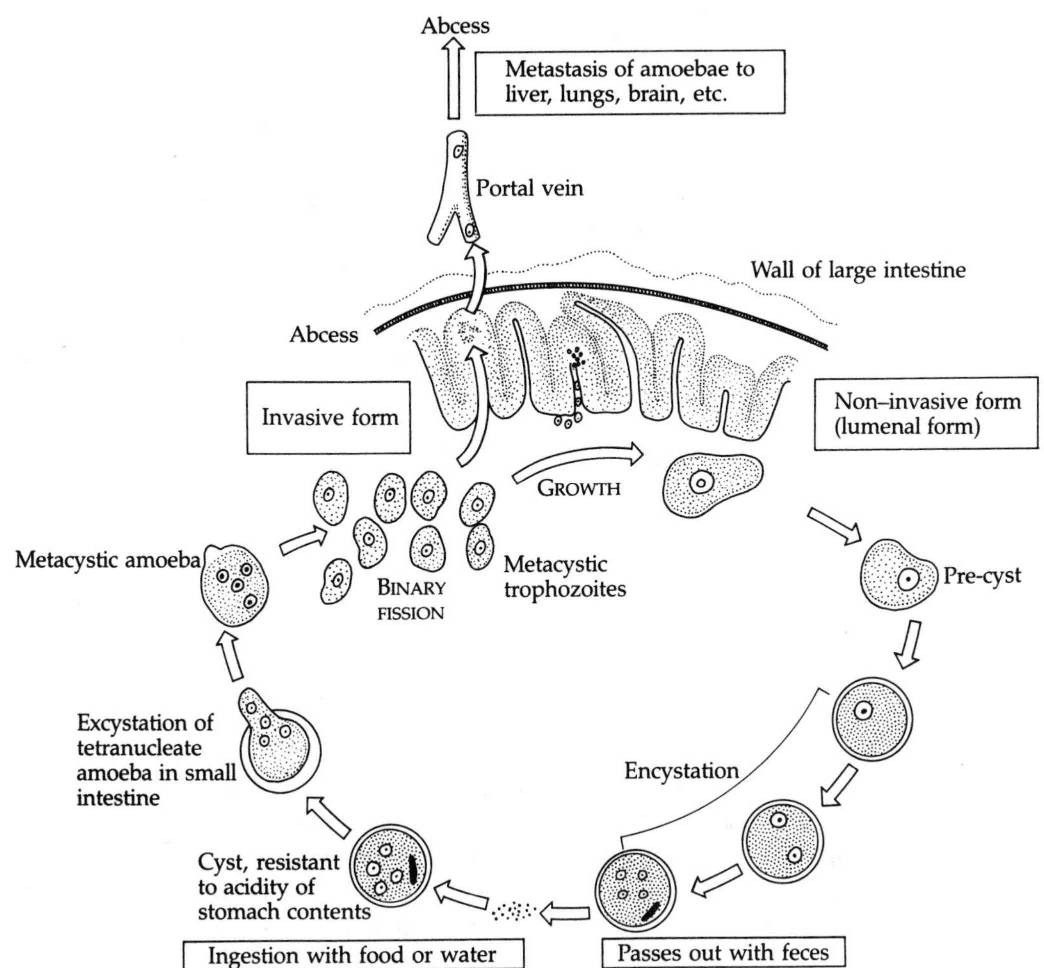

FIGURE 4-2
Life cycle of *Entamoeba histolytica*.

not confined to *E. histolytica* but is shared by other species of *Entamoeba*, notably *E. dispar*.

Under certain adverse environmental and/or physiological circumstances, trophozoites assume precystic characteristics by becoming more spherical and, as food vacuoles are extruded, shrinking in size. Pseudopodia, if formed, are sluggishly extended, and there appears to be no progressive movement. Encystation begins with the secretion by the precyst trophozoite of a thin, surrounding hyaline membrane to form a cyst wall. At this stage the cyst is usually spherical, averaging 12 μm in diameter (range, 10–20 μm), with a single nucleus. At times, glycogen masses and chromatoidal bars may be observed (Fig. 4-1b). The latter structures are considered to be deposits of nucleic acids that may vary in shape but always have smoothly rounded ends in *E. histolytica*. This characteristic distinguishes *E. histolytica* cysts from those of *E. coli*, in which the chromatoidal bars have jagged or splintered ends. The nucleus undergoes two mitotic divisions to produce four vesicular nuclei in the mature cyst of *E. histolytica* (Fig. 4-1c). Such cysts represent the infective form and pass out of the host in feces, after which the glycogen and chromatoidal substance are slowly metabolized and disappear.

Cysts of *E. histolytica* are highly resistant to desiccation and even to certain chemicals. Cysts in water can survive for a month, while those in feces on dry land can survive for more than 12 days; they tolerate temperatures up to 50°C.

When food or water contaminated with *E. histolytica* cysts is ingested by a host, the cysts pass through the stomach (protected from the harsh environment by the cyst wall) to the ileum, where excystation occurs. The neutral or slightly alkaline environment afforded by the small intestine is apparently requisite for excystation. However, *in vitro* studies suggest that excystation does not occur immediately; cysts placed in fresh culture medium at body temperature require 5–6 hours for excystation. Upon excystation, a single tetranucleate organism immediately undergoes mitosis, giving rise to eight small, metacystic trophozoites, which pass downward to the large intestine where they feed, grow, and reproduce. Reduction in intestinal peristalsis often allows the trophozoites to become established in the caecal area of the colon. The greater the number of organisms, the greater the likelihood that they will become established in the intestinal epithelium. Conversely, greater intestinal motility and/or large volumes of ingested food reduce the potential for establishment of the amoebae.

Multiplication of this species is thus seen to occur at two stages during the life cycle: by binary fission in the intestine-dwelling mature trophozoite stage and by nuclear division followed by binary fission in the metacystic stage.

Epidemiology

Entamoeba histolytica is cosmopolitan, with an estimated incidence of human infection exceeding 500 million cases. However, this figure is possibly misleading; up to 90% of reported human infections may be due to intestinal colonization with the morphologically identical *E. dispar*. *E. histolytica*, therefore, is probably responsible for only 50 million cases worldwide, with *E. dispar* accounting for the remainder. Although the prevalence of human infection varies widely, certain groups, such as patients in mental institutions, appear more susceptible than others. Transmission depends upon ingestion of contaminated food and/or drinking water. Areas with low standards of sanitation and those where human feces are used as fertilizer display the highest prevalence of human infections. The main source of infection is the cyst-passing, asymptomatic carrier or chronic patient. The infection in these individuals is called **luminal amoebiasis.** Acutely ill patients, those with **invasive amoebiasis**, are not significant transmitters; their diarrheic feces contain trophozoites, which are noninfective because, unlike cysts, they are unable to survive outside the intestinal environment. In addition, flies and cockroaches have been implicated as mechanical vectors in the spread of *E. histolytica* and other amoebae, since cysts can survive for lengthy periods in their digestive tracts, later to be regurgitated or passed out in feces upon human food.

The explanation for the apparent nonpathogenicity in certain human hosts remains elusive. In humans living in temperate zones, the organism often produces the nonpathogenic, luminal form of the disease, while in the tropics and subtropics the invasive form is more common.

Under pathogenic conditions, the food vacuoles of *E. histolytica* trophozoites characteristically contain host erythrocytes along with leukocytes and epithelial cells. At the height of its pathogenicity, the trophozoite attaches to the mucosal surface of the intestine. The attachment process is fostered by a cell-to-cell recognition between the trophozoite surface and the surface of the mucosal epithelium. The trophozoite secretes a battery of proteolytic enzymes, one of which is called histolysin, that enable the organism to invade submucosal tissue. In the infected individual who develops dysentery, the mucosal ulceration may penetrate deeper into the intestinal tissue, causing vast areas of tissue to be destroyed. The overlying mucosal epithelium then may be sloughed off, exposing these necrotic areas (Fig. 4-3). This destructive process is usually followed by a regenerative period, resulting in a thickening of the intestinal wall as a result of the deposition of fibrous connective tissue. Trophozoites also may be carried to the liver, chiefly by the hepatic portal system, causing

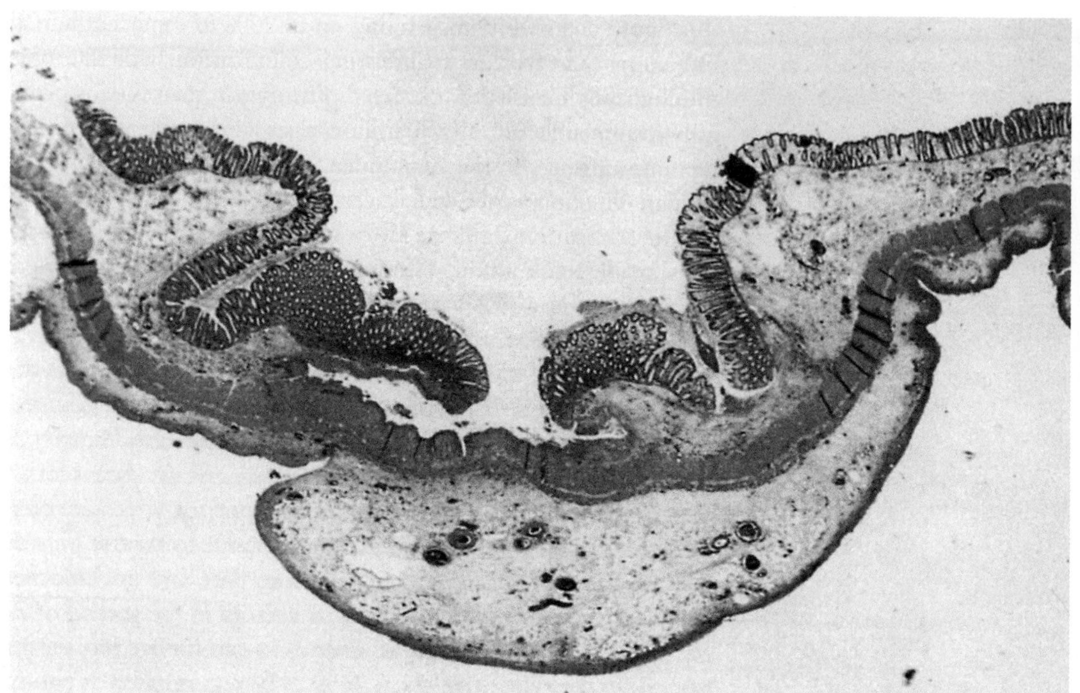

FIGURE 4-3
Section of human colon showing chronic amoebic ulcer.

hepatic amoebiasis and even amoebic hepatitis. The first sign of hepatic involvement is the formation of an early hepatic abscess containing a matrix of necrose hepatic cells, which eventually become liquefied. Hepatic abscesses may be single or multiple (Fig. 4-4). Although the liver appears to be the visceral organ most often affected (in about 5% of all cases), other organs such as the lungs, heart, brain, spleen, gonads, and skin may also be invaded, resulting in secondary amoebiasis. The reaction in the liver is due not only to the trophozoite and its secretions but also to emanation of toxic material resulting from the ulcerative changes in the intestine.

Second only to the liver in frequency as an extraintestinal site are the lungs. Pulmonary amoebiasis is relatively rare, however; when seen, it is probably a direct result of hepatic infection. Unlike most amoebic abscesses, which are bacteriologically sterile, pulmonary abscesses are often vulnerable to secondary bacterial infections.

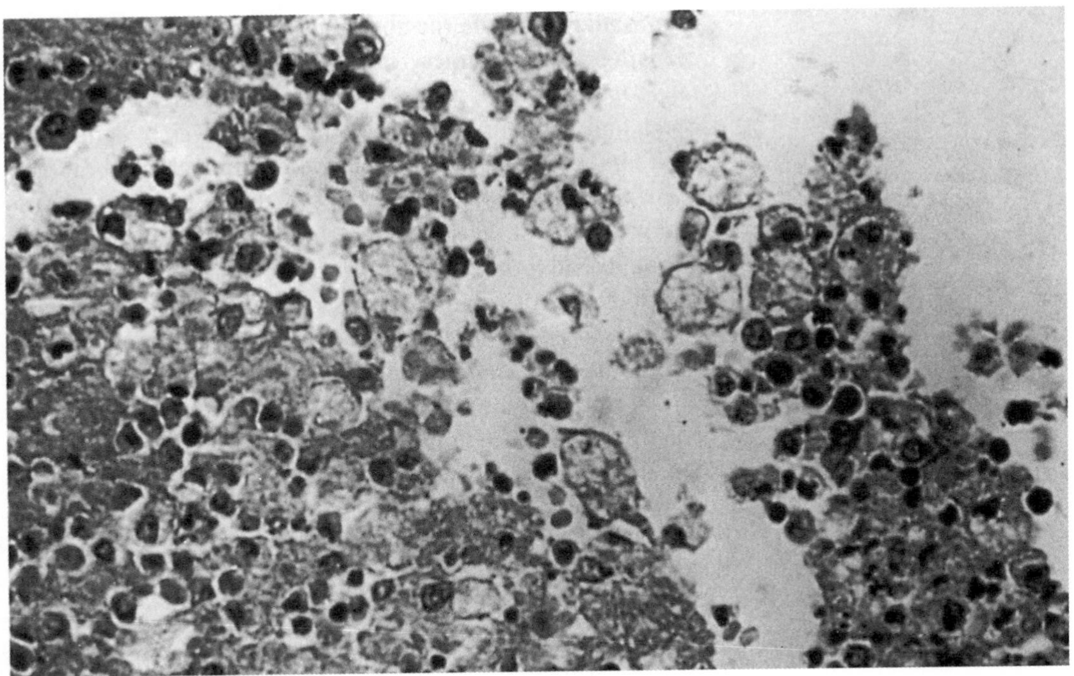

FIGURE 4-4
Abscess in human liver due to *Entamoeba histolytica.*

Symptomatology and Diagnosis

Victims of amoebiasis vary widely in their symptoms; in some individuals, even the more highly pathogenic, tropical forms can be symptomless. Pathogenic responses that do occur are highly variable, the severity depending upon the location and intensity of the infection.

Invasive amoebiasis may be manifested as **amoebic dysentery** (**acute intestinal amoebiasis**) or as **chronic amoebiasis.** In the former, severe diarrhea (i.e., blood and mucus in liquid feces) usually develops after an incubation period of 1–4 weeks and is commonly accompanied by a fever of 100–102°F. Diagnosis requires differentiation of amoebic dysentery from other types of dysentery and, ultimately, identification of the parasite; one diagnostic criterion is the presence of characteristic trophozoites and/or cysts in the stools. In the chronic form, on the other hand, there may be continuous attacks of diarrhea or recurrent attacks with intervening periods of milder intestinal problems. Hepatic amoebiasis is the most serious consequence of either form, because abscesses may perforate the abdominal wall or extend through the diaphragm into the lungs. Any of these manifestations may be fatal. *E. histolytica* has been incriminated in a few cases of cerebral, optic, and facial infections, often causing severely damaging or even fatal consequences. For instance, although cerebral amoebiasis occurs in fewer than 0.1% of patients, its onset is abrupt and usually fatal. In such cases, transmission of the organism is accomplished through direct, fecal contamination of the skin, eye socket, etc., rather than metastasis from the intestine or liver.

Laboratory diagnosis of amoebiasis depends upon identification of the cysts and/or trophozoites of *E. histolytica*. Examination of stools for intestinal forms requires both direct smears and concentration procedures such as zinc sulfate flotation or formalin-ether. Such examinations should be performed for three consecutive days unless positive results are obtained in a shorter period. The chance of finding cysts in infected persons almost triples after three days. Combining direct smears with concentration methods of detection more than doubles the diagnostic effectiveness of a single examination. At the present time, serious consideration is being given to the development of cost-effective means to differentiate *E. histolytica* infections from *E. dispar* infections in clinical laboratories. The monoclonal antibody-based enzyme-linked immunosorbent assay (ELISA) is currently considered the most appropriate test. Different diagnostic procedures are required for patients with extraintestinal amoebiasis, as stool specimens may not disclose the presence of the parasite. Trophozoites may be detected in sputum samples and tissue biopsies. Serological tests and X-ray scans may prove useful in revealing abscesses of the liver. It should be reemphasized at this point that positive identification of the parasite is requisite for an accurate diagnosis before chemotherapy is undertaken.

Treatment

Appropriate chemotherapy should be employed to destroy trophozoites, relieve symptoms, and control secondary bacterial infections. The drug of choice for the entire spectrum of symptoms is metronidazole or diiodohydroxyquin. Common sense dictates complete bed rest in cases of severe diarrhea accompanied by fever, regardless of the cause. In addition, a bland diet, low in carbohydrates such as sugar and high in liquids and proteins, is recommended. In symptomless carriers, it is essential that the trophozoites be destroyed, because they are the precursors of cysts that pass out of the host. Metronidazole is contraindicated for pregnant women, especially in their first trimester, as it is a known carcinogen and mutagen in rodents and bacteria.

To combat secondary bacterial infections, antibiotics such as tetracycline are used in combination with either metronidazole or, more recently, diiodohydroxyquin. The latter combination produces a high rate of cure for intestinal amoebiasis and may supplant the use of metronidazole. However, in cases of iodine sensitivity, diiodohydroxyquin is contraindicated.

Hepatic amoebiasis also responds well to metronidazole although the treatment is not totally effective. Emetine or dehydroemetine is used in instances when metronidazole treatment has been unsuccessful. Chloroquine can be used where there are contraindications for either of these two drugs, if it is kept in mind that chloroquine has no effect upon trophozoites in the intestine. Ornidazole, a drug closely akin to metronidazole, is reported to have cured hepatic amoebiasis with a single dose.

Physiology

Knowledge of the physiology of *E. histolytica* is fragmentary. When the metabolism of the organism is better understood, perhaps more effective chemotherapeutic methods will be developed. Because it grows best in an oxygen-free atmosphere, *E. histolytica* was once considered an obligate anaerobe. However, it has been shown that the organism can use oxygen in low concentrations even though it does not possess the usual organelles (i.e., mitochondria) or metabolic pathways, such as the cytochrome system or a functional Krebs cycle, normally associated with oxygen utilization. *In vitro*, an oxygen concentration of 10% or higher is lethal to the organism while carbon dioxide is required for growth, a characteristic *E. histolytica* shares with most intestine-dwelling organisms. Glucose and galactose are the major carbohydrates used by the organism, from which it produces ethanol, acetate, and carbon dioxide. In the presence of sublethal concentrations of oxygen, the same end products are produced but in different proportions.

Prevention

Food and water contaminated with feces containing the cysts of *E. histolytica* are the most common vehicles for transmission.

Prevention, therefore, depends upon interruption of the contamination–ingestion cycle. One such measure is the boiling or iodination of drinking water in endemic areas (1.25 grams of iodine per liter of drinking water; allow to stand 2–3 hours). In many areas, fruits and vegetables become contaminated when human excrement (night soil) is used as fertilizer. The rule of thumb for Westerners traveling in Third World countries is to drink only bottled water and avoid ice cubes, salads, and those fruits not peeled by the person consuming them. Broad education to improve sanitation coupled with a ban on the use of untreated human excrement as fertilizer are perhaps the most effective means for curbing transmission of pathogenic protozoa such as *E. histolytica*. Transmission of *E. histolytica* by infected food handlers can be controlled by local ordinances requiring periodic physical examinations, including stool examinations, for all food handlers.

ENTAMOEBA DISPAR

It is now generally accepted that *E. histolytica* is in reality a species complex with the pathogenic form retaining the species name of *E. histolytica*. On the basis of isoenzyme electrophoresis as well as clinical epidemiological evidence, *E. dispar*, although morphologically identical to *E. histolytica*, is considered its nonpathogenic equivalent. For instance, *E. histolytica*, whether symptomatic or asymptomatic, can elicit a serological response in humans while *E. dispar* cannot. Therefore, the presence of quadrinucleate cysts in feces combined with negative serological test results would indicate the presence of the nonpathogenic *E. dispar*.

ENTAMOEBA HARTMANNI

It has been reported that *E. histolytica* occurs in two forms, a "small race" with trophozoites measuring 12–15 μm in diameter and cysts 5–9 μm in diameter, and a "large race" with trophozoites measuring 20–30 μm in diameter and cysts 10–20 μm in diameter. Some investigators regard the small race of *E. histolytica* as a separate species, *E. hartmanni*, whose life cycle and overall morphology are very similar to those of *E. histolytica*. Because *E. hartmanni* is small and nonpathogenic, its vacuoles do not contain erythrocytes. As with *E. dispar*, it is important that diagnosticians differentiate between these organisms and *E. histolytica* to preclude unnecessary chemotherapy.

ENTAMOEBA COLI

This widely distributed intestinal amoeba (Fig. 4-5) is generally considered nonpathogenic in humans. The trophozoite averages 25 μm in diameter (range, 15–40 μm) and forms a cyst averaging 17 μm diameter (range, 10–33 μm). The prevalence of infection, like that for all parasites, varies with different localities and seasons. For example, it is reported to occur in 37.1% of a sampling of Tennesseans and 26.1% of the inhabitants of Wise Count, Virginia. Another study involving an extensive survey of all sections of the United States found infection rates exceeding 19%, making *E. coli* possibly the most common intestinal amoeba in the United States.

The trophozoite of *E. coli* does not ingest or invade host tissues. The food vacuoles observed in its heavily granulated cytoplasm usually contain bacteria, yeast, and fragments of intestinal debris. The nucleus may be visible in saline preparations. When stained, the nuclear envelope appears coarse with irregularly dispersed, peripheral chromatin on its inner surface, and there is a large, eccentric endosome. However, there is wide variation in this morphology. As in *E. histolytica*, cysts constitute the usual means of identification. The mature cyst characteristically contains eight vesicular nuclei, each with an eccentrically situated endosome. Younger cysts may contain one, two, or four nuclei. Chromatoidal bodies, when present in cysts, may be needlelike or irregular with distinctly splintered terminals. Cysts are found

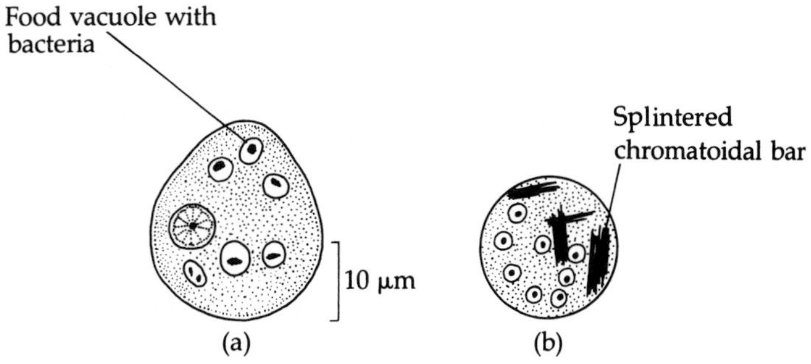

FIGURE 4-5
Entamoeba coli.
(a) Trophozoite. (b) Mature cyst with eight nuclei and splintered chromatoidal bars.

frequently in diarrheic stools, but there is no evidence that this amoeba is the cause of the diarrhea.

The life cycle of *E. coli* parallels that of *E. histolytica* (Fig. 4-2); it includes precystic, metacystic, and trophozoite stages. Infection of the host is initiated by ingestion of cysts.

ENTAMOEBA POLECKI

An intestinal amoeba rarely found in humans but usually reported in pigs, goats, monkeys, and dogs, this parasite can be confused with *E. histolytica*. In size, its trophozoite and cyst are intermediate between those of *E. histolytica* and *E. coli*, and the cyst is almost always uninucleate. Some investigators consider the parasite identical to *E. coli*, while others place it in a separate species. It is generally considered to be nonpathogenic.

ENTAMOEBA GINGIVALIS

Entamoeba gingivalis (Fig. 4-6) is cosmopolitan in distribution, commonly found in the tartar and debris associated with the gingival tissues of the mouth. It was the first parasitic amoeba reported in humans by Gros in 1849. There is little indication that it is pathogenic, and, while it abounds in people with unhealthy oral conditions (i.e., gingivitis or periodontitis), a cause-and-effect relationship has not been established. Food vacuoles may contain oral epithelial cells, leukocytes, occasional erythrocytes, and various microbial organisms. *E. gingivalis* does not form cysts; it is transmitted either directly (e.g., by kissing) or indirectly via trophozoite-contaminated food, chewing gum, toothpicks, etc.

IODAMOEBA BUTSCHLII

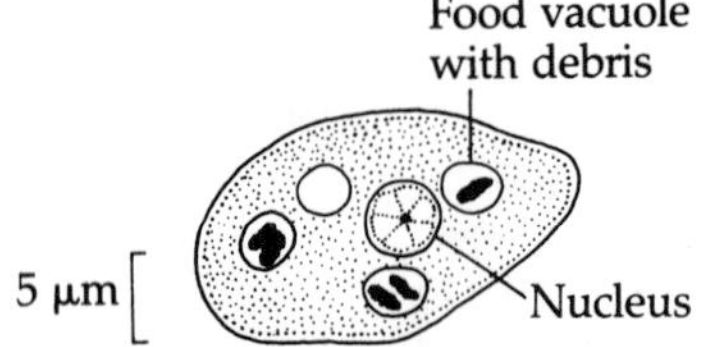

FIGURE 4-6
***Entamoeba gingivalis* trophozoite.**

Iodamoeba butschlii (Fig. 4-7) is transmitted by a cyst that is very distinctive, facilitating identification. It varies from a rounded to a somewhat angular shape, usually 10 µm in greatest diameter (range, 5–18 µm). The nucleus is large with a large, ovoid, usually eccentric endosome. Within the cyst is a large glycogen body, which stains deeply with iodine. The cyst and the emerged trophozoite are uninucleate. The amoeba escapes through a pore in the cyst wall and moves rapidly. Moisture and warmth are the

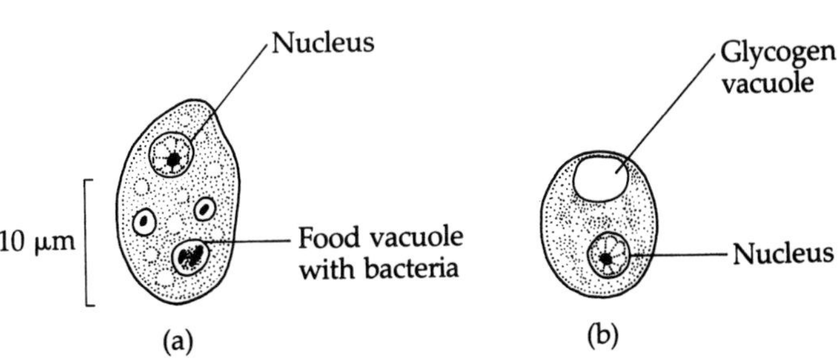

FIGURE 4-7 ***Iodamoeba butschlii.*** (a) Trophozoite. (b) Cyst.

only known requirements for excystation. Mature trophozoites average 10 μm in diameter (range, 6–25 μm) and reside in the large intestine, feeding on bacteria and yeast, as is evident from the contents of their food vacuoles. This species is not considered a pathogen. The large, vesicular nucleus is a prominent feature in both the trophozoite and the cyst.

ENDOLIMAX NANA

Endolimax nana (Fig. 4-8) is the smallest of the intestine-dwelling amoebae infecting humans; its trophozoite averages only 8 μm in diameter (range, 6–15 μm). The trophozoite lives in the host's colon and is generally considered to be nonpathogenic. According to some surveys, the prevalence of *E. nana* infections may be as high as 30% in some populations. The life cycle is identical to that of other cyst-forming amoebae, with the cyst being the infective stage. *E. nana* cysts can be distinguished from other cysts by their smaller size (9 μm in greatest diameter; range, 5–14 μm), ovoid shape, and one to four vesicular nuclei, each usually containing a large, eccentric endosome. The nuclear envelope is very thin and difficult to see even in stained preparations. A tetranucleate metacystic amoeba escapes through a pore in the cyst wall and undergoes a series of cytoplasmic divisions in which a portion of cytoplasm is passed on to each uninucleate product. Trophozoites actively feed upon bacteria and multiply rapidly by binary fission.

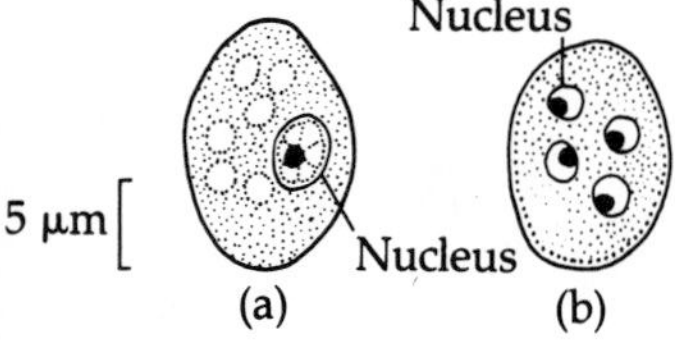

FIGURE 4-8 ***Endolimax nana.*** (a) Trophozoite. (b) Cyst.

PATHOGENIC FREE-LIVING AMOEBAE

In recent years, there has been a great deal of interest in a group of small, free-living amoebae belonging to the genera *Naegleria* and *Acanthamoeba*. These amoebae, normally free-living in fresh water and soil, are capable of facultative parasitism in humans and are highly pathogenic. Their pathogenicity in humans was first noted in 1965, when fatal cases of **primary amoebic meningoencephalitis** (**PAM**) were diagnosed simultaneously in Australia and Florida. Since then, more than 150 cases have been reported worldwide, including cases from many parts of the United States. Most victims have a history of recent exposure to stagnant, warm, fresh, or brackish water, such as that found in swimming pools, ponds, and lakes.

NAEGLERIA FOWLERI

Naegleria fowleri (Fig. 4-9) appears to be the principal causative agent for PAM. Its life cycle includes flagellated and amoeboid trophozoites and cysts, with rapid transformation from one form to the other. The flagellated trophozoite possesses two flagella, while the amoeboid trophozoite displays a single,

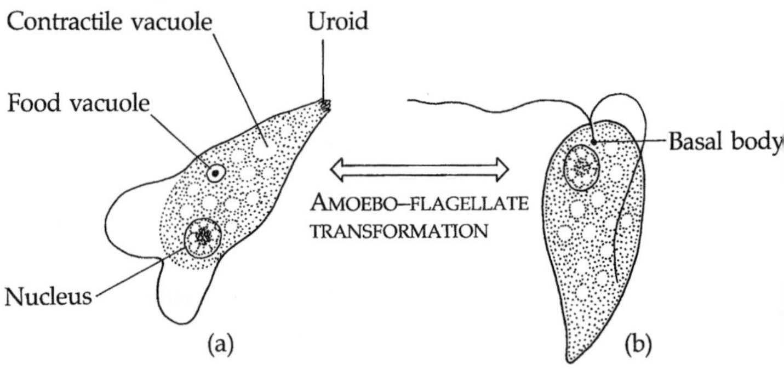

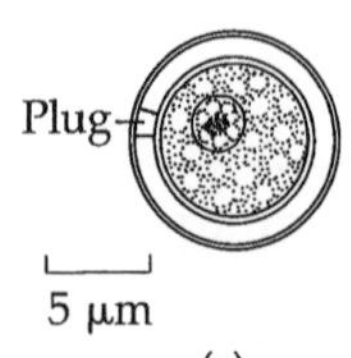

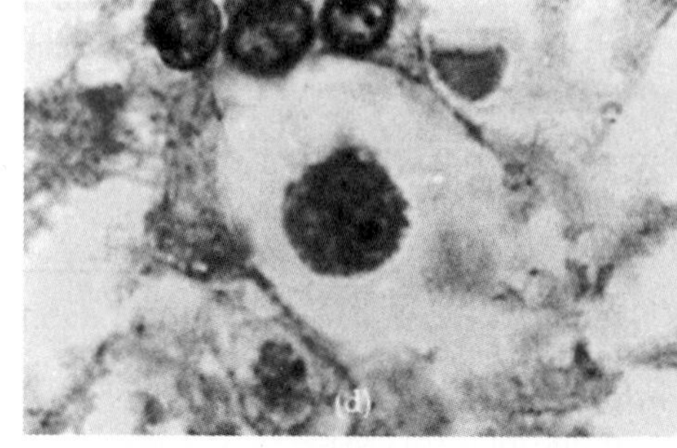

FIGURE 4-9
***Naegleria fowleri,* a soil amoeba sometimes pathogenic in humans.**
Under certain physiological/environmental conditions, the amoeboid form undergoes transformation into a flagellated form. (a) Amoeboid form. (b) Flagellated form. (c) Cyst. Scale only approximate. (d) Amoeboid form from cerebrospinal fluid (phase contrast).

blunt pseudopodium with minutely pointed extensions on its end. In the free-living state, the organisms have contractile vacuoles. Binary fission occurs only in the amoeboid trophozoite stage. The flagellated trophozoites are capable of rapid movement through the water, and transmission to humans most likely occurs when these forms invade the nasopharyngeal mucosa. The amoeboid trophozoite migrates through the nervous system via the cribriform plate to the brain, where inflammation occurs and death usually ensues. No cyst stage occurs in the human host, and flagellated trophozoites are observed only during the invasive stage. Diagnostic confirmation requires identification of the motile amoeboid trophozoite in cerebrospinal fluid, but since death may occur in 5–7 days, most cases are diagnosed at autopsy.

ACANTHAMOEBA

Four species of *Acanthamoeba* (Fig. 4-10) (*A. culbertsoni, A. polyphaga, A. castellanii,* and *A. rhysodes*) cause chronic PAM and have been positively implicated in human cases. It is possible that some of these may represent strains of a single species, *A. castellanii*, rather than separate species. Except for the absence of a flagellated trophozoite stage, the life cycle of *Acanthamoeba* is very similar to that of *Naegleria*. The amoeboid trophozoites of the two genera can be distinguished by their pseudopodia; the trophozoites of *Naegleria* form a single, lobose pseudopodium and move rapidly, while those of *Acanthamoeba* form small, pointed pseudopodia (acanthopodia) and move sluggishly. *Acanthamoeba* infections can be distinguished from those of *Naegleria* by the characteristic cysts of *Acanthamoeba* found in affected tissues. The cysts of *Naegleria* are round, while those of *Acanthamoeba* are square. Less common than *Naegleria*, *Acanthamoeba* is a facultative parasite of humans responsible for symptoms similar to but less severe than those of *Naegleria* infections. Central nervous system involvement, **granulomatous amoebic meningoencephalitis** (GAM), is relatively rare but usually fatal, especially in immunologically compromised patients. While there is no uniformly effective treatment for *Naegleria* infections, in a few cases there has been favorable response to intravenous administration of amphotericin B. New infections of *Acanthamoeba* respond favorably to sulfonamides, and estab-

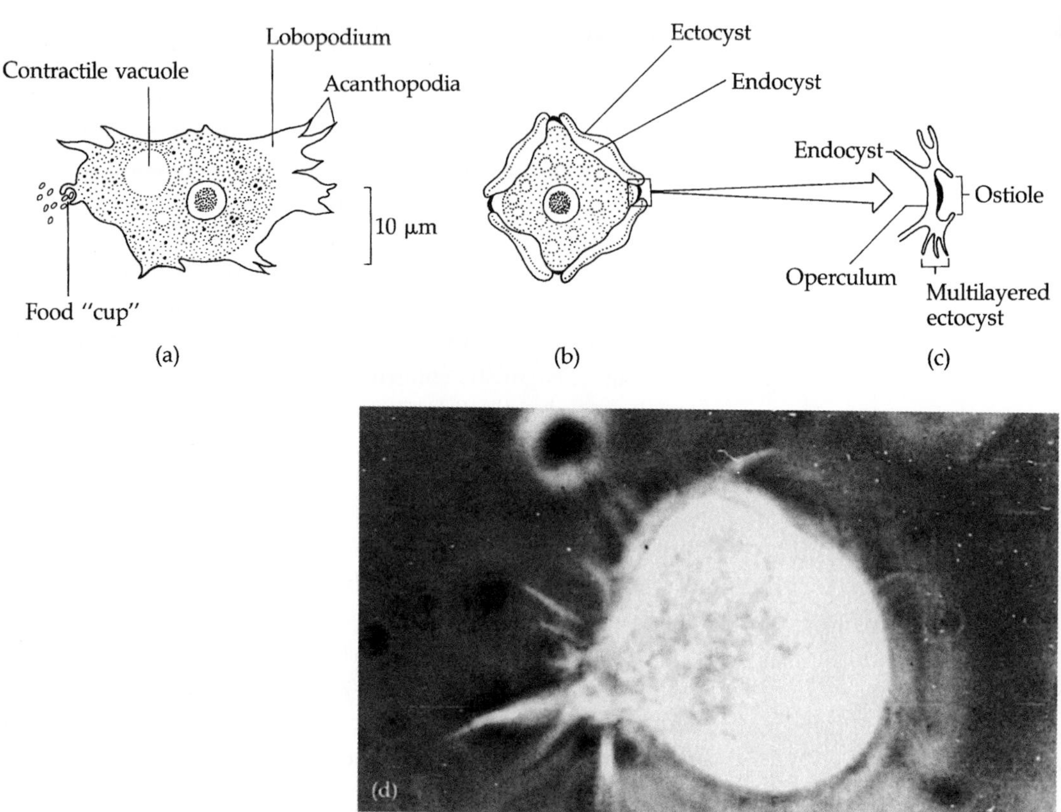

FIGURE 4-10
***Acanthamoeba castellanii*, a potentially pathogenic soil amoeba.**
(a) Trophozoite. (b) Cyst. (c) Ostiole enlarged. (d) Trophozoite from patient's eye (phase contrast).

lished infections appear to respond to amphotericin B. Ocular keratitis, attributed to *Acanthamoeba* infecting wearers of soft contact lenses, is refractory to these drugs. Patients with ocular keratitis have been treated successfully with intensive topical chemotherapy consisting of miconazole nitrate, gramicidin B, and propaminidine isethionate.

MICROSPORIDIANS

Several protistan species of the phylum Microspora parasitize a wide range of invertebrates and some vertebrates, including fish, birds, and mammals. Human infection was rare until the advent of AIDS. Since 1985, a number of microsporidia species have been reported in AIDS patients. Phylogenetically similar to prokaryotic cells, microsporidians lack mitochondria and Golgi complexes and have ribosomal RNA sequences like those of bacteria. They resemble eukaryotes in their nuclear organization. The life cycle consists of an intracellular, divisional phase followed by a spore-producing phase. When the infected cell dies, mature spores are released into the immediate environment. Morphologically unique, the spore is equipped with an extrusive polar tube by which sporoplasm can be inoculated into new host cells. *Enterocytozoon bieneusi* infects intestinal cells, causing chronic diarrhea, cramps, and nausea. In AIDS patients, it is associated with severe weight loss, malabsorption, and zinc deficiency. It is the most common microsporidium infecting AIDS patients, with a prevalence of 40%. Several other species belonging to the genus *Encephalitozoon* are capable of infecting a wide variety of cells, including macrophages, causing diarrhea, bronchitis, nephritis, hepatitis, and peritonitis among AIDS patients.

Immunodiagnosis, using either indirect immunofluorescent antibody tests or western blot techniques, is the most sensitive diagnostic technique available. Albendazole eradicates all *Encephalitozoon* species by disrupting microtubules, thereby inhibiting cell division. Fumagillin, 5-fluorouracil, and sparfloxacin are also effective against *Encephalitozoon* infections. No effective therapy against *E. bieneusi* has yet been developed, although Octreotide (Sandostatin) provides symptomatic relief.

CILIATES

Members of the phylum Ciliophora are protozoans possessing cilia in at least one stage of their life cycle and having two different types of nuclei: one macronucleus and one or more micronuclei. Only one ciliophoran, *Balantidium coli*, infects humans.

BALANTIDIUM COLI

A distinctive feature of *Balantidium coli* (Fig. 4-11) is the presence of a depression, or **peristome**, leading into the cytosome.

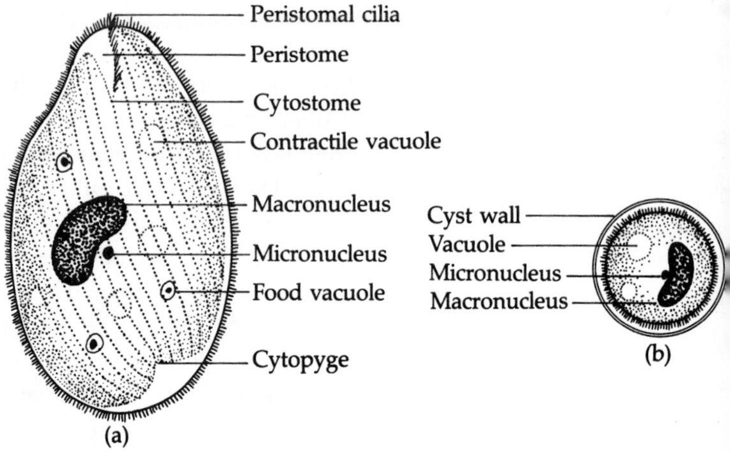

FIGURE 4-11
***Balantidium coli*, an intestinal parasite of pigs, monkeys, and humans.**
(a) Trophozoite. (b) Cyst.

Balantidium coli is commonly considered a pathogen of humans that also parasitizes pigs and monkeys. Some investigators, however, classify the organism that parasitizes pigs as a distinct species, *B. suis*.

Life Cycle

Both a motile trophozoite stage and a cyst stage occur in the life cycle of *B. coli*. The trophozoite inhabits the caecum and colon of humans and is the largest known protozoan parasite of humans, measuring 50–130 μm by 20–70 μm. The conspicuous vestibulum leads into a large cytosome at the anterior end of the cell, opposite to which lies a cytopyge. Coarse cilia line the peristomal area. The macronucleus is typically elongate and kidney-shaped, while the vesicular micronucleus is spherical. There are two prominent contractile vacuoles, one in the middle of the cell and the other near the posterior end. The presence of contractile vacuoles, unique among parasitic protozoa, indicates a degree of osmoregulatory capability. Food vacuoles in the cytoplasm contain debris, bacteria, starch granules, erythrocytes, and fragments of host epithelium. *B. coli* typically reproduces asexually by transverse fission, with the posterior daughter cell forming a new cytosome after division. Conjugation also occurs in this species.

Transmission of *B. coli* from one host to another is accomplished via the cyst. The cysts are round, measuring 40–60 μm in diameter, with a heavy cyst wall that may consist of two layers. Cilia, the large macronucleus, and contractile vacuoles are readily visible within the cyst. Encystation usually occurs in the large intestine but may also occur outside the body of the host. Cysts are common in the feces of infected hosts and are generally not considered sites of reproduction, although cysts containing two individuals are sometimes found. Infection occurs when cysts are ingested by the host. Excystation takes place in the small intestine.

Epidemiology

Balantidiosis is most often found in tropical regions throughout the world; with an infection rate of less than 1%, however, it is not a common human disease. In pigs, the parasite has a prevalence of 20–100%, although it is nonpathogenic. Human infection is most common where malnutrition is widespread, where pigs share habitation with human families, and where fecal contamination of food and water occurs.

Symptomatology and Diagnosis

The trophozoite resides in the caecal area and throughout the large intestine. It thrives in an environment rich in starch, such as the small intestine; in such an environment, however, the trophozoite does not invade the intestinal mucosa. This proclivity for starch may be the reason for the trophozoite's invasive character once it becomes established in the human caecal region, which is low in starch; in the pig's intestine, where starch is more abundant, the organism remains in the lumen. It is believed that the trophozoite secretes proteolytic enzymes that act upon the mucosal epithelium, facilitating invasion.

Results of infection range from asymptomatic to severe. Parasitic invasion of the mucosal epithelium is followed by hemorrhage and ulceration; hence, the name **balantidial dysentery** often given to this condition. While symptoms such as colitis and diarrhea may resemble amoebiasis in many respects, extraintestinal disease is rare. Occasionally, *B. coli* is transported by the blood into the spinal fluid. Fatalities are rare, although one case of fatal myocarditis in Russia has been attributed to *B. coli*. A few deaths have been reported in Mexico and Central America.

The usual diagnostic procedure consists of stool examination for the presence of trophozoites and cysts. The trophozoites are readily identified by their large size and the fact that *B. coli* is the only ciliophoran parasitic in humans. Cysts can be identified by their large size, heavy cyst wall, large macronucleus, and the presence of cilia within the cyst.

Treatment

The infection may disappear spontaneously, or the host may become asymptomatic, remaining as a carrier. Drug treatment usually consists of oral administration of oxytetracycline or, in some cases, 5-nitroimidazole. The usual course of treatment with oxytetracycline lasts about 10 days.

SELECTED READINGS

Blanc, D. S. 1992. Determination of taxonomic status of pathogenic and nonpathogenic *Entamoeba histolytica* zymodemes using isozyme analysis. *Journal of Protozoology* **39**, 471–479.

Canning, E. U., and Hollister, W. S. 1987. Microsporidia of mammals—Widespread pathogens or opportunistic curiosities? *Parasitology Today* **3**, 276–273.

Diamond, L. S., and Clark, C. G. 1993. A redescription of *Entamoeba histolytica* Schaudinn, 1903 (emended Walker, 1911) separating it from *Entamoeba dispar* Brumpt, 1925. *Journal of Eukaryotic Microbiology* **40**, 340–344.

Elsdon-Dew, R. 1968. The epidemiology of amoebiasis. *Advances in Parasitology* **6**, 1–62.

Gitler, C., and Mirelman, D. 1986. Factors contributing to the pathogenic behavior of *Entamoeba histolytica. Annual Reviews in Microbiology* **40**, 237–262.

Martinez-Palomo, A. 1987. The pathogenesis of amoebiasis. *Parasitology Today* **3**, 111–118.

Ravdin, J. I. 1990. Cell biology of *Entamoeba histolytica* and immunology of amoebiasis. In *Modern Parasite Biology: Cellular, Immunological and Molecular Aspects* (Wyler, D. G., Ed.), pp. 126–150. W. H. Freeman & Company, New York.

Reeves, R. E. 1984. Metabolism of *Entamoeba histolytica* Schaudinn, 1903. *Advances in Parasitology* **23**, 106–142.

Warhurst, D. C. 1985. Pathogenic free-living amoebae. *Parasitology Today* **1**, 24–28.

Chapter Five

VISCERAL PROTOZOA II: FLAGELLATES

Members of the subphylum Mastigophora, the flagellates infecting the digestive and reproductive systems of humans, belong to seven species of the orders Retortamonadida, Diplomonadida, and Trichomonadida. As is true of amoebae, only a few flagellates are pathogenic, but it is important to distinguish them from the nonpathogenic forms. The nonpathogenic species are *Chilomastix mesnili, Retortamonas intestinalis, Enteromonas hominis, Trichomonas tenax*, *Pentatrichomonas hominis*, and *Dientamoeba fragilis*; forms pathogenic in humans are *Giardia lamblia* and *Trichomonas vaginalis*. Of these eight species, all but two, *T. tenax* and *T. vaginalis*, are intestinal parasites.

NONTRICHOMONAD FLAGELLATES

GIARDIA DUODENALIS

The bilateral symmetry of members of this genus (Figs. 5-1, 5-2) is distinctive among the protozoa. The trophozoite is rounded at the posterior end, tapered posteriorly, and flattened dorsoventrally. It is 14 μm long (range, 8–16 μm) by 10 μm wide (range, 5–12 μm; Fig. 5-1). The dorsal surface is convex; the ventral surface is usually concave but is occasionally flat and is dominated by a large, adhesive disc with a nucleus in the center of each half (Fig. 5-2a). The rim of the adhesive disc is supported by microtubules and fascicles of microfilaments (Fig. 5-2b), and four pairs of flagella arise from basal bodies clustered between the two nuclei. One pair extends down the midline of the cell, emerging posteriorly as trailing flagella; the ventral pair emerges at the posterior edge of the adhesive disc. Of the remaining two pairs, one emerges anteriolaterally and one laterally. Two prominent, slightly curved **median bodies** are distinctive to the genus *Giardia*. Their function is unknown, although it has been suggested that they may act as supportive structures.

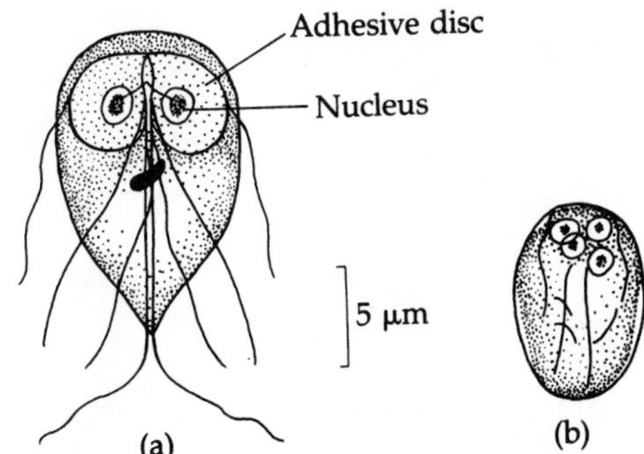

FIGURE 5-1
Giardia duodenalis.
(a) Trophozoite. (b) Cyst.

Life Cycle

The trophozoite of *G. duodenalis* reproduces by longitudinal fission. Its organelles undergo division in the following order: nuclei, adhesive disc, and cytoplasm. In the duodenum and bile duct of its host, the trophozoite can either maintain position by attaching its large adhesive disc to the epithelial cells (Fig. 5-2c) or use its flagella to swim rapidly in the lumen. Attachment is facilitated by the two ventral flagella working with the flexible rim of the disc. As trophozoites pass through the digestive tract, they usually encyst in the colon. The cystic transmission stage is typically ovoid and averages 11 μm long (range, 9–12 μm; Fig. 5-1). In saline smears, refractile granules can be seen in the cysts, and at times the cytoplasm appears to be detached from the cyst wall in several places. In cysts stained with iodine or hematoxylin, two to four nuclei are visible in addition to numerous fibrils (probably flagellar remnants) and median bodies.

In victims of giardiasis, massive infection is common. The presence of up to several billion trophozoites in a single diarrheic stool sample is not unusual. Cysts are rarely encountered in such stools, being found instead in either formed or partially formed stools. Infection results from ingestion of cyst-contaminated food or water or from direct hand-to-mouth contact. Ingestion of 100 or more cysts is considered infective. Following ingestion, cysts pass through the stomach to the small intestine where they excyst and begin the cycle anew.

Epidemiology

Giardia is the most prevalent intestinal parasite in humans. It is cosmopolitan and is common in children 6–10 years of age but is also seen often in older children and adults, with a high inci-

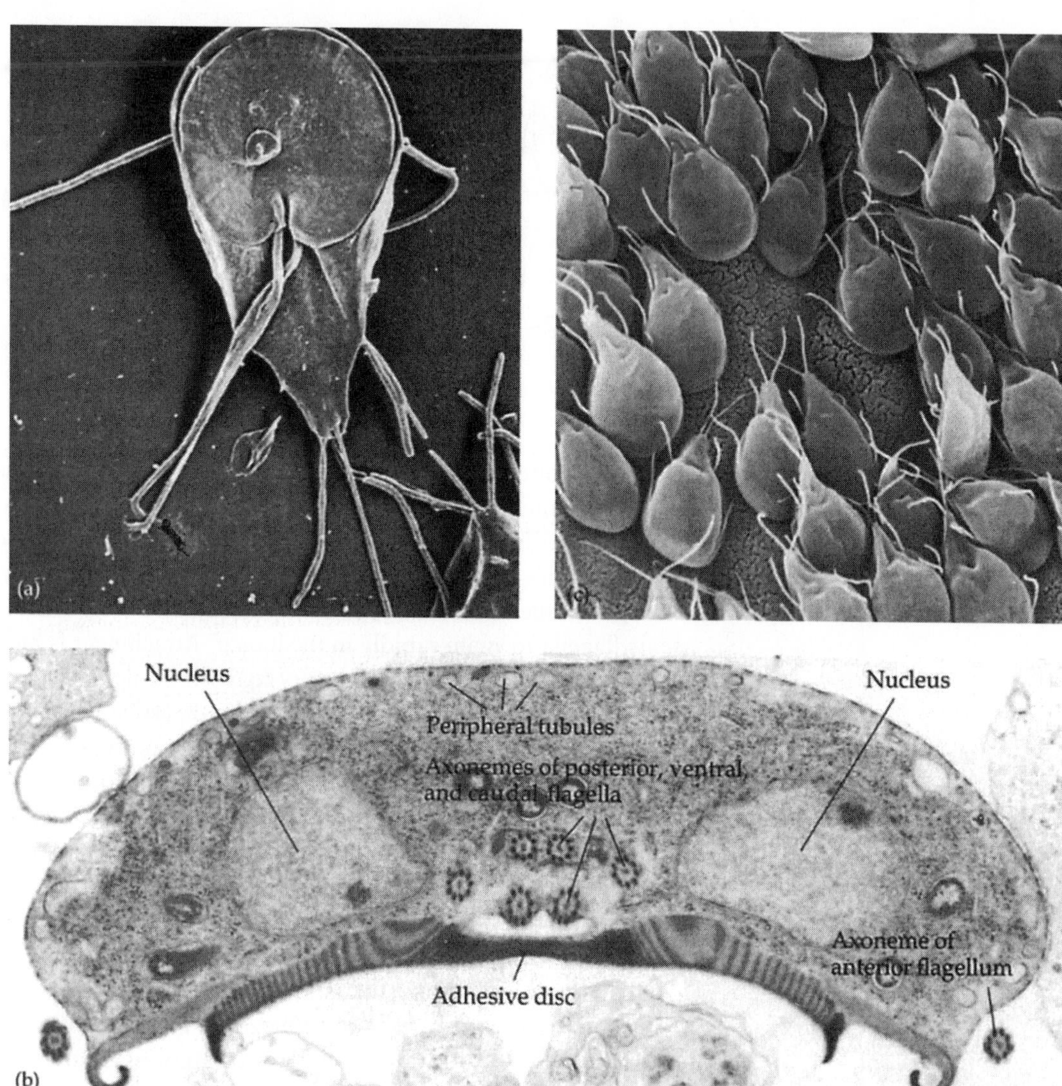

FIGURE 5-2
Giardia.
(a) Trophozoite of the *Giardia intestinalis* type. Scanning electron micrograph of the ventral surface showing the attachment organelle. Bar = 1 μm. (b) Transmission electron micrograph of a cross section of a *Giardia muris* trophozoite in the small intestine of an infected mouse. The marginal groove is the space between the striated rim of cytoplasm and the lateral ridge of the adhesive disc. This specimen bears endosymbionts, which are apparently bacteria. (× 15,350) (c) Scanning electron micrograph of an intestinal villus. The microvillus border of the epithelial cells is almost obscured by attached trophozoites.

dence in homosexual males. Outbreaks are frequent in daycare nurseries and other institutions where sanitation may be inadequate. An outbreak of giardiasis occurred in the ski resort town of Aspen, Colorado, when a water supply line was inadvertently crossed with a sewage line, and 11% of the skiers present that season became infected; 56 of the 59 infected persons experienced clinical symptoms of the disease. Giardiasis is common among tourists (an infection rate of approximately 23%) returning from Russia. An increase in *Giardia* infection has been noted among wilderness campers in the United States, probably due to drinking polluted water in areas where human contamination is unlikely. The term "Backpackers' Disease" has been coined in reference to the disease contracted by this group. Such outbreaks have led epidemiologists to suspect that wild animals may harbor species of *Giardia* capable of infecting humans. Surveys have implicated beavers, dogs, and sheep as potential reservoirs for human infections. Significant differences in size and structure among species of the genus *Giardia* have led to the assumption that each host species has a different parasite species. It now appears more likely that the variable morphology of *Giardia* is due to host diet rather than genetic variation, so that many of the described "species" are invalid distinctions.

Symptomatology and Diagnosis

Giardia duodenalis infection causes severe intestinal disorders, most commonly diarrhea and related sysmptoms due to malabsorption. Attachment of the trophozoite to the mucosal surface by means of its adhesive disc (Fig. 5-2c) causes shortening of the villi of the small intestine, inflammation of the crypts and lamina propria, and lesions on mucosal cells. In rare instances, trophozoites may penetrate the mucosa. Because *Giardia* has not been known to produce toxins, it appears that symptoms result from combined mechanical and chemical factors. Severe *Giardia* infections produce a malabsorption syndrome characterized by the inability of the small intestine to absorb such essential, fat-soluble substances as carotene, vitamin B_{12}, and folate. These absorptive abnormalities may be accompanied by reduced secretion of a number of intestinal digestive enzymes, such as disaccharidase. Additional symptoms of infection are diarrheic stools, steatorrhea, abdominal distension, nausea, flatulence, and eventual weight loss. Occasionally, bile duct and gallbladder involvement may produce jaundice and colic.

Identification of characteristic cysts in the stool is used in diagnosis of this parasite. Either saline or iodine smears can be employed for initial diagnosis, but a concentration method is commonly used to enhance detection. Examination for trophozoites is rare, since their detection depends upon almost immediate inspection or fixation of diarrheic stool samples. Duodenal aspiration, either by intubation or by the enteric capsule method, is an alternative and more satisfactory technique for trophozoite detection, especially in early stages of infection.

Treatment

Treatment with metronidazole is recommended. Complete cure is usually effected within a week after treatment begins. However, if the bile duct or gallbladder is infected, "relapses" may occur for years. Tinidazole is a one-dose treatment that is highly effective but is not approved for use in the United States at this time. Because of the ease with which the cyst is transmitted, all members of the household should be treated simultaneously.

Physiology

Little is known of the physiology of *Giardia*, due in large measure to the inadequancy of *in vitro* culture methods. An *in vivo* study to determine the method of uptake of macromolecular markers such as ferritin by *Giardia* indicates rapid transfer of the marker from the host's intestinal lumen into vacuoles close to the surface of the protozoan, suggesting a means by which *Giardia* obtains nutrients. Other studies using radiolabeled sugars show that *Giardia* is capable of incorporating certain monosaccharides into glycogen. *Giardia* has no mitochondria but can use oxygen when available. There is no evidence of either an electron transport system or a Krebs cycle. The organism relies on substrate-level phosphorylation as its major means of obtaining ATP; ethanol, CO_2, and acetate are principal end products of carbohydrate metabolism in *Giardia*. The organism excretes mostly acetate in the presence of oxygen and ethanol in the absence of oxygen.

Prevention

Generally, preventive measures recommended for *E. histolytica* are applicable to *G. duodenalis* as well. The prescribed amount of iodine added to drinking water should be doubled to insure killing of *G. duodenalis* cysts.

CHILOMASTIX MESNILI

Cosmopolitan in distribution, this organism (Fig. 5-3) infects about 6% of the world's human population. *C. mesnili* is usually considered nonpathogenic but may cause intestinal disorders, most commonly diarrhea, when present in sufficient numbers. The stage found in the human colon, the motile, pyriform trophozoite, averages 12 μm long (range, 5–20 μm) and has a blunt anterior end from which extend three free flagella. A spiral groove extends the length of the cell, terminating at the pointed posterior end. A prominent cytostome enclosing a fourth, recurrent flagellum is located in the anterior portion of the cell, as is the large nucleus. A prominent, curved, supporting fibrillar structure, the so-called Shepherd's Crook, lies just under the cytostome wall.

The parasite utilizes a resistant cyst stage for transmission. The lemon-shaped, relatively thick-walled cyst is approximately 8 μm in diameter. It is identifiable by its single nucleus and the cytostome, which contains the remnant of the recurrent flagellum and Shepherd's Crook. Staining the cyst reveals four basal bodies, one for each of the flagella.

RETORTAMONAS INTESTINALIS

This nonpathogen (Fig. 5-4) closely resembles *Chilomastix mesnili*, although it is only about one-third as large. The trophozoite has one free, anterior flagellum and a recurrent, cytostomal flagellum that emerges as a free, posteriorly trailing flagellum. As in *C. mesnili*, the trophozoite resides in the colon, and a cyst, approximately 6 μm long by 3 μm wide, serves as the transmission stage.

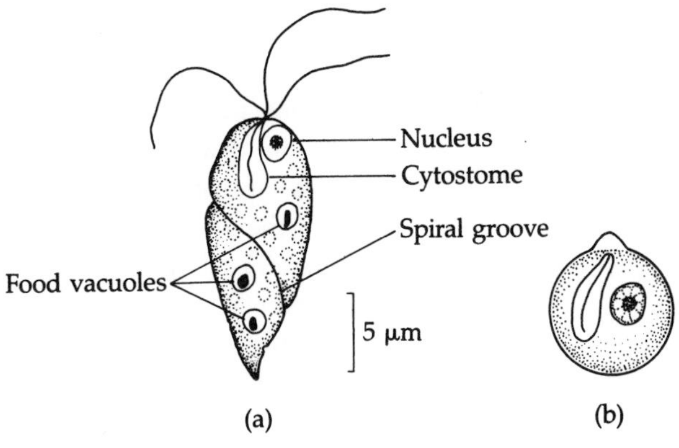

FIGURE 5-3
Chilomastix mesnili.
(a) Trophozoite. (b) Cyst.

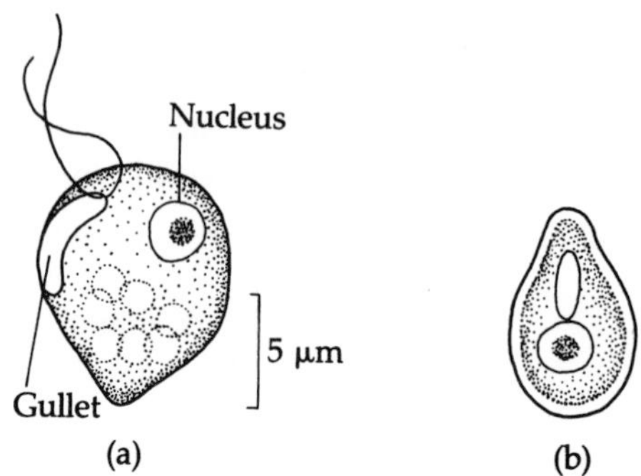

FIGURE 5-4
Retortamonas intestinalis.
(a) Trophozoite. (b) Cyst.

ENTEROMONAS HOMINIS

This rare human intestinal parasite (Fig. 5-5) also has trophozoite and cyst stages, but human hosts experience no clinical symptoms with the infection. The pyriform trophozoite, 4–10 μm long by 3–6 μm wide, has three anterior flagella and one recurrent flagellum, the latter extending posteriorly along one side and trailing free. The mature cyst, approximately 7 μm by 4 μm, is ovoid with two to four nuclei, which are usually situated at the ends of the cyst. Most cysts are binucleate.

DIENTAMOEBA FRAGILIS

The current system for classifying the Protozoa places *Dientamoeba fragilis* (Fig. 5-6) in the class Zoomastigophorea, which includes certain amoeboid forms that may or may not possess flagella. Although *D. fragilis* exists only in the amoeboid form, it is assigned to this class on the basis of ultrastructural and immunological affinities.

Dientamoeba fragilis occurs worldwide. While it is often considered nonpathogenic and has not been shown to cause intestinal lesions, patients with gastrointestinal disturbances experience relief from discomfort when *D. fragilis* is destroyed by chemotherapy. Fibrosis of the appendiceal wall in all *D. fragilis* infections of the appendix constitutes further strong evidence of this organism's pathogenic potential. Also, *D. fragilis* shows a decided preference for erythrocytes when they are available.

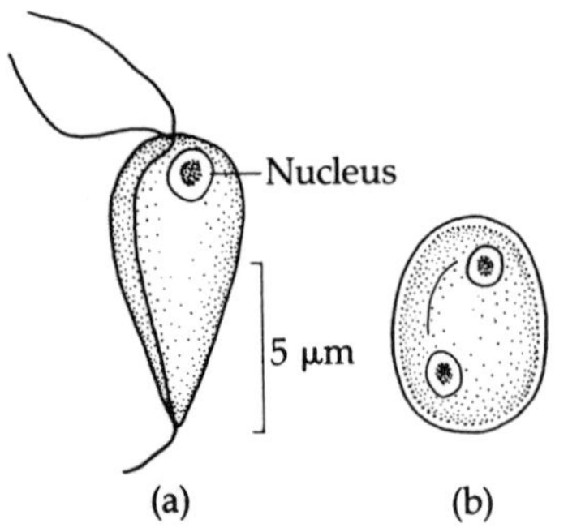

FIGURE 5-5
Enteromonas hominis.
(a) Trophozoite. (b) Cyst.

The trophozoite, which measures 6–12 μm in diameter, lives in the cecal area of the large intestine and moves sluggishly by

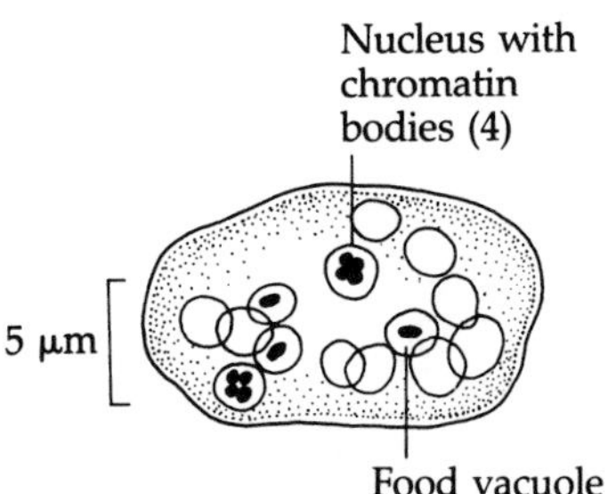

FIGURE 5-6
Binucleate form of *Dientamoeba fragilis*.

means of thin, leaflike pseudopodia. It is frequently binucleate, with a thin nuclear envelope visible only after staining. The prominent endosome is surrounded by minute clumps of chromatin, giving it a beaded appearance. Because no cyst form has been reported, the mechanism of transmission is unknown, although eggs of the intestinal nematode *Enterobius* have been suggested as possible carriers. While the trophozoite is highly viable and is capable of motility up to 48 hours after leaving the host in feces, it cannot survive the digestive juices in the upper regions of the digestive tract.

Approximately 20–80% of the trophozoites recovered from human feces are binucleate, a condition that may represent merely an arrested telophase stage of mitosis. Identification of the trophozoite in the feces serves as diagnosis of infection. When placed in water, the trophozoite swells and then returns to normal size. In the swollen state, numerous cytoplasmic granules exhibit Brownian movement. This feature, called the "Hakansson Phenomenon," is peculiar to *D. fragilis* and occasionally is used in its identification.

THE GENUS *TRICHOMONAS* AND RELATED FORMS

Of the trichomonads that infect humans, two species, *Trichomonas tenax* and *T. vaginalis*, possess four free, anterior flagella. A third species, formerly called *T. hominis*, has five free, anterior flagella and is accordingly placed in the genus *Pentatrichomonas*. All trichomonads possess certain common features (Fig. 5-7), among which are three to five anterior flagella and a recurrent flagellum in the form of an undulating membrane. All flagella in these forms originate from anteriorly situated basal bodies. The costa, which also originates from the region of the basal bodies, extends along the base of the undulating membrane. All three species have a row of granules called **hydrogenosomes** (paracostal or paraxostylar granules) associated with the costa and/or axostyle. An axostyle extending the length of the trichomonad appears to protrude from the organism's posterior end, although it is covered by the plasma membrane. A prominent Golgi complex (parabasal body) lies anteri-

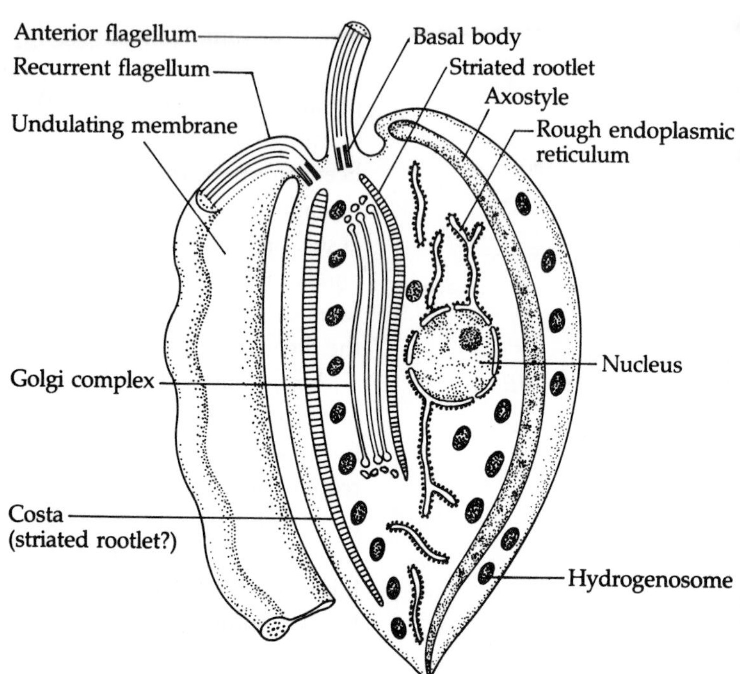

***FIGURE 5-7* Ultrastructural morphology of a generalized trichomonad.**

orly near the single nucleus. There are no known cyst stages in the life cycles of these organisms; while venereal or oral contact are obvious methods of transmission for *T. vaginalis* and *T. tenax*, that of *P. hominis* remains obscure.

TRICHOMONAS TENAX

This flagellate (Fig. 5-8a) is commonly found in the tartar and gums of the mouth, as well as in the nasopharyngeal region. Trophozoites are very small (5–16 μm by 2–15 μm), with four free flagella and a fifth flagellum recurved as an undulating membrane that extends about two-thirds of the length of the cell. The costa runs parallel to the undulating membrane. Transmission is necessarily by direct contact, usually through kissing or using contaminated eating utensils. Drinking contaminated water from a community source may be another means of transmission, since some investigators have shown that this flagellate can live in drinking water for several hours. The organism is not considered pathogenic and can be avoided through proper oral hygiene. Like *Entamoeba gingivalis*, it tends to flourish in unhealthy environ-

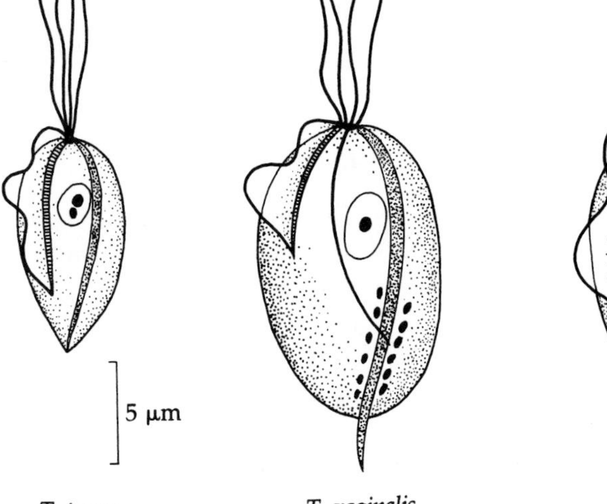

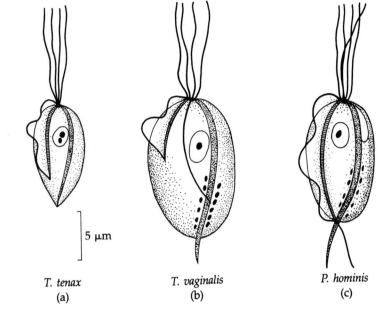

FIGURE 5-8
(a) *Trichomonas tenax*. (b) *Trichomonas vaginalis*. (c) *Pentatrichomonas hominis*.

ments fostered by poor oral hygiene and is most easily found in patients who practice poor hygiene.

TRICHOMONAS VAGINALIS

Of the three human-infecting trichomonads, *T. vaginalis* (Fig. 5-8b) is the only pathogen, although a heavy infection of *Pentatrichomonas hominis* may cause diarrhea. *T. vaginalis* inhabits the vagina in the female and the urethra, epididymis, and prostate gland in the male. Morphologically, it is distinguishable from the other two trichomonads by its larger size (7–32 μm by 5–12 μm) and its shorter undulating membrane, which extends only one-third the length of the cell. The trophozoite occasionally produces pseudopodia. Clusters of hydrogenosomes extend along both the costa and the axostyle.

Life Cycle

Typical of flagellates, *T. vaginalis* reproduces by longitudinal binary fission. The optimum pH range for the organism to reproduce is approximately 5–6. While the normal pH of the vagina is

4–4.5, when the level of acidity is disturbed, an environment is created in which *T. vaginalis* thrives. The pH of the vagina is normally maintained by the activity of a group of lactic acid-producing bacteria, but *T. vaginalis* can disrupt such bacteria, causing the pH to rise above 4.9.

Epidemiology

The prevalence of *T. vaginalis* infection among women is approximately 10–25%, varying inversely with the level of hygiene practiced. While about 15% of infected women with trichomoniasis complain of symptoms, altered vaginal secretions are evident in many more. In infected households, the recorded incidence of infection among men is much lower than among women from the same household. This statistic is misleading, however, since the flagellate is much more difficult to detect in men; in fact, positive identification sometimes requires the examination of prostate exudate. Transmission is by direct contact, usually through sexual intercourse. Damp washcloths and similar items also are sources of infection among children and adults, as viable trophozoites can be recovered from wet washcloths 24 hours after contamination. Trichomoniasis among newborns indicates that the fetus can acquire the organism while passing through the birth canal.

Symptomatology and Diagnosis

Trichomonas vaginalis produces deterioration of the cells of the vaginal mucosa, resulting in low-grade inflammation and persistent vaginitis. The condition is characterized by a yellowish discharge accompanied by persistent itching and burning. In males, symptoms are much less noticeable, although there may be urethritis and swelling of the prostate gland. These symptoms are sometimes confused with those of gonorrhea.

Diagnosis in females is confirmed by microscopical identification of motile trophozoites in vaginal discharge smears. Examination of the urine in both sexes and of prostate secretions in males following prostate massage are also helpful diagnostic procedures.

Treatment

Metronidazole is the most effective drug, although it is contraindicated in pregnant patients. Restoration of the normal pH of the vagina by periodic douches with a dilute solution of vinegar is an effective preventive method and can control mild infections. It is recommended that sexual partners be treated simultaneously.

Physiology

Trichomonads are anaerobic organisms, deriving much of their energy from the incomplete degradation of simple sugars accompanied by the production of short-chain organic acids such as lactic acid and acetic acid; the presence of oxygen has little effect on this process. Glucose and maltose are the most effective growth stimuli *in vitro*. Acetic acid is produced in the hydrogenosome from part of the pyruvic acid pool. The latter compound is produced in the cytoplasm via glycolysis, and a portion enters the hydrogenosome while the remainder is reduced to lactic acid in the cytoplasm and excreted. ATP is formed in the cytoplasm and in the hydrogenosome by substrate-level phosphorylation. Trichomonads lack mitochondria; however, it has been suggested that the hydrogenosome may be a modified mitochondrion, since it shows morphological and functional similarities to mitochondria, such as a double membrane and regulation of cell calcium. The hydrogenosome also considered by some to be a specialized microbody.

In culture, *T. vaginalis* feeds on bacteria and, occasionally, erythrocytes. The predilection for bacteria suggests a mechanism for the breakdown of the normal pH of the infected vagina, since the lactic acid bacilli act to maintain normal pH levels.

PENTATRICHOMONAS (TRICHOMONAS) HOMINIS

This trichomonad (Fig. 5-8c) is a smaller (5–14 μm by 7–10 μm), highly motile organism with an anterior cytostome and three to five free flagella. Typically, four flagella beat synchronously, while the fifth beats independently. A sixth, recurrent flagellum is associated with the undulating membrane and extends the length of the cell; it protrudes beyond the posterior end as a trailing flagellum. *P. hominis* is generally considered a nonpathogen of the human colon, and while it is often associated with diarrhea, there is no definite evidence that it causes the condition. *P. hominis* has no cyst stage; hence, transmission must occur via trophozoites, and flies may be implicated as mechanical vectors. The ability of trophozoites to survive for at least 24 hours in feces-contaminated milk suggests that transmission may occur through contaminated food and drink and that trophozoites are able to withstand the acidic environment of the stomach en route to the intestine. Reproduction is by longitudinal fission. *P. hominis* infects dogs, cats, and mice and other rodents, with such hosts serving as reservoirs in nature.

Identification of trophozoites in fresh fecal preparations provides the most accurate means of diagnosis. It is important that only fresh samples be used, since old stools may contain atypical or degenerating trophozoites resembling amoebae, which could result in their misidentification.

SELECTED READINGS

Adam, R. D. 1991. The biology of *Giardia* spp. *Microbiology Reviews* **55**, 706–732.

Camp, R. R., Mattern, C. F. T., and Honigberg, B. M. 1974. Study of *Dientamoeba fragilis* Jepps and Dobell. I. Electronmicroscopic observations of the binucleate stages. II. Taxonomic position and revision of the genus. *Journal of Protozoolgy* **21**, 69–82.

Flanagan, P. A. 1992. *Giardia* diagnosis, clinical course and epidemiology: A review. *Epidemiology and Infection* **109**, 1–22.

Honigberg, B. M. 1978. Trichomonads of importance in human medicine. In *Parasitic Protozoa* (Kreier, J. P., Ed.), Vol. 3. Academic, New York.

Kabnick, K. S., and Peattie, D. A. 1991. *Giardia*: A missing link between prokaryotes and eukaryotes. *American Scientist* **79**, 34–43.

Chapter Six

BLOOD AND TISSUE PROTOZOA I: HEMOFLAGELLATES

Humans are infected by hemoflagellates belonging to two genera of the family Trypanosomatidae, *Leishmania* and *Trypanosoma*. Both require blood-feeding insect vectors in their life cycles. The term **hemoflagellate** denotes the protozoan's site of residence in the human host: the blood and/or closely related tissues such as the spleen and liver. During their life cycle, hemoflagellates may assume as many as four distinct morphologic forms. While these forms appear to be successive stages, there is no specific sequential pattern of progression from one form to the next. Indeed, it appears that any of the forms is capable of developing into any other. Each of the forms is discussed in detail in the following text. Certain organelles are common to all forms. Underlying the plasma membrane is a system of microtubules, the **subpellicular microtubular network**, which forms a spiral framework just beneath the surface of the pellicle and provides limited structural support (see Fig. 3-5). However, this subpellicular network is not associated with the lining of the **flagellar pocket**, the site of uptake of exogenous macromolecules (Fig. 6-1). A flagellum arises from a basal body in close association with a prominent **kinetoplast**, a structure characteristic of members of the order Kinetoplastida, forming a kinetoplast-basal body complex (see Fig. 6-7). The organelle is rich in DNA that resembles mitochondrial DNA of other organisms, being composed of a limited number of nucleotides arranged in linked circlets. Kinetoplast DNA (kDNA) appears to be responsible for the elaboration of mitochondria in many of the forms as well as for the metamorphosis of one stage into another.

MORPHOLOGIC FORMS

AMASTIGOTE

The amastigote (Fig. 6-2) is ovoid and usually develops in vertebrate host cells. It is characterized by a single prominent nucle-

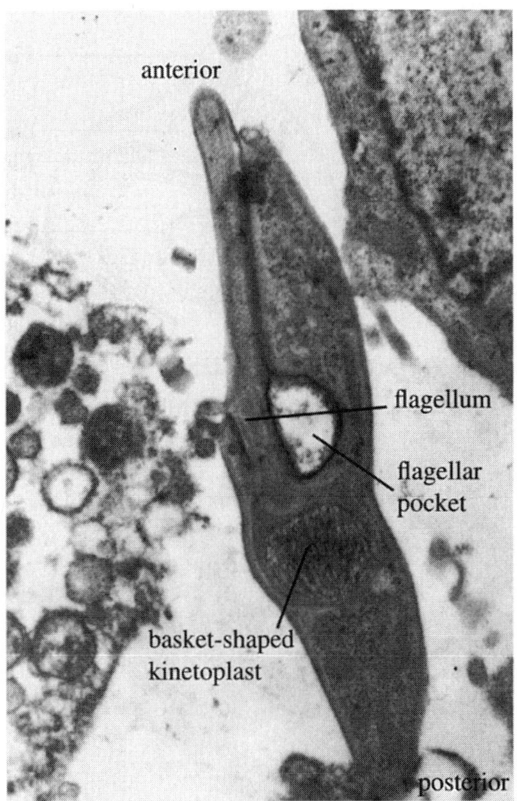

FIGURE 6-1
Transmission electron micrograph of a developing trypomastigote exposed to exogenous protein.
Note the accumulation of protein in the flagellar pocket.

us and a very short flagellum that projects barely (if at all) beyond the cell surface.

PROMASTIGOTE

The promastigote (Fig. 6-3) occurs only in the insect vector and differs morphologically from the amastigote in two significant aspects: (1) it is more elongated, and (2) its long flagellum is free anteriorly and serves the function of both locomotion through the medium and attachment to the insect gut wall. In addition, protruding from the kinetoplast of the promastigote are two mitochondrial branches: a prominent posterior one, often extending the length of the cell, and a shorter, anterior one.

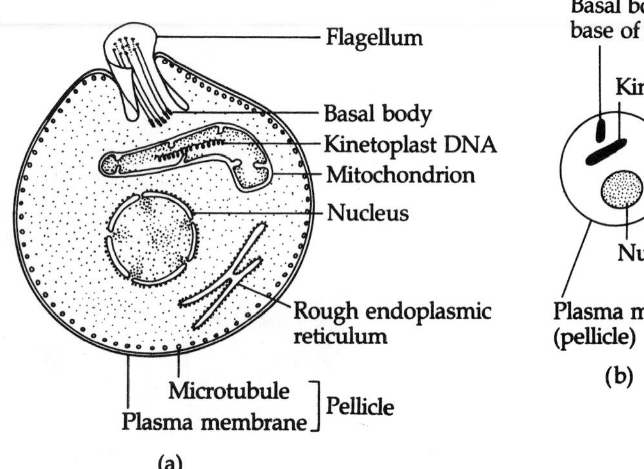

FIGURE 6-2
(a) Ultrastructure of a hemoflagellate amastigote. (b) Amastigote as it would appear by light microscopy.

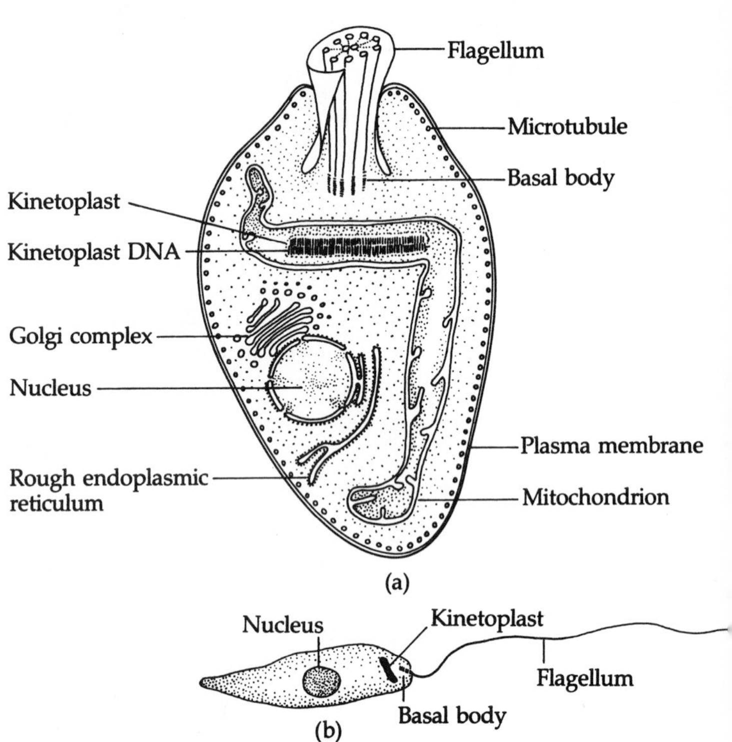

FIGURE 6-3
(a) Ultrastructure of a hemoflagellate promastigote. (b) Promastigote as it would appear by light microscopy.

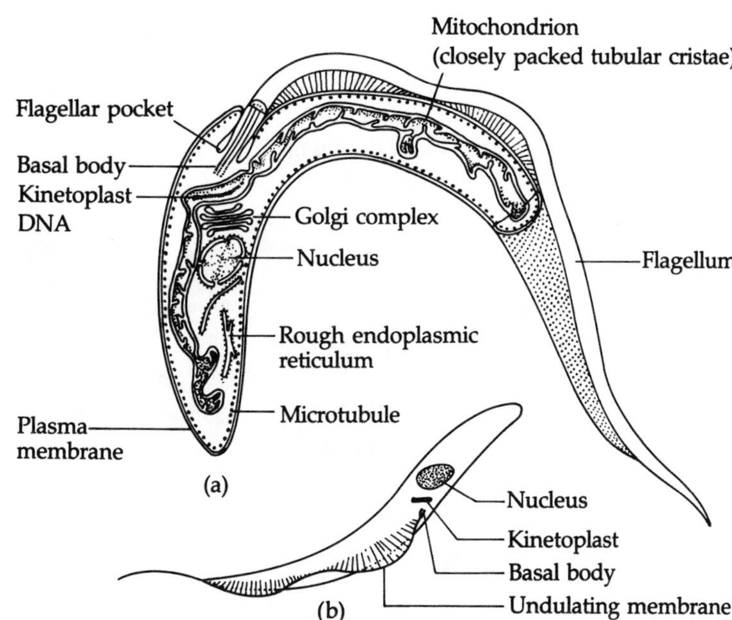

FIGURE 6-4
(a) Ultrastructure of a hemoflagellate epimastigote. (b) Epimastigote as it would appear by light microscopy.

EPIMASTIGOTE

In this form (Fig. 6-4), the kinetoplast–basal body complex is situated more posteriorly but remains anterior to the nucleus. From its point of origin near the kinetoplast–basal body complex to its emergence at the anterior tip of the cell, the flagellum is attached to the pellicle, producing an undulating membrane. The distal, free portion of the flagellum projects anteriorly, and anterior and posterior mitochondrial branches remain well developed.

TRYPOMASTIGOTE

The fourth morphological form discernible among hemoflagellates, the trypomastigote (Fig. 6-5), exhibits varying degrees of polymorphism. One type, the **long, slender trypomastigote** (Fig. 6-6) is characterized by (1) lengthening of the body, (2) elongation of the undulating membrane and flagellum, and (3) migration of the kinetoplast–basal body complex to a site posterior to the nucleus (Fig. 6-7). In this type, mito-

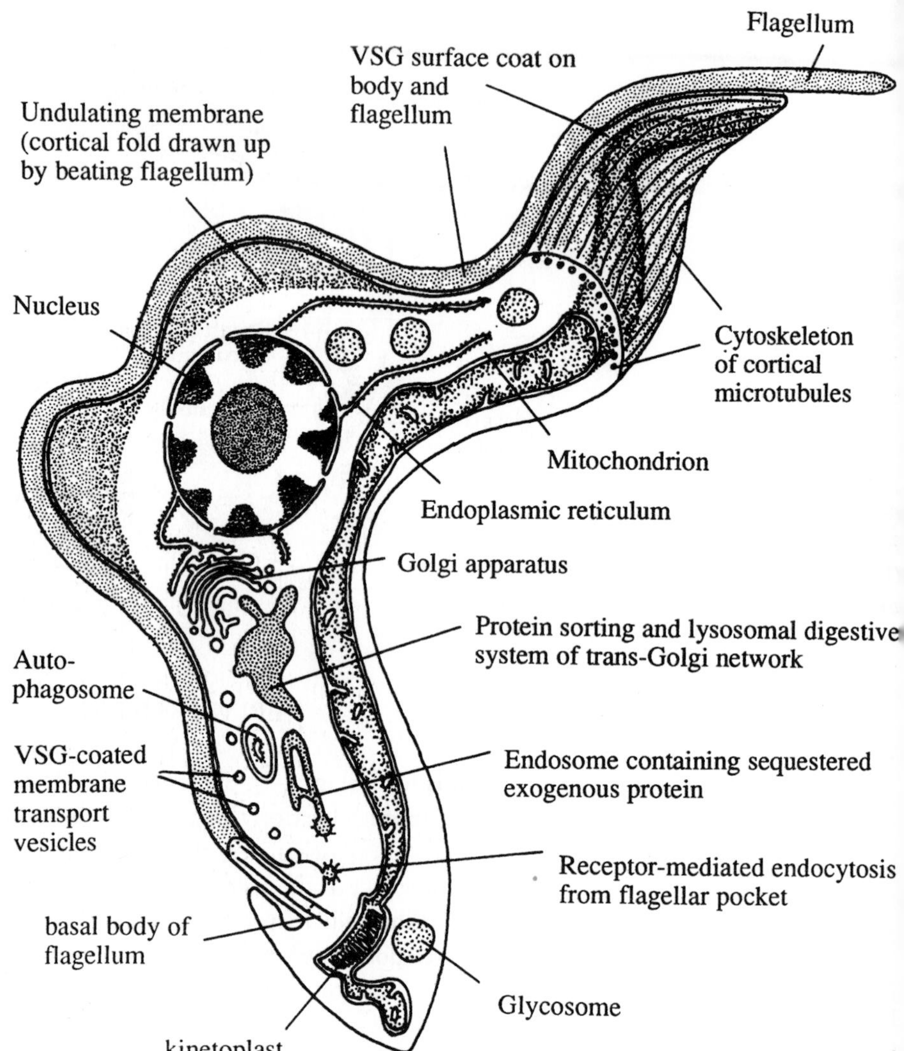

FIGURE 6-5 **Ultrastructure of a hemoflagellate trypomastigote.**

chondria are greatly diminished in function, and glycosomes, membrane-bound, microbody-like organelles that sometimes contain crystalline cores, are numerous in the cytoplasm. Another type, the **stumpy trypomastigote** (Fig. 6-6), is shorter and thicker and its free flagellum is either shorter or absent. The significance of polymorphism in the trypomastigote will be considered later.

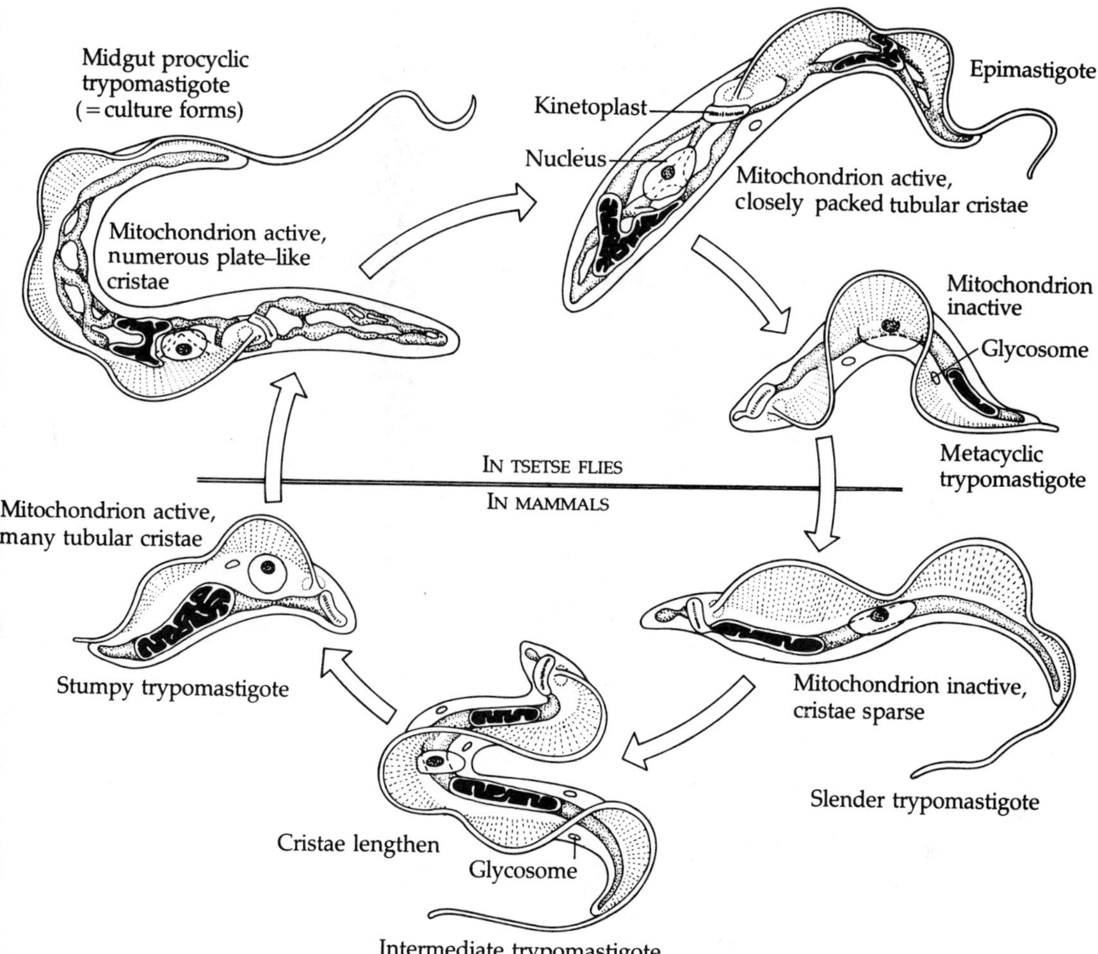

FIGURE 6-6
Form and metabolic activity of the mitochondrion of *Trypanosoma brucei brucei* at various stages of its life cycle.

GENUS *LEISHMANIA*

Through the use of molecular and immunological techniques, a number of species and subspecies of *Leishmania* have been partially characterized (Table 6-1). Those that infect humans produce only three clinical manifestations: **visceral, cutaneous,** and **mucocutaneous leishmaniasis.** While the infective species have identical life

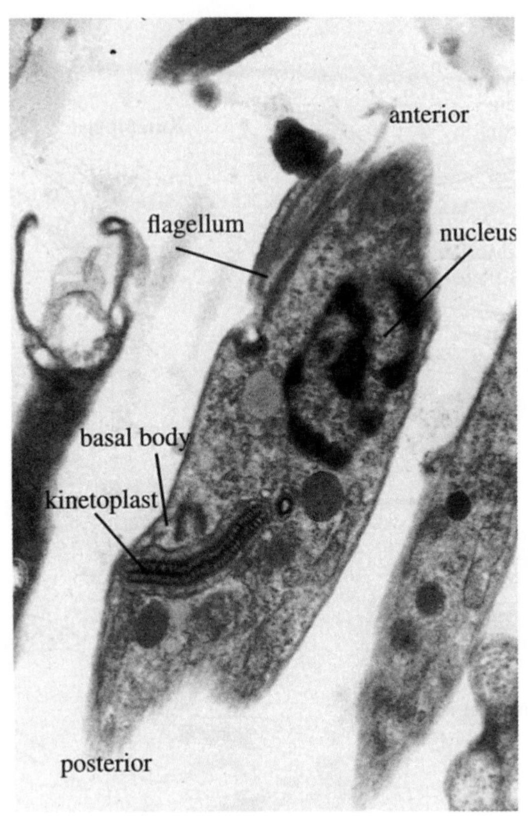

FIGURE 6-7
Transmission electron micrograph of a developing trypomastigote.
Note the position of the basal body/kinetoplast complex just posterior to the nucleus.

cycles and are morphologically indistinguishable, they differ in the type and location of the primary lesions they produce in humans.

LIFE CYCLE

Paradoxically, all species of *Leishmania* produce amastigotes that infect macrophages, the very cells of the mammalian host that constitute its primary defense against invasion by foreign organisms (Fig. 6-8). Upon entering a macrophage, the parasite establishes itself in an endocytotic vacuole called a **parasitophorous vacuole.** Lysosomes fuse with this vacuole, producing a type of secondary lysosome (digestive vacuole). Impervious to the lytic action of the lysosomal enzymes, the amastigote lives and reproduces within the parasitophorous vacuole. A number of mammals act as natural reservoir hosts for the parasite, the most

TABLE 6-1
***Leishmania* Species and Forms of Human Leishmaniasis**

Old World forms
- *L. major* "wet" cutaneous: widespread in rural areas of Asia and Africa
- *L. tropica* "dry" cutaneous: uncommon; urban areas of Europe, Asia, and North Africa
- *L. aethiopica* "diffuse" cutaneous: Ethiopia and Kenya, associated with rock rabbits
- *L. donovani donovani* visceral (kala-azar): Africa and Asia
- *L. donovani infantum* infantile visceral: Mediterranean region

New World forms
- *L. donovani chagasi* cutaneous: South America
- *L. braziliensis braziliensis* mucocutaneous: South America, especially Brazil
- *L. braziliensis guyanensis* cutaneous: South America
- *L. braziliensis panamensis* cutaneous: South and Central America
- *L. mexicana mexicana*, *L. mexicana amazonensis*, *L. mexicana pifanoi* cutaneous: South and Central America
- *L. peruviana* cutaneous: South America, mainly Andean region

common being canines, both wild and domestic, and rodents. Leishmaniasis in humans is therefore a **zoonosis.**

While obtaining a blood meal from a mammalian host, any of a wide variety of species of sandflies belonging to the genera *Phlebotomus* and *Lutzomyia* ingests cells containing the amastigotes. Following ingestion by the insect, the amastigote transforms into a promastigote in the insect's gut. If the insect is a suitable vector, the promastigote attaches to the midgut epithelium; otherwise, the promastigote passes out of the gut. This attachment retains the parasite in the insect's gut during the passage of food, and it is essential for the transformation of the promastigote into the mammalian infective stage, the metacyclic promastigote. While attached to the wall of the gut, the promastigotes multiply by longitudinal binary fission. The reproductive rate is so rapid that after 1–3 weeks, the anterior gut and pharynx of the insect become clogged with promastigotes. As they transform into infective metacyclic promastigotes, the promastigotes detach from the gut wall and are subsequently deposited in the skin of the mammal when the sandfly feeds again. Macrophages of the mammalian host quickly engulf the promastigotes, which then revert

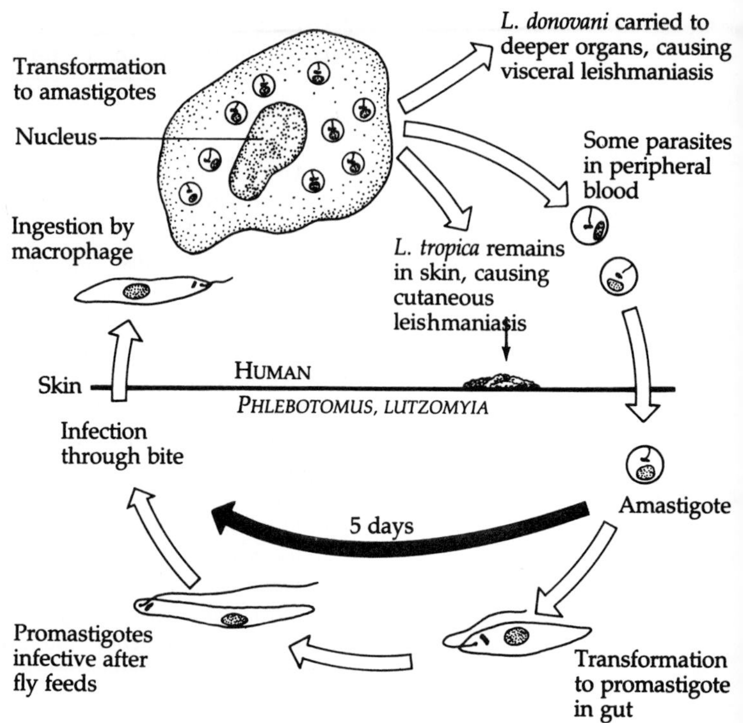

FIGURE 6-8
Life cycles of *Leishmania donovani* and *L. tropica*.

to the intracellular amastigote form. Reproduction of the amastigotes by longitudinal binary fission, followed by rupture of the infected host cells, produces large numbers of amastigotes, which are engulfed by other phagocytic cells, thus spreading the infection. Factors such as the species of *Leishmania* involved, temperature, immune status of the host, and even behavioral characteristics of the insect vector may determine the extent and site of infection in the mammalian host.

Reservoir hosts play an important role in the prevalence of leishmaniasis. In many regions of the world, dogs and other domestic reservoir hosts serve as a link between the sylvatic, or wild, reservoir hosts and the human population, via the sandfly vector. The reservoir hosts are usually unaffected by the parasites; thus, they provide a constant source of infection for humans. Where such reservoir hosts are present, they, rather than other infected humans, serve as primary sources of human infection via the bite of infected sandflies.

PHYSIOLOGY

Carbohydrate metabolism in members of the genus *Leishmania* is inextricably linked to the kinetoplast, the mitochondrion, and glycosomes of the amastigote and promastigote forms. For example, because the poorly developed mitochondrion of the amastigote includes neither a cytochrome system nor a functional Krebs cycle, the amastigote processes carbohydrates incompletely by anaerobic metabolism. This process occurs in glycosomes and the cytosol, producing short-chain organic acids as end products and ATP by substrate-level phosphorylation. When the amastigote is ingested by the sandfly or subjected to *in vitro* conditions simulating those within the vector, the amastigote transforms into a promastigote. With this transformation, the mitochondrion grows, acquires more cristae, and becomes functionally and morphologically well developed, with an active cytochrome system and a functional Krebs cycle. Under such conditions, the cell utilizes aerobic metabolism, producing ATP by oxidative phosphorylation. Such mitochondrial growth is controlled by kinetoplastic DNA.

The chemical components of the amastigote pellicle apparently protect the cell from the hydrolytic action of the macrophage lysosomal enzymes. Knowledge of the physiology of these organisms has not led to the development of effective chemotherapeutic agents or vaccines. However, the pentavalent antimony compound, antimony sodium gluconate (Pentostam), is currently being used effectively against most forms of cutaneous leishmaniasis, although its mode of action is not yet understood.

VISCERAL LEISHMANIASIS (*LEISHMANIA DONOVANI*)

Leishmania donovani is the causative agent for visceral leishmaniasis, also known as **dumdum fever** or **kala-azar**, an often fatal disease of humans. In the mammalian host, amastigote-infected cells are found at numerous sites, including the spleen, liver, bone marrow, lymph glands, and intestinal mucosa.

Epidemiology

Recent epidemiologic and clinical studies reveal the existence of at least three varieties or strains of *L. donovani*. The Mediterranean–Middle Asian variety occurs throughout the Mediterranean Basin and extends through southern Russia to China. The common sandfly vectors are *Phlebotomus major*, *P. chinensis*, *P. perniciosus*, and *P. longicuspis*. A number of canines serve as both sylvatic and domestic reservoir hosts, and because young children are the most frequent human victims, the disease is known as **infantile kala-azar.**

A second variety, classic kala-azar, occurs in northeast India and Bangladesh. The usual vector for this strain is *Phlebotomus argentipes*. The amastigote mainly infects adult and adolescent humans and involves no reservoir hosts. A more virulent but clinically similar variety is transmitted by different *Phlebotomus* species in east Africa and employs wild rodents as reservoirs.

A third variety, widespread in Central and South America, uses *Phlebotomus longipalpis* as the vector and canines as both sylvatic and domestic reservoir hosts.

Symptomatology and Diagnosis

Because leishmaniasis is primarily a disease of the reticulo–endothelial (macrophage) system, replacement of infected cells produces hyperplasia and consequent enlargement of visceral organs associated with the system, such as the spleen (splenomegaly) and liver (hepatomegaly). A concomitant decrease in red and white blood cell production results in anemia and leukopenia, facilitating secondary bacterial infection. Without medical treatment, the condition is usually fatal. Surviving individuals commonly acquire long-lasting immunity, however.

In India, a **post-kala-azar dermal leishmanoid** may develop in which numerous parasite-laden nodules appear in the skin. Such nodules are found in no more than 10% of fully recovered kala-azar patients.

In endemic areas, classic initial symptoms of kala-azar are fever and chills, which may persist for several weeks. The fever chart typically shows two fever spikes per day, a pattern called a "dromedary" curve that provides a useful diagnostic tool. In more advanced cases, enlargement of the liver and spleen produces abdominal distention. Definitive diagnosis is the positive identification of intracellular amastigotes in blood or tissue smears. When such smears are inconclusive, other diagnostic techniques must be employed. One technique is **xenodiagnosis**, that is, the direct inoculation of laboratory animals, such as hamsters, with tissue homogenates from the patient. Signs of infection in the animal within one month constitute positive diagnosis. Biopsy and punctures of organs such as the spleen, liver, or sternum to reveal parasites are also useful diagnostic procedures. Immunological tests are used but are difficult to evaluate, since postrecovery cases are indistinguishable from active cases. Further, such tests cannot differentiate among the various species of *Leishmania* and *Trypanosoma cruzi.*

Treatment

Proper nursing care and complete bed rest are essential, especially in more acute cases; blood transfusions are frequently required. Chemotherapy consists of closely monitored intramuscular or intravenous injection of pentavalent antimony compounds such as antimony sodium gluconate. Extreme caution is essential in the administration of such treatment, since not only can antimony produce serious side effects, but insufficient treatment may result in relapses or post-kala-azar dermal leishmanoid.

CUTANEOUS LEISHMANIASIS (*LEISHMANIA TROPICA AND LEISHMANIA MEXICANA*)

Cutaneous leishmaniasis, a relatively mild skin disease commonly known as **oriental sore**, is caused by *Leishmania tropica* in the Old World and *Leishmania mexicana* in the New World. Unlike the amastigote of *L. donovani*, those of *L. tropica* and *L. mexicana* are found primarily in macrophages around cutaneous sores. Sandflies must feed at these sites in order to acquire the infective amastigotes.

Epidemiology

L. tropica is endemic to those countries of Europe and North Africa bordering the Mediterranean Sea and to the Asian countries of Syria, Israel, southern Russia, China, Vietnam, and India. *L. mexicana* has been reported from Peru, Bolivia, Brazil, the Guianas, and Mexico. A variant clinical form of cutaneous leishmaniasis occurring in South and Central America and Ethiopia is referred to as **diffuse cutaneous leishmaniasis**.

The vectors for *L. tropica* and *L. mexicana* are members of the sandfly genera *Phlebotomus* and *Lutzomyia*, respectively. The life cycles of *L. tropica* and *L. mexicana* parallel that of *L. donovani.* In addition to humans, *L. tropica* infects dogs and cats in China and a few Mediterranean countries. Natural infections are known to occur in monkeys, bullocks, brown bears, horses, and gerbils in the Middle East. In some areas of the Middle East, the infection is endemic among rodents in whose burrows the sandflies live and breed. Humans who intrude into these areas are readily infected. In the Western Hemisphere, dogs serve as the primary domestic reservoir, while armadillos and arboreal rodents may also serve as sylvatic reservoirs.

Symptomatology and Diagnosis

In humans, the initial sign of infection is the appearance of a vascularized papule or nodule on the skin at the feeding site of the insect. After a few weeks, the papule becomes ulcerated, erupts, and spreads, forming cutaneous lesions most commonly on the hands, feet, legs, and face (Fig. 6-9). The usual incubation period varies from as short as 1–2 weeks to as long as several months or even, in rare instances, several years. Two types of oriental sore are produced by different strains of the protozoan: (1) the chronic, dry (or urban) type, with delayed ulceration and numerous amastigotes, is produced by *L. minor* (often considered a differ-

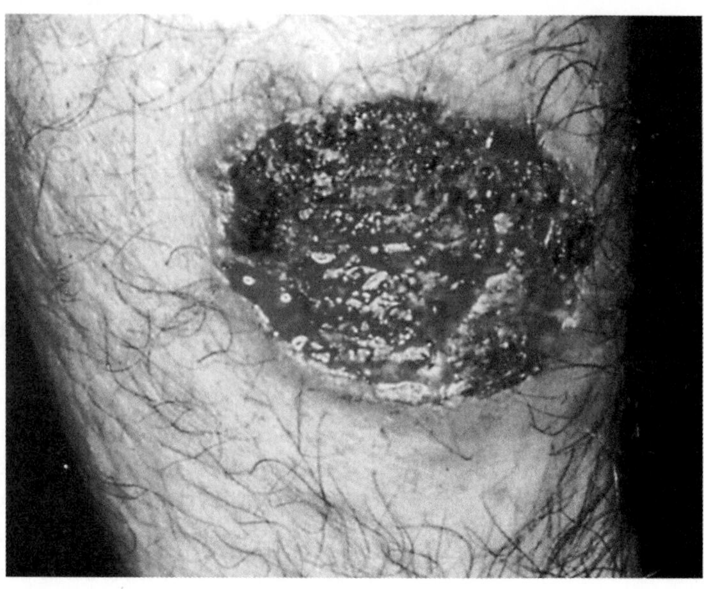

FIGURE 6-9
Oriental sore, or cutaneous leishmaniasis.

ent species); and (2) the acute, moist (or rural) type, characterized by early ulceration and few amastigotes, is produced by *L. major*.

In the absence of secondary bacterial contamination, sores tend to heal within a year, but disfiguring scars often remain. The lesions in diffuse cutaneous leishmaniasis, however, differ from those accompanying the usual infection in that they are disseminated as multiple nodules under the skin and contain numerous parasites in the associated macrophages, in this manner resembling lepromatous leprosy. This form of cutaneous leishmaniasis is found in patients with a specific deficiency in their cell-mediated immune processes.

Characteristic features of the lesions of cutaneous leishmaniasis, such as an elevated and hardened rim of the ulcer, are useful in diagnosis. Positive diagnosis requires identification of amastigotes in infected cells. The most reliable diagnosis is achieved by *in vitro* culturing of lesion scrapings or aspirates and subsequent identification of promastigotes in the medium. An immunological test is available, but, as in *L. donovani*, its diagnostic value is limited.

Treatment

Healing may eventually occur without chemotherapy, but the process is long and can produce disfiguring scars, especially if proper hygienic practices are not strictly observed. Secondary microbial infections are a constant danger as long as the ulcer is open. The treatment of choice is a daily intramuscular injection of pentavalent antimony compounds for approximately one week. A second or third course of treatment may be required. Concomitant topical antibiotic treatment is employed in cases of microbial contamination of skin lesions.

MUCOCUTANEOUS LEISHMANIASIS (*LEISHMANIA BRAZILIENSIS*)

Leishmania braziliensis causes mucocutaneous leishmaniasis. Amastigotes are found in macrophages in ulcerations at mucocutaneous junctures of the skin. This disease is also known by various other names, including **American leishmaniasis, espundia, uta, pian bois,** and **chiclero ulcer.**

Epidemiology

The disease is common in humans in an area extending from the Yucatan peninsula in Mexico south to Argentina. While human infections have also occurred in the Sudan, Kenya, Italy, China, and India, the disease is far more common in the Western Hemisphere—hence the name American leishmaniasis. Interestingly, the disease does not occur in the high Andes Mountains, since the parasite's vector is not found there.

A primary skin lesion appears following the bite of an infected sandfly of the genus *Lutzomyia*. Geographic location determines the site of secondary lesions. In Mexico and Central America, for instance, the secondary lesion usually appears on the ear, causing chiclero ulcer, a condition common among chicleros, the forest-dwelling natives who harvest the gum of chicle trees. Recent investigations suggest that the variety of the parasite that causes chiclero ulcer may be a separate species, *L. mexicana*. This variation of the disease, like many forms of leishmaniasis, is zoonotic, and various forest rodents, dogs, cats, and kinkajous serve as reservoirs. Mucocutaneous involvement is seldom seen in the geographic region where *L. mexicana* is acknowledged as the causative agent.

In its southern range, the disease caused by *L. braziliensis* follows a different course. The secondary lesions erupt at the mucocutaneous junctures of the skin, with nasal and buccal tissues most often affected (Fig. 6-10). In these geographic areas the disease is commonly called espundia or uta.

Symptomatology and Diagnosis

As indicated earlier, clinical manifestations of the disease in the Western Hemisphere vary so widely that considerable confusion exists about the identity of the parasite responsible (Table 6-1). Some investigators attribute the entire battery of symptoms occurring at multiple loci to a single species, *L. tropica*; others list four or more species. Regardless, introduction of promastigotes into humans by the sandfly typically results in a small red papule on the skin, the **primary lesion**, which ulcerates in 1–4 weeks and heals in 6–15 months. In Venezuela and Paraguay, primary lesions often appear as flat, ulcerated plaques that remain open and ooze. The disease is termed *pian bois* in these areas. A secondary lesion invariably appears elsewhere on the body. The sites of secondary lesions are usually distinctive. For instance, chiclero ulcer

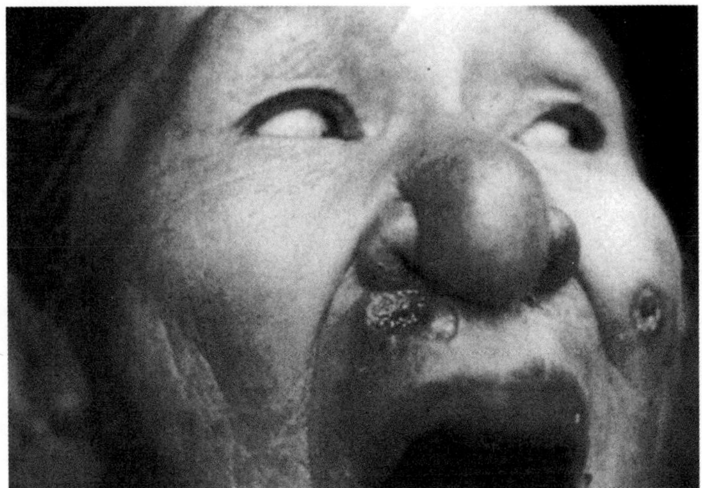

FIGURE 6-10
Mucocutaneous leishmaniasis.
Lesions caused by *Leishmania braziliensis.*

is associated with degeneration of the pinna of the ear, while espundia and uta are characterized by degeneration of the cartilaginous and soft tissues of the nasal and buccal areas. Occasionally, infections metastasize to adjacent tissues, forming satellite lesions. Secondary bacterial and fungal infections are common.

For accurate diagnosis, it is essential to distinguish the lesions of leishmaniasis from those of other skin diseases, such as yaws, syphilis, and chronic skin diseases. The surest diagnosis is identification of the protozoan in infected cells and cultures. Material collected by either aspiration or scrapings from the edges of lesions is suitable for such diagnostic studies. Histological examination of biopsy material is the most efficient method and provides the most accurate results. When possible, it is preferable to examine early lesions, since they yield more parasites than older lesions. The same problems exist with immunological diagnostic procedures for this form of leishmaniasis as are encountered in *L. donovani* and *L. tropica* infections.

Treatment

Generally, treatment with pentavalent antimony compounds is also used for this form of leishmaniasis. When there is mucocutaneous involvement, more extensive chemotherapy is indicated, since these lesions are most resistant to the usual regimen. For the most intractable cases, daily intravenous injections of amphotericin B for up to 10 days is recommended. Amphotericin B is toxic to some patients, and its administration should be closely monitored. If treatment is insufficient or is discontinued too soon, the parasite may remain dormant for many years and then reemerge to cause relapse. Once complete cure is effected, however, lifetime immunity is conferred.

GENUS *TRYPANOSOMA*

Members of the genus *Trypanosoma* that infect humans can be divided into two major groups according to their geographic distribution and characteristic pathogenicity. The African varieties, indigenous to that continent, cause a disease commonly known as **African sleeping sickness**. The other variety, confined to the Western Hemisphere, causes **American trypanosomiasis**, or **Chagas' disease**. The New World disease involves intracellular parasitism; although the parasite also affects blood and other tissue fluids.

AFRICAN TRYPANOSOMIASIS (*TRYPANOSOMA BRUCEI RHODESIENSE* AND *TRYPANOSOMA BRUCEI GAMBIENSE*)

The two organisms responsible for African sleeping sickness are subspecies of *Trypanosoma brucei*, namely *Trypanosoma brucei rhodesiense* and *T. b. gambiense*. The life cycles of the organisms are essentially identical, the major differences being (1) the species of the insect genus *Glossina* that serve as vectors, (2) the vertebrate host, (3) the time required for development within host and vector, and (4) the time required for evolution of the disease in the vertebrate host. The following generalized life cycle therefore can be used for both organisms.

Life Cycle

Introduction of the infective stage of the protozoan into the human host occurs with the bite of an infected tsetse fly vector belonging to the genus *Glossina* (Fig. 6-11). As the insect secretes

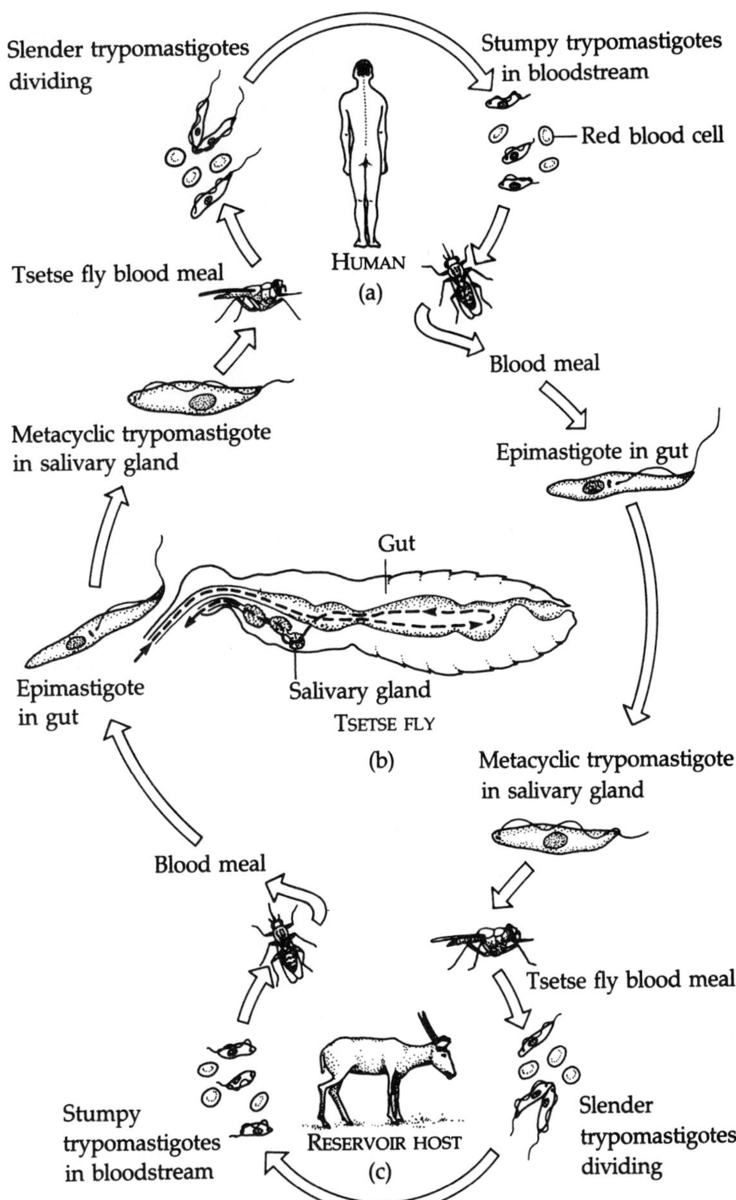

FIGURE 6-11
Life cycles of *Trypanosoma brucei gambiense* and *T. b. rhodesiense*.
(a) Development of trypanosomes in the peripheral blood of humans: infection of central nervous system. (b) Development in tsetse flies (*Glossina* spp.). (c) Development similar to (a) in the peripheral blood of the reservoir host (for example, an antelope).

saliva into the dermis of its victim to dilate the blood vessels and prevent coagulation of the blood, it simultaneously introduces the **metacyclic trypomastigote,** the infective form of the protozoan. The morphology and physiology of the mitochondrion dis-

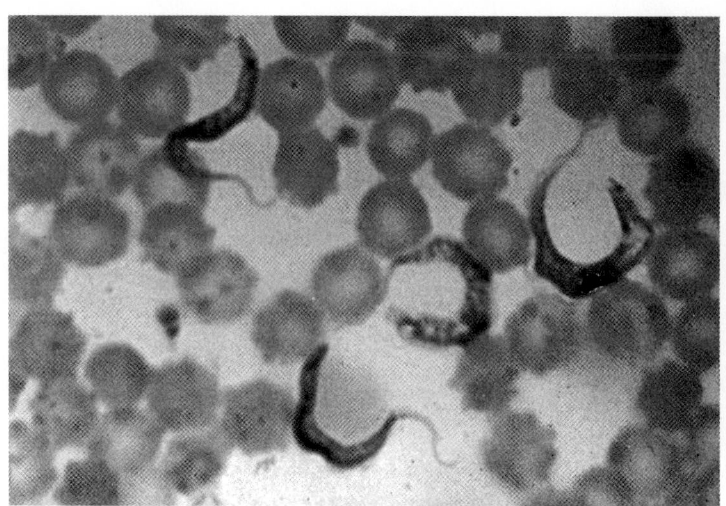

FIGURE 6-12
Slender form of *Trypanosoma brucei gambiense*, found in the bloodstream of its mammalian host.

tinguish the metacyclic trypomastigote from most of the other life cycle forms that occur in the insect vector: the mitochondrion has few cristae and contains no intermediates for electron transport. Also, the metacyclic trypomastigote is blunt, with a short free flagellum. Once introduced into the mammalian bloodstream, the trypomastigotes spread rapidly within the host and eventually migrate to the cerebrospinal fluid. In the bloodstream, trypomastigotes exhibit three forms (Fig. 6-6): (1) a long, slender form with a free flagellum extending from the undulating membrane (Fig. 6-12); (2) a short, stumpy form lacking a prominent free flagellum; and (3) a form intermediate between the two.

In order for the parasite's life cycle to be completed and for the tsetse fly to transmit sleeping sickness, the insect must ingest in its blood meal the short, stumpy trypomastigote, which is physiologically adapted for existence within the insect vector. The presence of a mitochondrion with prominent cristae and a functional electron transport system enables this form to live in the insect midgut, where food may be scarcer than in the vertebrate host's bloodstream. Once ingested by the insect, the stumpy trypomastigotes elongate, lose their surface coats and antigenic identity, and become **procyclic trypomastigotes**. The parasites then multiply by longitudinal binary fission and invade the extraperitrophic spaces. As their numbers increase, they migrate anteriorly, and by the tenth day after ingestion, they enter the proventriculus.

Metamorphosis during this migration to the insect's foregut produces the **epimastigote**, the dominant form in the esophagus and buccal cavity of the fly. By the twentieth day, the epimastigotes move into the salivary gland ducts, attach to the epithelium by their flagella, and multiply. By the end of the third week, they transform into metacyclic trypomastigotes and detach into the lumen of the gland. Thus, two distinct forms—the trypomastigote, with its morphological and physiological variants, and the epimastigote—are essential for completion of the life cycle of trypanosomes that cause African sleeping sickness.

Epidemiology

African sleeping sickness has probably plagued human inhabitants of Africa since humans first encroached upon the domain of the tsetse fly. At the turn of the twentieth century, three quarters of a million people died in Central Africa from African trypanosomiasis. Subsequently, the colonial regimes in Africa were very successful in curbing the disease and almost eradicating it. However, since the era of independence in the 1960s, control measures have deteriorated in many African nations. Since 1990, the rate of infection has risen 10-fold and may now surpass one million cases each year. The pathological effects of African trypanosomiasis on humans and domestic animals (primarily cattle) have sometimes brought productive activity in certain areas to a virtual standstill. So devastating is the disease that most of Africa between 15° N and 15° S latitude (an area approximately the size of the continental United States), with the potential for supporting 125 million head of livestock, still remains essentially useless for cattle production (Fig. 6-13). The toll in human victims is staggering: more than 20,000 new cases diagnosed annually, about half of them fatal and many of the rest resulting in permanent brain damage. The disease has reached epidemic proportions in the Democratic Republic of the Congo and in Angola. Because the disease also affects cattle, sheep, and goats in a region where human diet has historically been acutely deficient in protein, its effects are compounded. A related disease in domestic animals, called **nagana**, is caused by similar organisms, *Trypanosoma brucei brucei*, *T. vivax*, and *T. congolense*. Authorities disagree as to whether humans are susceptible to *T. b. brucei*. Fortunately for the rest of the world, the tsetse fly appears to be the only insect capable of transmitting African trypanosomiasis that

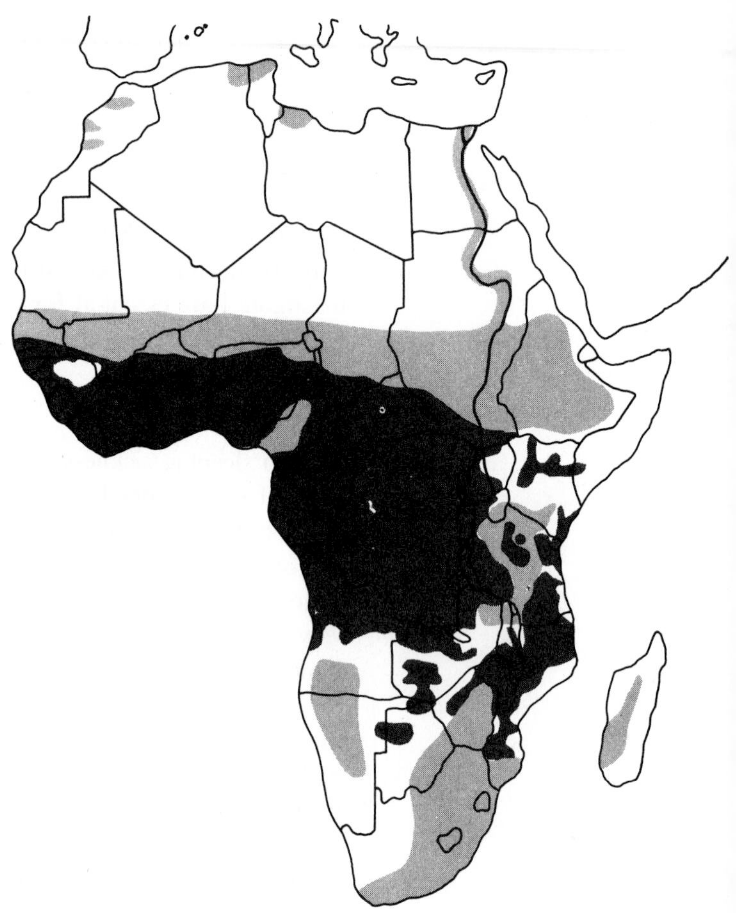

FIGURE 6-13
Africa's cattle-raising country (light shading) and tsetse fly-infested areas (dark shading) show virtually no overlap. Trypanosomiasis spread by tsetse flies has kept 10 million square kilometers of grazing land out of production.

causes human sleeping sickness, and Africa appears to provide its only habitat.

Trypanosoma brucei rhodesiense causes **East African** or **Rhodesian** sleeping sickness, a more virulent form that is usually transmitted by *Glossina morsitans*. In addition to human hosts, wild game and domestic animals in which this parasite is endemic may serve as reservoir hosts. The disease runs its course so rapidly (2–6 months) in humans that person-to-person transmission via the tsetse fly is uncommon.

Trypanosoma brucei gambiense causes **West African, Equatorial African**, or **Gambian** sleeping sickness, a more chronic form of the disease. Domestic and wild animals, such as pigs, an-

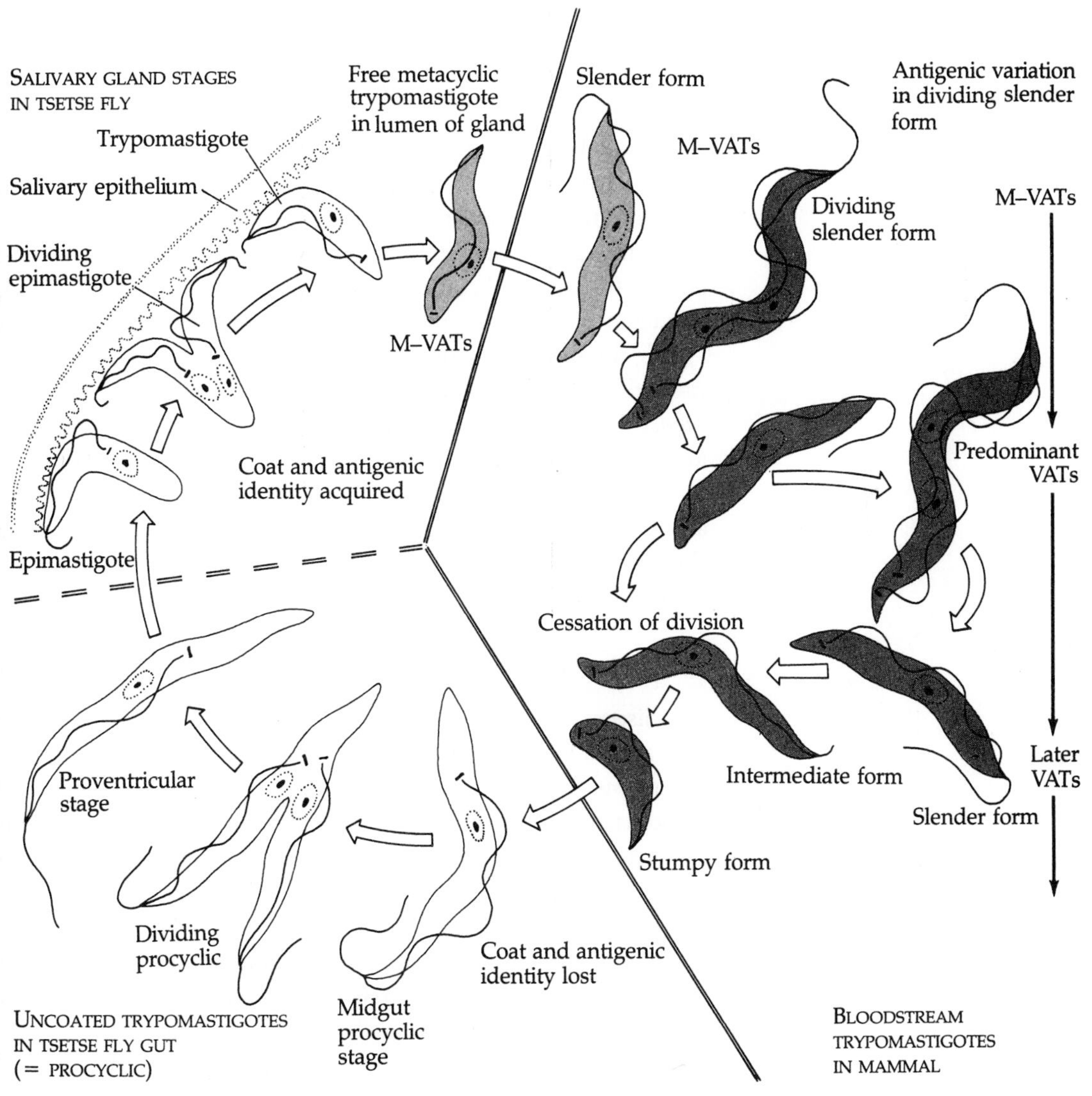

FIGURE 6-14
Life cycle of *Trypanosoma brucei brucei* showing phases of multiplication.
Shaded stages possess the variable antigen-containing surface coat (VAT). The coat is acquired in the salivary glands of the tsetse fly, when free-swimming metacyclic trypomastigotes arise from vector-attached trypomastigotes. Only the coated metacyclic stage can infect the mammal. After ingestion by the vector, the stumpy trypomastigotes transform into procyclic trypomastigotes, simultaneously losing the variable antigen coat.

telopes, buffaloes, and reed bucks, may serve as reservoir hosts. The insect vectors are *Glossina palpalis* and *G. tachinoides*. Human-to-human transmission via the bite of the tsetse fly is common, since the trypomastigotes can remain in circulating blood for 2–4 years, providing ample opportunity for vectors to transmit them.

In Gambian sleeping sickness, fluctuation in the number of parasites in the blood is common, producing periods of remission that alternate with periods when the parasite census is high. These fluctuations are attributed to the ability of the organism to change the chemical composition of its surface coat (glycocalyx), producing a veritable parade of successive **variant antigenic types** (VATs) in the vertebrate host (Fig. 6-14). It is estimated that more than 1,000 variants are theoretically possible for *T. b. gambiense*. With each alteration of the coat, the immunological mechanism of the vertebrate host is activated, gradually depleting the ability of the host immune system to respond. The antigenic variability of these parasites makes the search for an effective vaccine that confers lasting protection an unpromising avenue for the control of this disease.

Symptomatology and Diagnosis

The diseases caused by *T. b. rhodesiense* and *T. b. gambiense* are very similar except for the interval required for their development in humans. In general, shortly after the introduction of metacyclic trypomastigotes through the bite of the tsetse fly, an inflammatory reaction of 1–2 days' duration occurs at the site of the bite. The characteristic reaction, a **trypanosomal chancre**, includes reddening of the skin, a swelling 1–5 cm in diameter, and enlargement of adjacent lymph nodes. When the blood and lymph are invaded, headache and irregular fever develop. These symptoms are accompanied by further enlargement of lymph nodes, especially in the neck and supraclavicular areas. During this period, the patient may show a number of neurological symptoms, such as tremors of the tongue and eyelids and some mental dullness manifested as progressive apathy. From this point, neurological symptoms dominate the clinical picture along with increased apathy, loss of appetite, extended daytime sleeping, and concurrent involvement of the muscular system, progressing to paralysis. Classic symptoms are rapid weight loss due to anorexia, anemia induced by malnutrition, drowsiness, and, finally, irreversible coma.

Typically, diagnosis of the disease is a multistep procedure.

Step 1 is clinical assessment, especially when there are telltale neurological signs and/or mental dullness accompanied by enlarged and sensitive cervical lymph nodes (known as **Winterbottom's sign**). Step 2 is examination of blood smears, marrow, or cerebrospinal fluid for trypomastigotes. If results from steps 1 and 2 are inconclusive, step 3 is testing for specific antibodies in the blood. A complete history of the patient is also required for verification of contact with known tsetse fly habitats. It is estimated that this diagnostic regimen produces accurate results in more than 80% of cases.

Treatment

In his search for a successful trypanocidal agent, Paul Ehrlich, a pioneer in therapeutic research and immunology in the early twentieth century, developed a series of compounds such as trypan blue and trypan red. These compounds were used as chemotherapeutic agents for some time until it was discovered that their level of toxicity in humans was too great to justify their continued use. Suramin sodium, one of the current drugs of choice (see the following), evolved from these earlier agents. The research by Ehrlich, in spite of its failure at the time to produce a satisfactory drug for curing African sleeping sickness, proved that chemotherapeutic agents could be effective against disease-producing organisms; Ehrlich eventually succeeded in developing salvarsan, one of the first drugs to treat syphilis.

At the present time, therapeutic drugs are most effective against African sleeping sickness when treatment is initiated early in the course of the disease, prior to central nervous system involvement, since most effective agents do not pass the blood–brain barrier. Chemotherapy begun later becomes increasingly complex and has diminished effects. During the hemolymphatic stage, it is recommended that six intravenous injections of suramin sodium be administered over a 3-week interval. For the late, central nervous system stage, the arsenic-containing compound Melarsoprol is administered intravenously for several weeks. These two drugs, as well as a number of alternatives, can cause various toxic side effects. Severe reactions are rare, however, and the usually mild adverse effects are not sufficient to contraindicate treatment when weighed against the virulence of a disease that is almost invariably fatal when left untreated. In field tests in Africa, a new drug, difluoromethylornithine, has shown promise against *T. b. gambiense* infection during the late, central nervous system stage.

Physiology

The physiology of the long, slender trypomastigote found in the circulatory system of the vertebrate host differs from that of the epimastigote observed in the insect vector. Morphological changes related to metabolic characteristics occur in the mitochondrion of each form. For example, with its well-developed mitochondrion, the epimastigote synthesizes ATP through oxidative phosphorylation as well as glycolysis. A dearth of metabolizable substrates in the lumen of the insect gut dictates that the epimastigote must use an efficient system to synthesize energy-rich compounds. On the other hand, the long, slender trypomastigote, which lives in the organic cornucopia of the mammalian bloodstream, derives no selective advantage from substrate conservation; it obtains energy-rich compounds by the far less efficient system of substrate-level phosphorylation via glycolysis. Regardless of the morphological stage of the parasite, glycolysis occurs in specialized organelles called **glycosomes**. Reduced nicotinamide adenosine dinucleotide (NAD) is oxidized indirectly in the glycosome by an α-glycerophosphate oxidase system, part of which is localized in the mitochondrion.

AMERICAN TRYPANOSOMIASIS (*TRYPANOSOMA CRUZI*)

In 1909, the Brazilian physician and scientist Carlos Chagas found that thatched-roof huts in a small village in Brazil were infested with large, blood-sucking insects whose digestive tracts were laden with flagellates able to infect laboratory animals. Diseased children inhabiting these infested huts were found later to harbor the same flagellates. Today, this disease is recognized as an American form of trypanosomiasis caused by *Trypanosoma cruzi*. The disease is named Chagas' disease in recognition of its discoverer.

Life Cycle

The stage of *T. cruzi* infective to humans, the metacyclic trypomastigote, develops in the hindgut of the cone-nosed insect, or

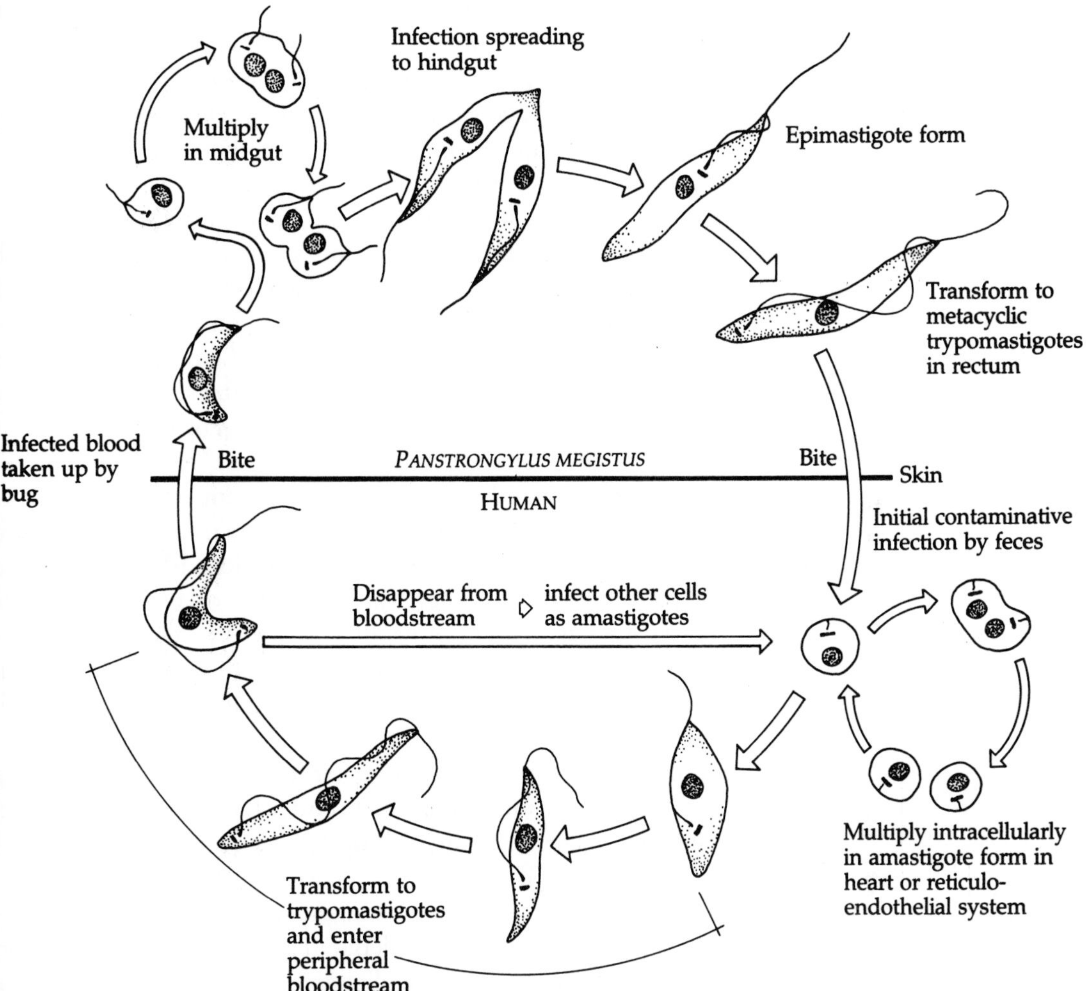

FIGURE 6-15
Life cycle of *Trypanosoma cruzi* in humans and in the insect *Panstrongylus (Triatoma) megistus.*

"kissing bug," *Panstrongylus megistus* (Fig. 6-15) and many related hemipteran insects. Because development to infectivity occurs in the hindgut rather than the salivary glands, *T. cruzi* is placed in the section Stercoraria. Metacyclic forms are passed with the feces of the bug, usually as it is taking a blood meal from a vertebrate host, and infection occurs when infected fecal material is rubbed into the bite wound, eyes, or mucous membranes.

Mammalian reservoir hosts may become infected by ingestion of infected insects or small mammals.

Upon entering the bloodstream of the vertebrate host, metacyclic trypomastigotes invade a variety of cells, including macrophages, and rapidly transform into the amastigote form. The amastigote evades the lysosome system by escaping from the parasitophorous vacuole into the cytosol of the infected cell. The organs most vulnerable to infection are the spleen, liver, lymph glands, and all types of muscle. When a cluster of amastigotes occurs in a cardiac muscle fiber, the aggregate is termed a **pseudocyst.** Other areas, such as the nervous and reproductive systems and bone marrow, may also be invaded. After repeated divisions, amastigotes may differentiate to trypomastigotes about 24 hours prior to cell rupture and parasite escape. The released trypomastigotes enter the circulatory system and may infect other cells. Unlike the African trypanosomes, the trypomastigote form of *T. cruzi* never reproduces in mammalian blood plasma. In chronic cases, since they appear unable to produce variable surface antigens and can be effectively destroyed by circulating antibodies, trypomastigotes of *T. cruzi* are rarely observed in the blood. Amastigotes in various host cells, on the other hand, are apparently protected thereby from antibody reactions. Trypomastigotes of *T. cruzi* also differ morphologically from those of African trypanosomes, being shorter (about 20 μm long) and showing a characteristic "U" or "C" shape in stained preparations (Fig. 6-16).

Insects become infected by ingesting blood containing trypomastigotes, which then undergo repeated longitudinal fission during passage through the digestive tract of the insect. By the time they reach the midgut, they have metamorphosed to the epimastigote stage. Still replicating, the epimastigotes pass into the hindgut, where they attach by their flagella to the epithelium of the rectal gland. As they transform to the metacyclic trypomastigote form, they lose flagellar–epithelial attachment. By the tenth day after ingestion, the infective metacyclic trypomastigotes appear free in the lumen of the rectum.

Epidemiology

Trypanosoma cruzi infection is prevalent throughout Latin America, affecting an estimated 24 million people, with approximately 100 million people at risk of contracting the infec-

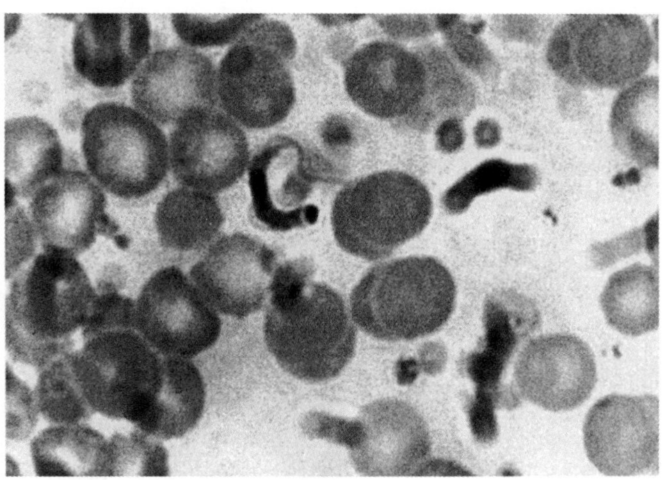

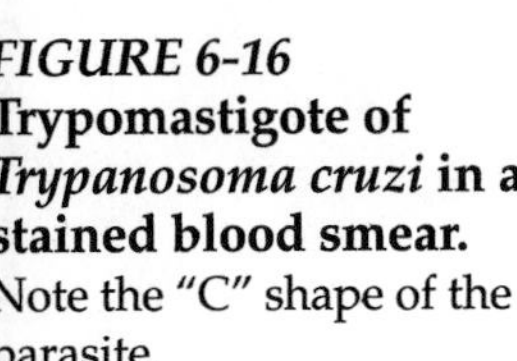

FIGURE 6-16
Trypomastigote of *Trypanosoma cruzi* in a stained blood smear.
Note the "C" shape of the parasite.

tion. The most common modes of acquiring *T. cruzi* infection are through the blood-sucking triatomine bug and blood transfusion. The incidence of infection is greatest in rural areas, especially among the poor, whose primitive living conditions facilitate bites by the insect vectors. American trypanosomiasis is a typical zoonotic disease that affects dogs, cats, bats, armadillos, rodents, and other mammalian reservoir hosts. Rodent infections also occur in the southwestern United States and in raccoons as far north as Maryland and Illinois. However, only a few cases of naturally acquired human infections have been reported in the United States, and those occurred only in Texas and California. Several explanations have been advanced to account for the dearth of human infection in the United States. One is that the insect vectors are **zoophilic**; that is, they prefer animal hosts to human hosts (the converse is **anthropophilic**). Another explanation is that defecation by northern insect vectors may not occur until well after a blood meal, thereby reducing the probability of infection.

Symptomatology and Diagnosis

Upon introduction into the human, the parasites invade macrophages of the subcutaneous tissue at the site of infection, causing a local, edematous swelling called a **chagoma**. In endemic areas, human patients often exhibit edematous patches over the body as the disease progresses; these patches occur most frequently on

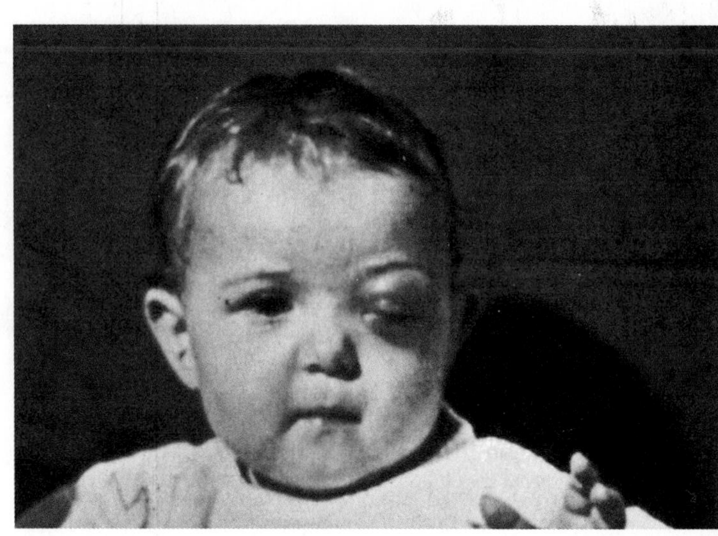

FIGURE 6-17
Romaña's sign.

one side of the face. This unilateral edema is often periorbital and associated with conjunctivitis, a syndrome known as **Romaña's sign** (Fig. 6-17). In early stages of the disease, parasites abound in infected tissues as well as in the circulating blood. As the infection becomes more chronic, the number of parasites in the circulation diminishes greatly, to the extent that they are almost impossible to find. Approximately 1–3 weeks after infection, fever, headaches, malaise, and prostration may develop. Enlargement of the liver and spleen as well as myocardial damage may follow, but cardiac involvement and gastrointestinal symptoms may not become apparent until many years after the primary infection.

Examination of fresh blood within the first month or two following infection may reveal *T. cruzi* trypomastigotes, particularly if the blood is drawn during a fever episode. Blood cultures may also yield incriminating organisms, and serological tests and clinical examinations sometimes provide accurate diagnosis. Direct agglutination tests with the IgM serum fraction are sensitive enough for diagnosis in the acute cases, when infectious organisms are scarce. Normally, however, antibodies do not develop until several months following initial infection, rendering other serological tests, such as complement fixation and immunofluorescence, impractical. A simple but practical method employed in public health surveys is **xenodiagnosis,** in which a laboratory-raised vector is allowed to feed on a suspected patient; the insect is dissected after 2–3 weeks and examined for intestinal flagellates.

Modern molecular technology as a diagnostic tool is in its infancy at this time. A **polymerase chain reaction** (PCR) technique has been developed, but because it is expensive and slow, it has not come into general use.

Treatment

Current lack of an effective chemotherapeutic agent makes treatment of Chagas' disease extremely difficult. A Bayer product, Nifurtimox, has shown promise in treating early chronic and acute cases. Once the protozoan invades host cells, it apparently is shielded from the action of any drug. Limited success against the bloodstream form has been achieved by treatment with the antimalarial drug primaquine phosphate. It is felt that, even though the intracellular amastigotes are shielded from drug activity, any reduction in the number of circulating infective trypomastigotes is beneficial in that it reduces the number of potential cell invaders.

Physiology

Trypanosoma cruzi differs physiologically from the African trypanosomes. For instance, the occurrence of well-developed mitochondrial cristae in all stages of the life cycle of *T. cruzi* suggests that there is little difference in oxygen metabolism in the various stages. Indeed, recent data indicate that oxygen consumption is the same in the intracellular amastigote, the bloodstream trypomastigote, and the insect stages. A complete glycolytic pathway has been reported in all stages, with glucose being the major carbohydrate. Also, at least some intermediates of a functional Krebs cycle have been reported in all stages. Of the glucose that is consumed, some is oxidized to carbon dioxide while some is incompletely oxidized to organic acids, such as succinic acid and acetic acid.

SELECTED READINGS

Alexander, J., and Russell, D. G. 1992. The interaction of *Leishmania* species with macrophages. *Advances in Parasitology* **31,** 176–254.

Barry, J. D. 1986. Surface antigens of African trypanosomes in the tsetse fly. *Parasitology Today* **2,** 143–145.

Bloom, B. R. 1979. Games parasites play: How parasites evade immun surveillance. *Nature* **279,** 21–26.

Donelson, J. E., and Turner, M. J. 1985. How the trypanosome change its coat. *Scientific American* **252,** 44–51.

Hide, G., Mattram, J. C., Coombs, G. H., and Holmes, P. H. (Eds.) 1997 *Trypanosomiasis and Leishmaniasis.* Oxford University Press, Ox ford, England.

Nantulya, V. M. 1986. Immunological approaches to the control of an imal trypanosomiasis. *Parasitology Today* **2,** 168–173.

Turner, M. J., and Donelson, J. E. 1990. Cell biology of African try panosomes. In *Modern Parasite Biology: Cellular, Immunologica and Molecular Aspects* (Wyler, D. J., Ed.) pp. 51–63. W. H. Freema & Company, New York.

Webster, B., and Russel, D. G. 1993. The flagellar pocket of trypano somatids. *Parasitology Today* **9,** 201–206.

Chapter Seven

BLOOD AND TISSUE PROTOZOA II: HUMAN MALARIA

The organisms that cause human malaria, babesiosis, toxoplasmosis, cryptosporidiosis, isosporiasis, cyclosporidiosis, and *Pneumocystis carinii* pneumonia belong to the phylum Apicomplexa. This taxonomic group was established to accommodate protozoans possessing structures known collectively as the **apical complex** (Fig. 7-1). This complex of organelles is found in the sporozoite and merozoite stages of the life cycles of these organisms. Immediately beneath the plasma membrane at the protozoan's anterior end are one or two electron-dense structures called **polar rings** (Fig. 7-1). In certain members of the suborder Eimeriina (including *Toxoplasma gondii*, the causative agent of toxoplasmosis), a truncated cone of spirally arranged fibrillar structures (the **conoid**) lies within the polar rings. The **rhoptries** (singular, rhoptry) are two or more electron-dense bodies located within the polar rings (and within the conoid, when present) and extending posteriorly from the plasma membrane.

Except in members of the genus *Babesia*, subpellicular microtubules radiate from the polar rings parallel to the long axis of the cell. These organelles probably serve as support elements and may facilitate the limited motility of these parasitic cells. A group of smaller, more convoluted structures, called **micronemes**, lies parallel to the rhoptries and appears to merge with them at the apex of the cell. The function of the rhoptries and micronemes has not been firmly established, but they appear to secrete proteins that probably alter the host cell's plasma membrane, facilitating the parasite's incorporation into the host cell.

Located at the lateral edges of the parasite are one or more **micropores**. These organelles are analogous to cytostomes as they seem to be the sites of endocytosis of nutrients during the intracellular life of the organism. At the edges of each micropore are two concentric, electron-dense rings, situated directly beneath the plasma membrane. Host cytoplasm is drawn through the microporal rings and into a food vacuole that pinches off from the plasma membrane; the vesicle is the site of intracellular digestion. Once a sporozoite or merozoite has been incorporated into a host cell and transformed into a trophozoite, all of its organelles ex-

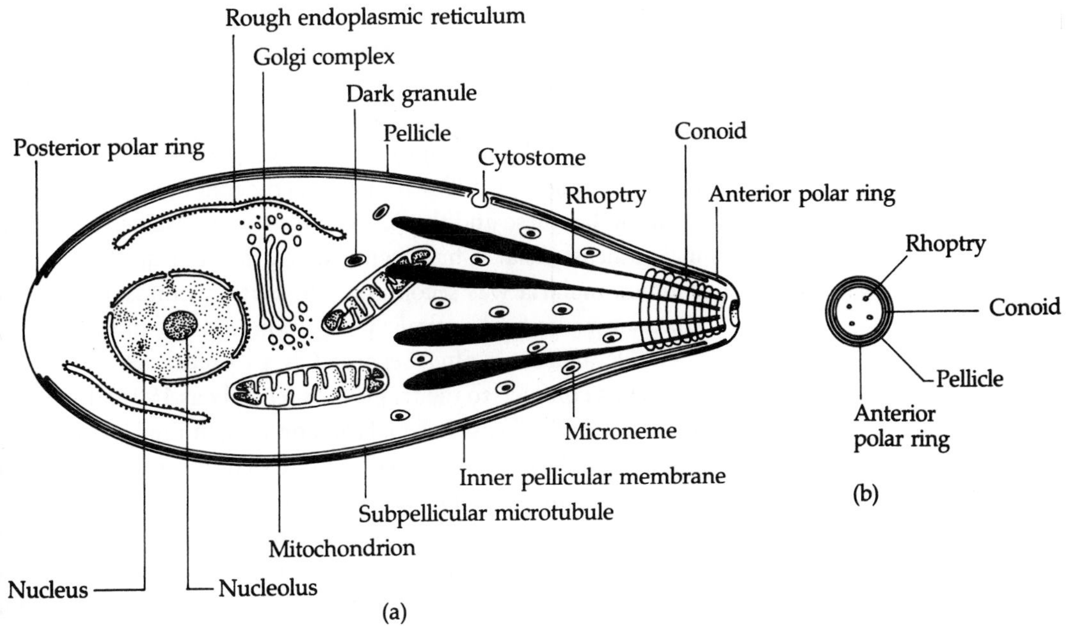

FIGURE 7-1
(a) Apicomplexan sporozoite or merozoite showing constituents of apical complex. (b) Cross section through anterior polar ring.

cept the micropores lose their physical integrity and disappear; the micropores persist through all succeeding stages.

PLASMODIUM AND HUMAN MALARIA

Malaria, one of the most prevalent and debilitating diseases afflicting humans, has played a major role in shaping history and civilizations. Its ravages probably contributed to the fall of the ancient Greek and Roman Empires. In medieval times, crusaders often fell victim to malaria during their expeditions, and probably more of their casualties can be attributed to the disease than to the "infidels" they fought. The manner in which malaria was introduced into the Western Hemisphere is uncertain. Writings from ancient civilizations, such as the Mayan, make no reference to any malaria-like diseases. It appears most likely that the Spanish conquistadors and their African slaves first brought the parasite to the New World. United States troops in both the American Civil War and the Spanish-American War were severely incapacitated by this disease; more than one-quarter of all persons admitted to hospitals during those conflicts were malaria patients. During World War II, malaria epidemics critically affected both the Japanese and the Allied forces in the Pacific Islands and in Southeast Asia. It has been claimed that during the Vietnam conflict, malaria was second only to battle wounds as the most common cause for hospitalization among American forces.

While malaria is often regarded as a tropical disease, it is by no means confined to the tropics. As recently as 1937, there were at least 1 million cases of malaria annually in the United States. The disease has been reported in more than 90 countries, inhabited by 2.4 billion people. However, more than 90% of all malaria cases are from 52 of the 58 countries in mostly sub-Saharan Africa, and two-thirds of the remaining cases are concentrated in India, Brazil, Sri Lanka, Vietnam, Colombia, and the Solomon Islands. At present, there are an estimated 300–500 million clinical cases each year, producing an annual death toll of 1.5–2.7 million. Although control programs sponsored by several cooperating nations and the World Health Organization of the United Nations have made great inroads in the fight against this disease, it obviously remains a major health problem in many parts of the world.

The more than fifty species of *Plasmodium* included in the suborder Haemosporina infect a wide variety of animals, but only four, *P. vivax*, *P. falciparum*, *P. malariae*, and *P. ovale*, commonly cause malaria in humans. Certain facets of the disease, such as the life cycle of the infective organism, chemotherapy, and epidemiology, are similar enough across species that the following discussion will make no distinction among the four species except where dissimilarities are medically significant.

LIFE CYCLE

Ronald Ross received the Nobel Prize in Medicine in 1902 for his studies on the life cycle of the malaria-producing organism. A number of other investigators, including Manson, Lavern, Bignami, and Grassi, made significant contributions. The entire life span of the four species of *Plasmodium* that infect humans is spent in two hosts: the insect vector, a female mosquito belonging to the genus *Anopheles*; and a human host (Fig. 7-2). Only female mosquitoes serve as vectors. The mouthparts of males cannot penetrate human skin; hence, males feed solely on plant juices. Females, on the other hand, also feed on blood, which is usually required for oviposition. A significant feature of the life cycle is the alternation of sexual and asexual phases in the two hosts. One asexual phase, termed **schizogony**, occurs in the human. The sexual phase, **gamogony**, occurs mainly in the mosquito as does a second asexual phase, termed **sporogony**. The infective form in humans is the slender, elongated **sporozoite**, about 10–55 μm in length and about 1 μm in diameter.

During feeding, the mosquito secretes sporozoite-bearing saliva beneath the epidermis of the human victim, thus inoculating the sporozoites into the bloodstream. After approximately one hour, the sporozoite disappears from the circulation, reemerging 24–48 hours later in the parenchymal cells of the liver, where the **exoerythrocytic schizogonic phase** begins. The specificity of the relationship between the sporozoite and hepatocytes rather than other cells is due, in part, to the recognition of the surface coat of the sporozoite (**circumsporozoite coat**) by receptors on the surface of the hepatocytes. Electron microscopy has confirmed that sporozoites and merozoites interact with the plasma membrane of the host cell and actively participate in their incorporation (Fig. 7-3). During this process, rhoptries and micronemes are believed to secrete surface-active molecules that cause the host-cell plasma membrane to expand and then invaginate forming a **parasitophorous vacuole** that envelops the parasite.

Once inside the hepatocyte, the sporozoite develops into a trophozoite, feeding on host cytoplasm with its now functional micropore. There is evidence that additional nutrients enter the trophozoite by pinocytosis. After 1–2 weeks (depending upon the species of *Plasmodium*), the nucleus of the trophozoite divides several times, followed by division of the cytoplasm. This multiple fission process produces thousands of merozoites, each approximately 2.5 μm in length and 1.5 μm in diameter. The merozoites erupt from the host cell, enter the blood circulation, and invade red blood cells, initiating the **erythrocytic schizogonic phase.** As with the engulfment of the sporozoite by the hepatocyte, the endocytosis of the merozoite into the red blood cell is dependent on surface recognition between the two cells. Studies of *P. vivax* show that the membrane receptor site for the invasion

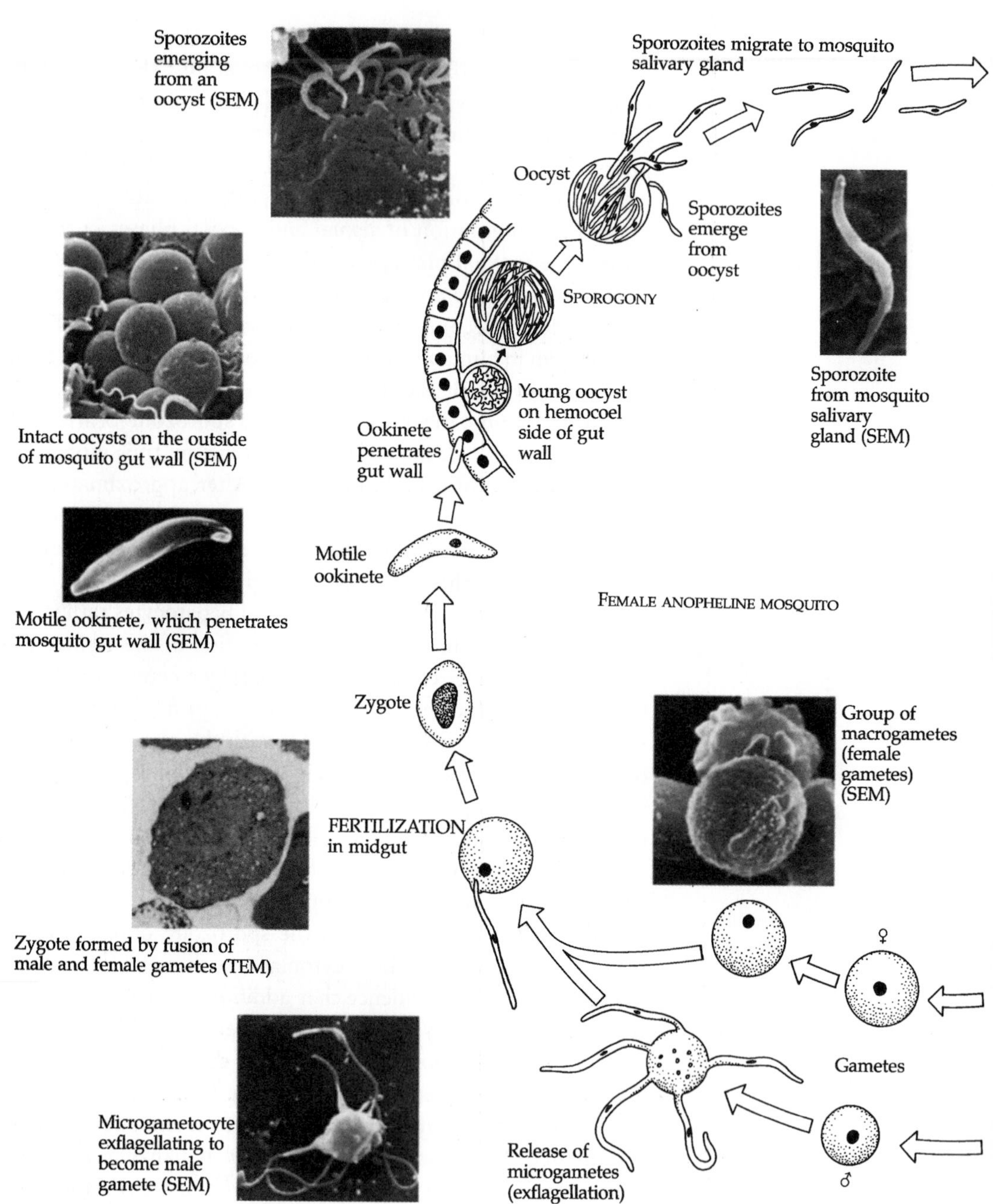
Sporozoites emerging from an oocyst (SEM)
Sporozoites migrate to mosquito salivary gland
Oocyst
Sporozoites emerge from oocyst
SPOROGONY
Intact oocysts on the outside of mosquito gut wall (SEM)
Young oocyst on hemocoel side of gut wall
Ookinete penetrates gut wall
Sporozoite from mosquito salivary gland (SEM)
Motile ookinete
Motile ookinete, which penetrates mosquito gut wall (SEM)
FEMALE ANOPHELINE MOSQUITO
Zygote
Group of macrogametes (female gametes) (SEM)
FERTILIZATION in midgut
Zygote formed by fusion of male and female gametes (TEM)
♀
Gametes
Microgametocyte exflagellating to become male gamete (SEM)
Release of microgametes (exflagellation)
♂

FIGURE 7-2
Life cycle of *Plasmodium* spp.

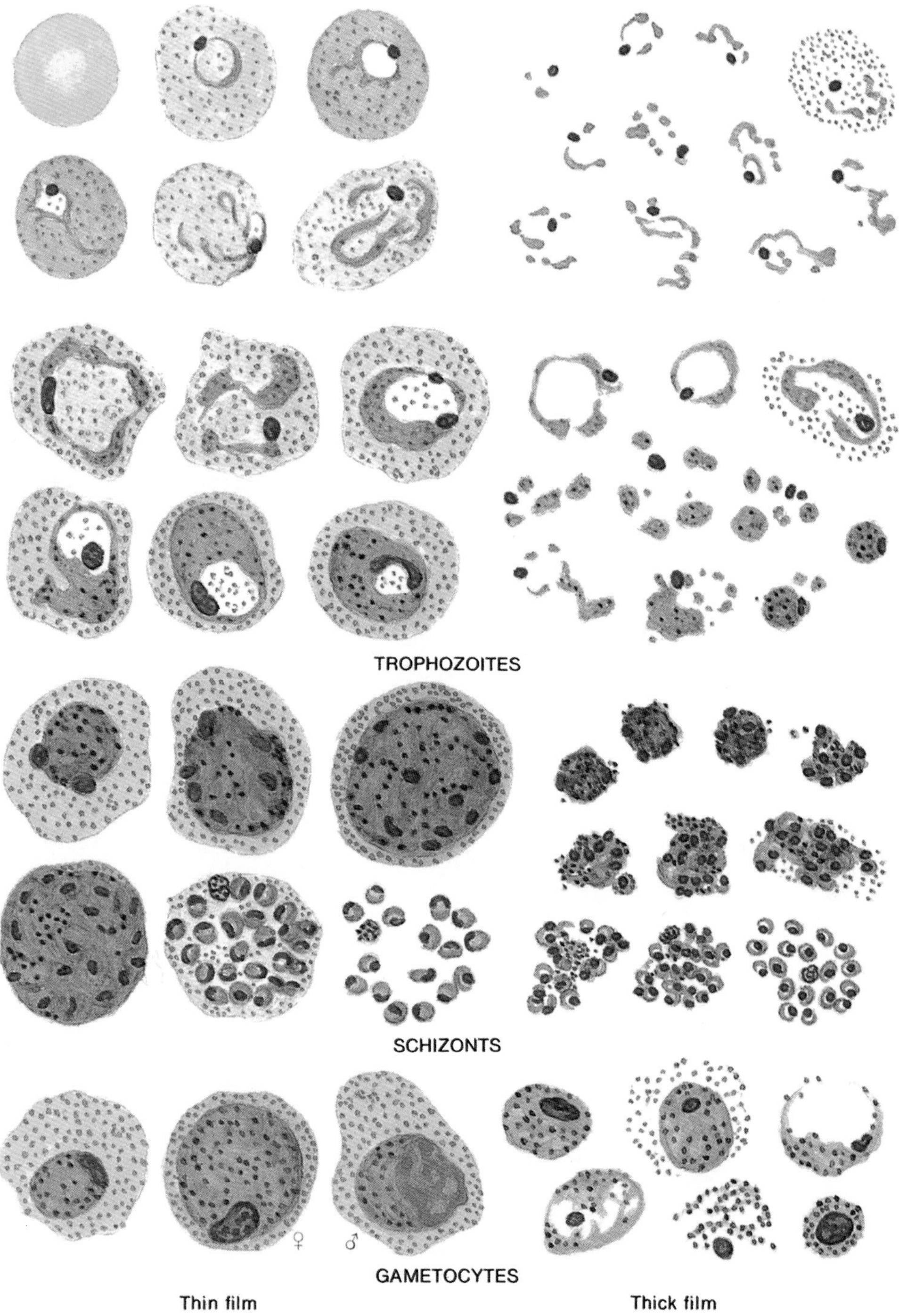

PLATE 1. Plasmodium vivax. Appearance of parasite stages in Giemsa-stained thin and thick blood films. See Chapter 7, page 137 for relevant discussion.

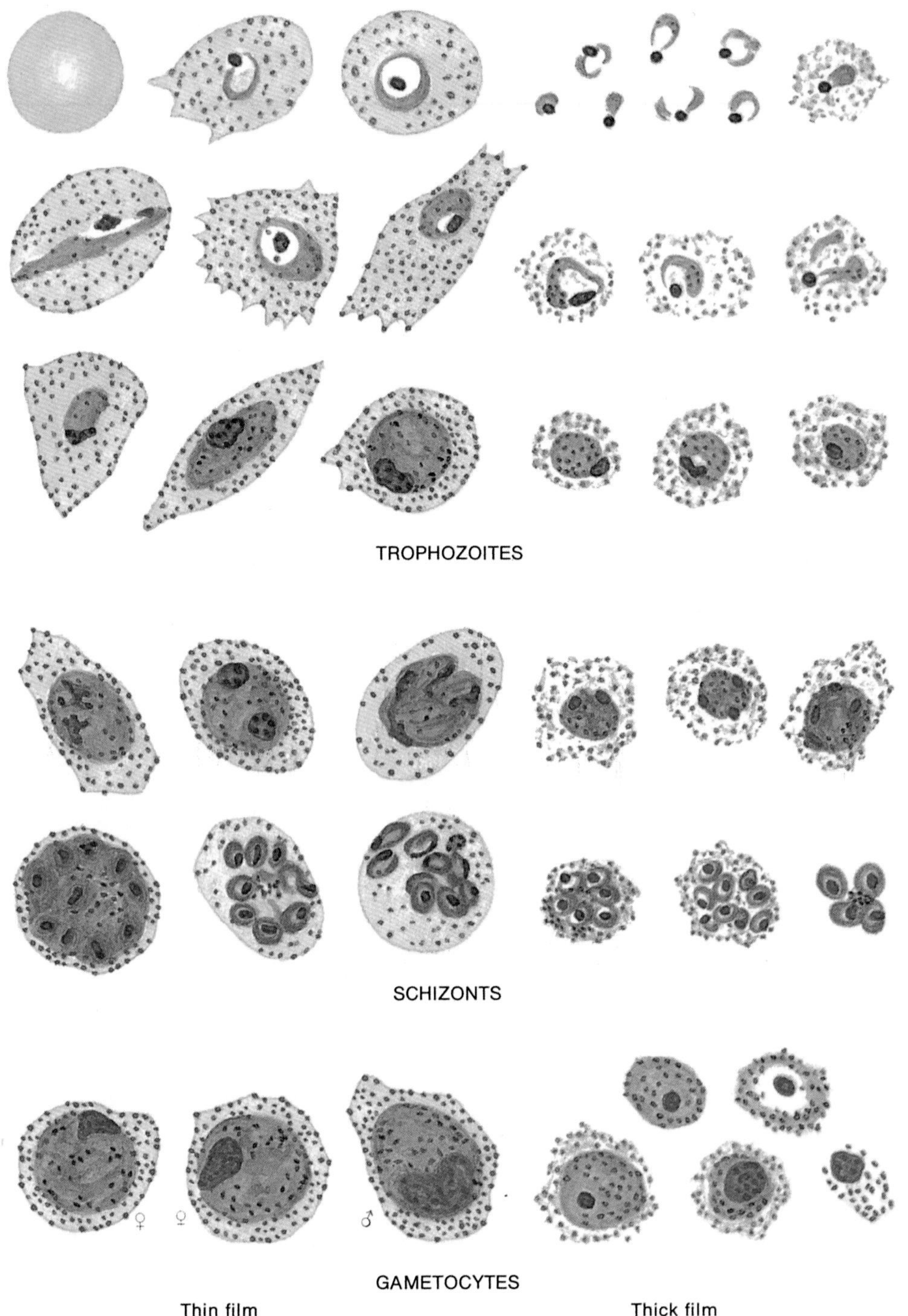

PLATE 2. ***Plasmodium ovale.*** Appearance of parasite stages in Giemsa-stained thin and thick blood films. See Chapter 7, page 137 for relevant discussion.

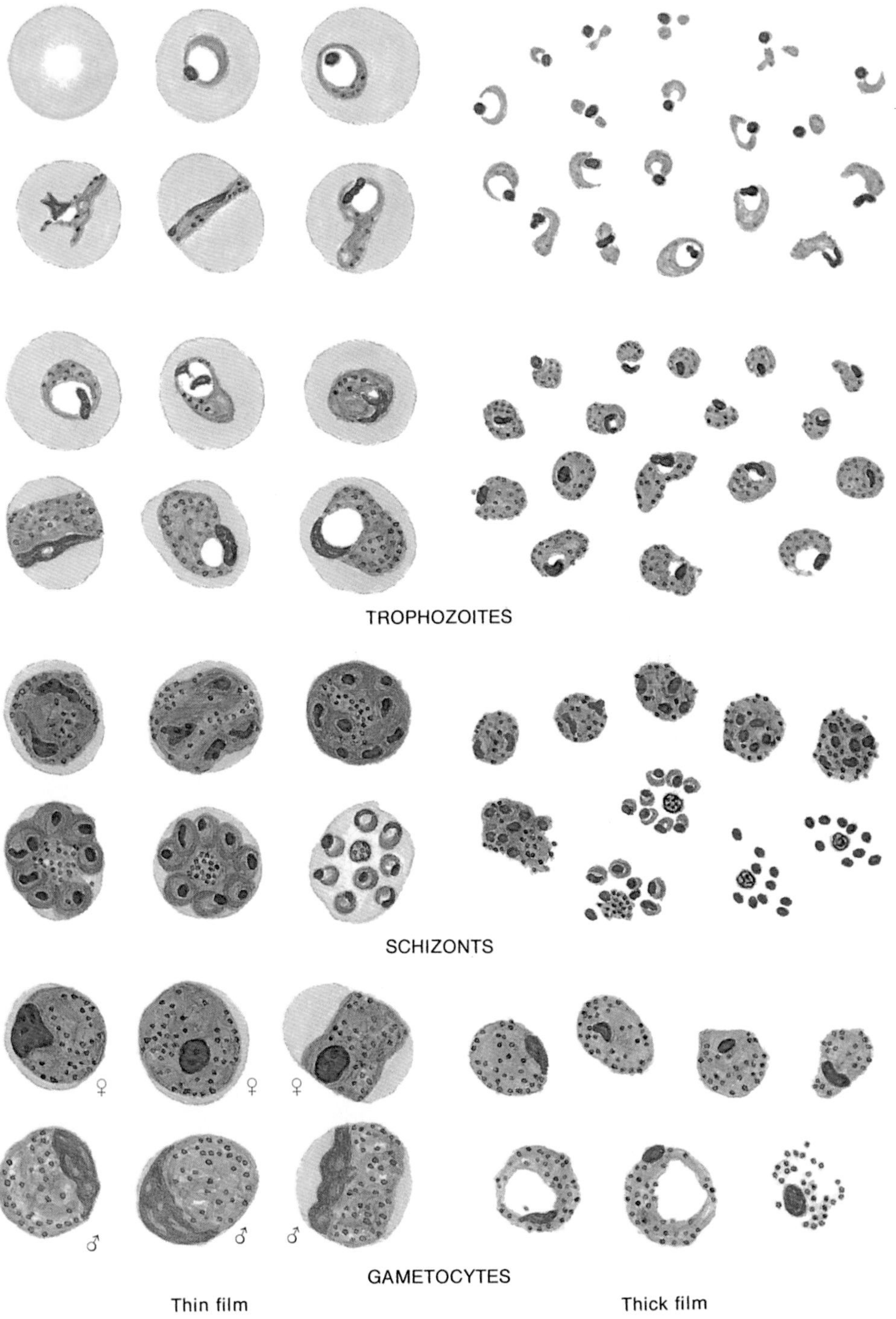

PLATE 3. Plasmodium malariae. Appearance of parasite stages in Giemsa-stained thin and thick blood films. See Chapter 7, page 139 for relevant discussion.

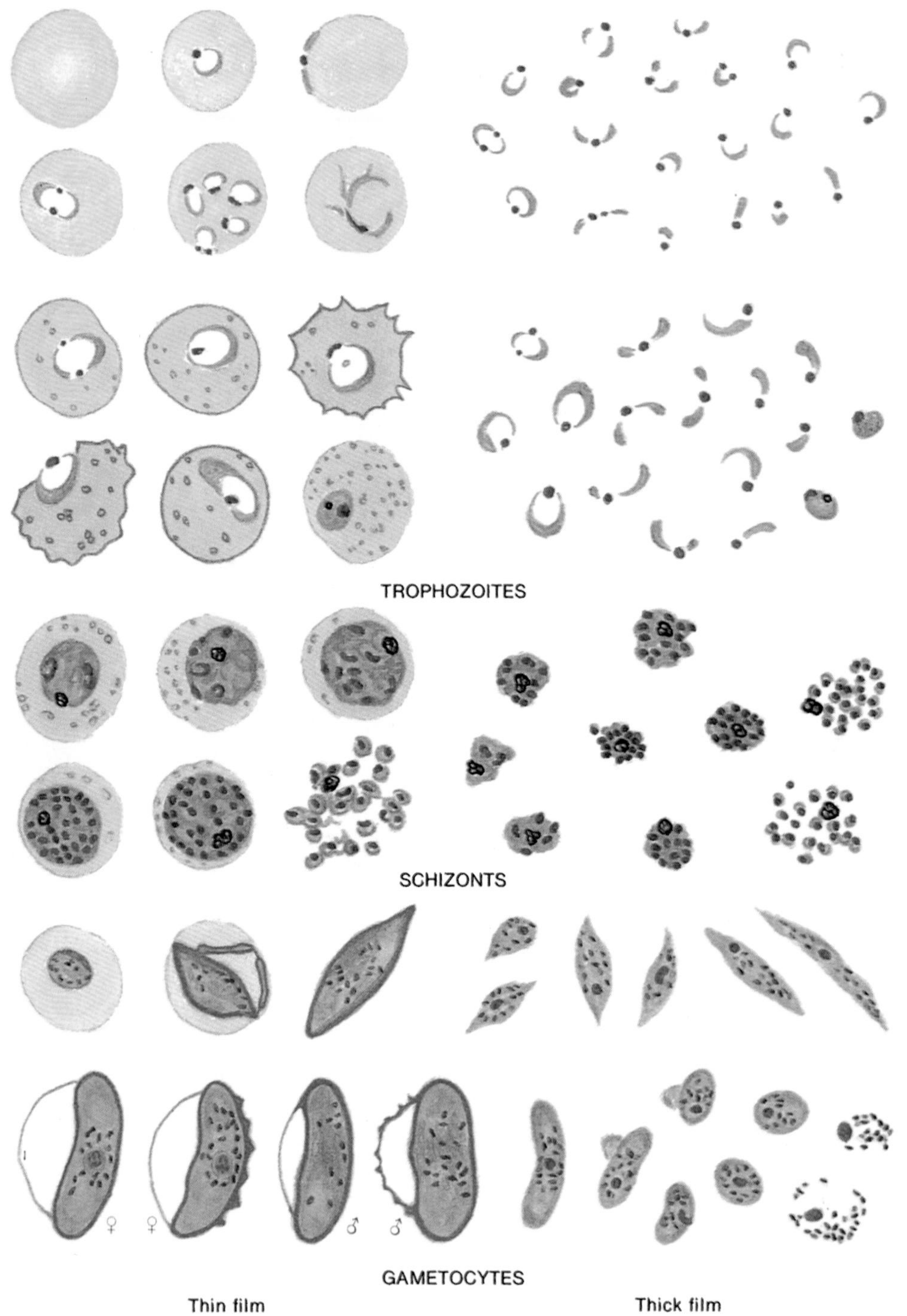

PLATE 4. ***Plasmodium falciparum.*** Appearance of parasite stages in Giemsa-stained thin and thick blood films. See Chapter 7, page 139 for relevant discussion.

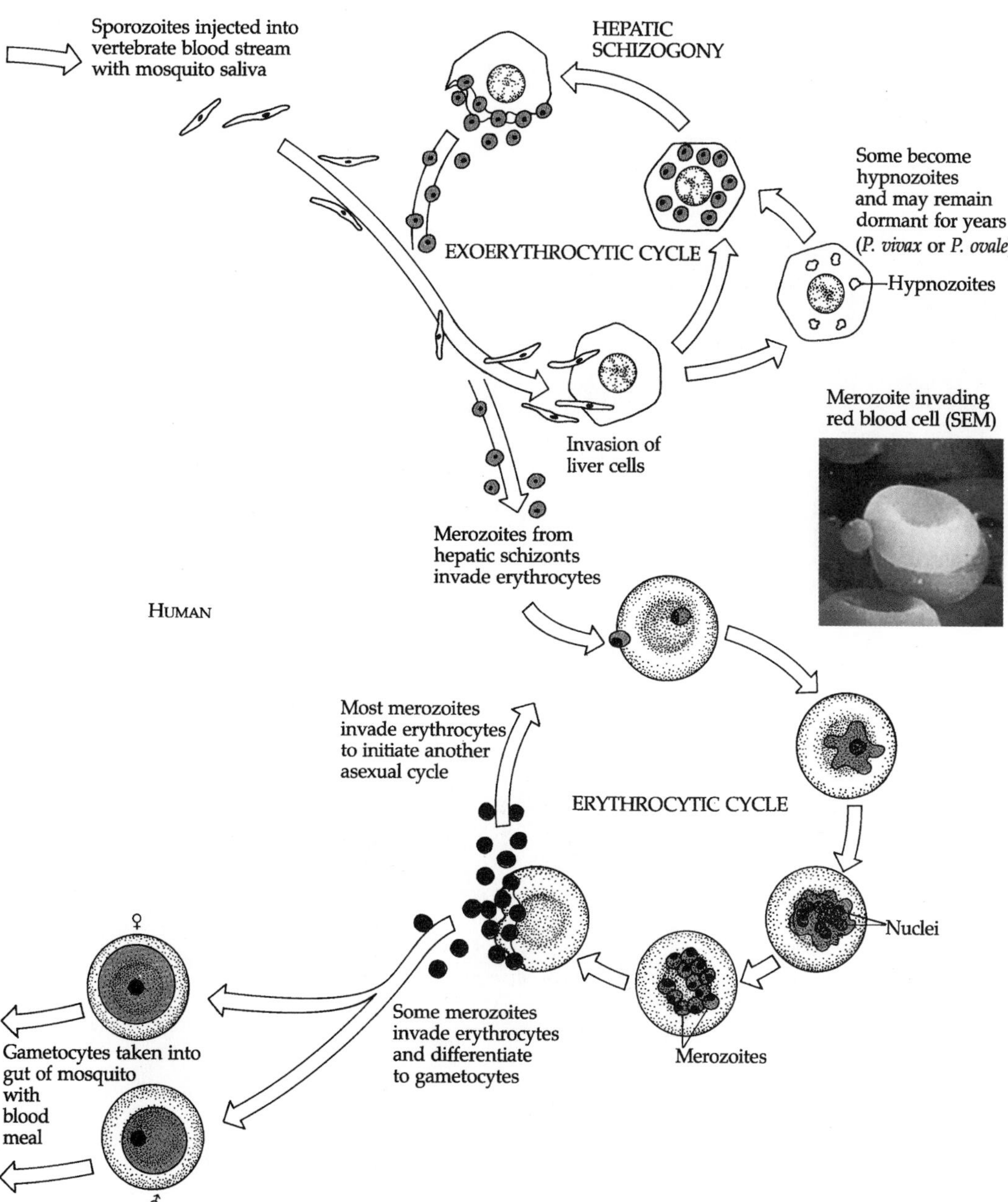
Sporozoites injected into vertebrate blood stream with mosquito saliva
HEPATIC SCHIZOGONY
Some become hypnozoites and may remain dormant for years (P. vivax or P. ovale)
EXOERYTHROCYTIC CYCLE
Hypnozoites
Invasion of liver cells
Merozoite invading red blood cell (SEM)
Merozoites from hepatic schizonts invade erythrocytes
HUMAN
Most merozoites invade erythrocytes to initiate another asexual cycle
ERYTHROCYTIC CYCLE
Nuclei
♀
Gametocytes taken into gut of mosquito with blood meal
Some merozoites invade erythrocytes and differentiate to gametocytes
Merozoites
♂

FIGURE 7-2
Continued.

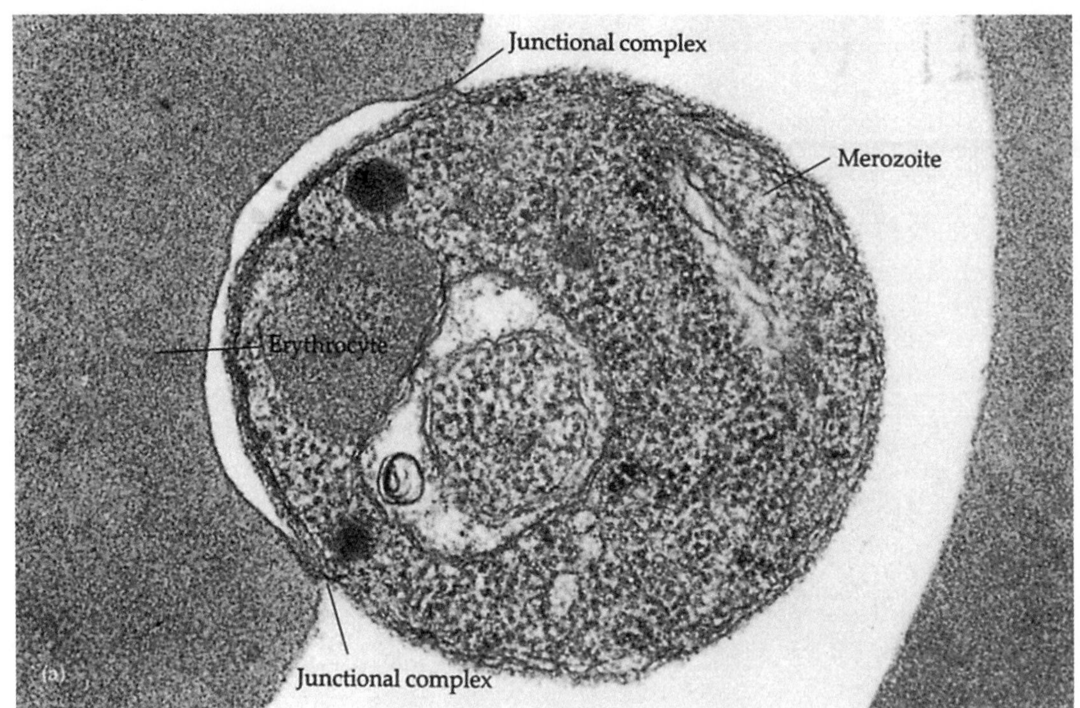

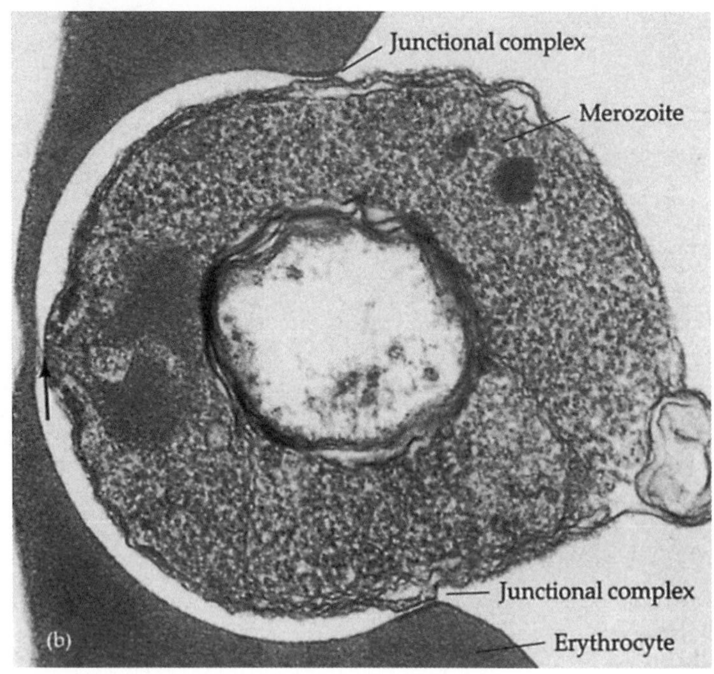

FIGURE 7-3

(a) Merozoite entering erythrocyte.

Note the junctional complexes at each side of entry.

(b) Merozoite further along in penetrating erythrocyte.

The arrow points to a projection connecting the merozoite's apical end and the erythrocyte membrane. Again, note the junctional complexes.

phenomenon is determined by the type of antigen present on the surface of the red blood cell. For instance, merozoite engulfment requires at least one of two Duffy antigens (Fy^{a+} or Fy^{b+}). Humans lacking the Duffy antigens, including practically all West Africans and approximately 70% of American blacks, are resistant to vivax malaria. *Plasmodium falciparum* and *P. malariae* malarias, on the other hand, are not influenced by Duffy antigens, thus accounting for their prevalence in West Africa.

Inside the erythrocyte, the merozoite grows to the early trophozoite stage. Under light microscopy, the early trophozoite appears to consist of a ring of cytoplasm and a dotlike nucleus. Due to its resemblance to a finger ring, this stage is called the **signet ring stage**. In reality, the ring stage trophozoite is cup-shaped; it has a large vacuole filled with host hemoglobin in varying stages of digestion (Fig. 7-4). This early form develops to the mature trophozoite stage and then undergoes multiple fission into schizonts, producing a characteristic number of a new generation of merozoites in each infected erythrocyte. As in the liver, each of these merozoites is capable of infecting a new erythrocyte. One of two fates awaits this new penetrant; it may become another signet ring trophozoite and begin schizogony anew, or it may become a male **microgametocyte** or a female **macrogametocyte**. What determines which course these parasites take has not yet been identified.

The sexual phase occurs in the female *Anopheles* and begins when the mosquito takes a blood meal that contains macrogametocytes and microgametocytes. These stages are unaffected by the digestive juices of the insect. Lysis of the surrounding erythrocytic material releases gametocytes into the lumen of the stomach. There, microgametocytes undergo a maturation process known as **exflagellation**, during which the nucleus undergoes three mitotic divisions, producing 6–8 nuclei that migrate to the periphery of the gametocyte. Accompanying the nuclear divisions are centriolar divisions; one centriolar portion joins each nuclear segment to become a basal body, providing the center from which the axoneme subsequently arises. Almost simultaneously, the nucleus, axoneme, and a small amount of adhering cytoplasm form a **microgamete**, which detaches from the mass and swims to the macrogametocyte. During this period, the macrogametocyte develops into a female **macrogamete** and forms a membrane-derived fertilization cone, which is penetrated by the microgamete.

The fusion of male and female pronuclei (**syngamy**) produces

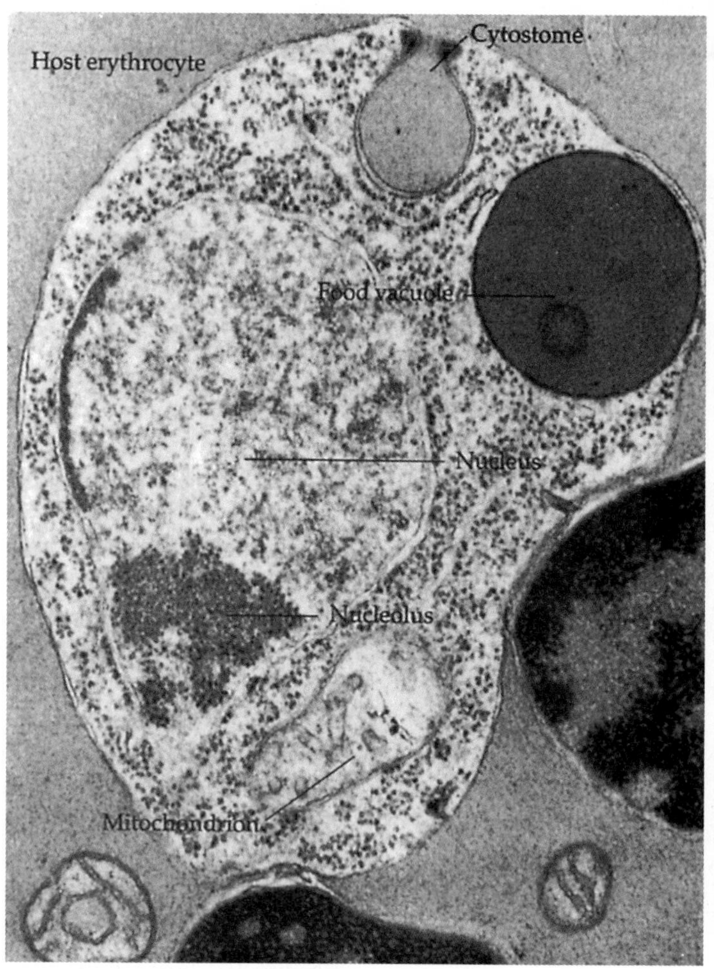

FIGURE 7-4
An erythrocytic trophozoite of *Plasmodium gallinaceum* showing host cell hemoglobin being ingested at cytostome site.
The bulge is prominently limited by a double membrane, whereas the food vacuole near the cytostome is limited by a single membrane. The content of the food vacuole is dark compared to the host cell contents, indicating that digestion is taking place. A mitochondrion, endoplasmic reticulum, ribosomes, and a large nucleus with a nucleolus are also present in the parasite. (×22,500)

a diploid zygote that, after 12–24 hours, elongates into a motile, microscopic, wormlike **ookinete**. The ookinete penetrates the gut wall of the mosquito to the area between the epithelium and basal lamina, where it develops into a rounded **oocyst**. Formation of the oocyst occurs approximately 40 hours after the mosquito has taken its blood meal. The oocyst then grows to 4–5 times its original diameter, appearing as a bulge on the hemocoel side of the gut. Growth of the oocyst is due, in part, to the proliferation of haploid cells, called **sporoblasts**, within the oocyst. Sporoblast nuclei undergo numerous divisions, producing thousands of sporozoites enclosed within the sporoblast membranes. As the membranes rupture, sporozoites enter the cavity of the oocyst.

Within 10–24 days after the mosquito ingests the gametocytes, the sporozoite-filled oocysts themselves rupture, releasing the sporozoites into the hemocoel. The sporozoites are carried to the salivary gland ducts of the insect and are then ready to be injected into the next person from whom the mosquito draws a blood meal.

LIFE CYCLE VARIATIONS

While the life cycles of the various species of *Plasmodium* that infect humans are basically similar, there are a number of differences, some of which are important in clinical diagnosis. These differences are summarized in Table 7-1.

Plasmodium vivax and Plasmodium ovale (Benign Tertian Malaria)

Plasmodium vivax was first described by Grassi and Feletti in 1890 and is the most common species of the genus in the Americas. *Plasmodium ovale* was first described by Stephens in 1922 (see Color Plates 1 and 2). Both species have a predilection for immature erythrocytes (reticulocytes). Less than 1% of the total erythrocyte population in each victim is parasitized by *P. vivax* or *P. ovale*. A diagnostically significant characteristic is the larger size of these infected erythrocytes, probably due to a preferential invasion of relatively larger reticulocytes by the parasite. This enlargement of infected cells is less pronounced in ovale malaria than in vivax infections. Cells infected with *P. ovale* also tend to be somewhat ellipsoid in shape. In all *Plasmodium*-infected erythrocytes, two types of granules are found. One type (**Schuffner's dots** in *P. vivax* and *P. ovale*) is distributed throughout the cytoplasm of the erythrocyte and usually stains pink or red when subjected to traditional hematological stains, such as Giemsa's, Wright's, or Romanovsky's. Electron microscope studies indicate that such pigmented granules are small surface invaginations surrounded by small vesicles. The source of these granules in infected cells is uncertain; they may be products of degenerative changes in the infected erythrocyte. The second type is the coarser, dark **hemozoin** granules, the by-products of hemoglobin degradation by the parasite. Hemozoin is usually found more closely associated with the parasite than with erythrocytic cytoplasm.

The cytoplasm of the trophozoite stages is very irregular and displays active amoeboid movement, which is the basis of the

TABLE 7-1
Diagnostic Differences among the Four Species of Human-Infecting *Plasmodium*

	Plasmodium vivax	***Plasmodium malariae***	***Plasmodium ovale***	***Plasmodium falciparum***
Duration of schizogony	48 hours	72 hours	49–50 hours	36–48 hours
Motility	Active amoeboid until about half grown	Trophozoite slightly amoeboid	Trophozoite slightly amoeboid	Trophozoite active amoeboid
Pigment (hematin)	Yellowish-brown; fine granules and minute rods	Dark brown to black; coarse granules	Dark brown; coarse granules	Dark brown; coarse granules
Stages found in peripheral blood	Trophozoites, schizonts, gametocytes	Trophozoites, schizonts, gametocytes	Trophozoites, schizonts, gametocytes	Trophozoites, gametocytes
Multiple infection in erythrocyte	Common	Very rare	Rare	Very common
Appearance of infected erythrocyte	Greatly enlarged; pale with red Schüffner's dots	Not enlarged; normal appearance with Ziemann's dots	Slightly enlarged; outline oval to irregular, with Schüffner's dots	Normal size; greenish; basophilic Maurer's clefts and dots
Trophozoites (ring forms)	Amoeboid; small and large rings with vacuole and usually one chromatin dot	Small and large rings with vacuole and usually one chromatin dot; also young band forms	Amoeboid; small and large rings with vacuole	Very small and large rings with vacuole, commonly with two chromatin dots; amoeboid
Segmented schizonts	Fills enlarged RBC; 12–24 merozoites irregularly arranged around mass of pigment	Almost fills normal-sized RBC; 6–12 merozoites regularly arranged around central pigment mass	Fills approx. ¾ of RBC; 6–12 merozoites around centric or eccentric pigment mass	Not usually seen in peripheral blood
Gametocytes	Round; fills RBC; chromatin undistributed in cytoplasm	Round; fills RBC; chromatin undistributed in cytoplasm	Round; fills ¾ of RBC; chromatin undistributed in cytoplasm	Crescentic- or kidney-shaped; chromatin undistributed in cytoplasm

species name, *P. vivax* (from Latin meaning "vigorous"). During schizogony, 12–24 (average, 16) merozoites are produced, each measuring about 1.5 μm in diameter. These rupture from the infected erythrocyte synchronously at 48-hour intervals, with accompanying fever. The designation *tertian* is derived from the ancient Roman custom of counting the days of an event in sequence; therefore, the first day of the fever peak is designated "day one," the intervening day is "day 2," and the day of the next fever episode is "day three." In vivax malaria, the time interval between peaks is only 48 hours, so "day three" then becomes "day one" when counting the next interval.

Gametocytes begin to appear in approximately 4 days. Macrogametocytes, which outnumber their somewhat smaller male counterparts about two to one, measure about 10 μm in diameter, each almost completely filling the infected erythrocyte.

Plasmodium malariae (Quartan Malaria)

Plasmodium malariae, the first parasite to be recognized as a cause of malaria, was described in 1880 by a French army physician, Charles Louis Alphonse Laveran (see Color Plate 3). While *P. vivax* and *P. ovale* selectively parasitize young cells, *P. malariae* shows an affinity for older cells, parasitizing about 0.2% of the victim's total erythrocyte population.

Following incorporation into erythrocytes, early trophozoites begin to accumulate hemozoin and the pink-staining **Ziemann's dots**. The cytoplasm of the trophozoite is compact, often appearing as a band across the infected cell. Morphologically, mature trophozoites resemble macrogametocytes and are, therefore, difficult to distinguish. No change in diameter is evident in the infected erythrocyte, probably due to the parasite's affinity for older erythrocytes.

Following schizogony, the number of merozoites varies from 6 to 12 (average, 8). Hemozoin usually accumulates as a dense mass in the center of the schizont. Merozoites rupture from the infected cell synchronously every 72 hours with an accompanying fever paroxysm (quartan malaria). Recrudescence (see pp. 142–144) has been reported as long as 53 years after initial infection.

Plasmodium falciparum (Malignant Tertian Malaria)

Plasmodium falciparum is responsible for 80% of cases of human malaria worldwide and is deeply entrenched in tropical

Africa (see Color Plate 4). Examination of blood smears of infected patients, originally described by William Welch in 1897, shows that *P. falciparum* differs significantly from the preceding three species. Typically, only ring trophozoites and gametocytes are seen in the peripheral circulation, the later stages of schizogony being trapped in capillaries of muscle and visceral organs. The plasma membranes of infected erythrocytes undergo an alteration that causes them to adhere to the walls of capillaries. Infected erythrocytes are not enlarged and represent about 10% of the total erythrocyte population. *P. falciparum* infects erythrocytes of any age indiscriminately. Multiple infections of single erythrocytes are common, and the presence of more than one ring trophozoite in a cell is not unusual. Double nuclei also occur frequently in the ring stage. The schizonts, rarely seen in peripheral blood, produce 8–32 (average, 20) merozoites. Rupture of merozoites from infected erythrocytes is erratic, with accompanying fever paroxysms occurring at intervals of 48–72 hours. Gametocytes are elongated or crescent-shaped cells that stretch the erythrocyte but remain inside it. Macrogametocytes are slightly longer than microgametocytes, the two measuring 12–14 and 9–11 μm long, respectively. Pigment granules characteristic of *P. falciparum*-infected erythrocytes, **Maurer's dots** or **clefts**, tend to aggregate around the nuclear region of gametocytes, as does hemozoin.

EPIDEMIOLOGY

Endemicity of human malaria is usually determined by the geographic distribution of its arthropod vector, an anopheline mosquito. Areas where the vector is not present, including Hawaii, many southeastern Pacific islands, and New Zealand, are free of the disease (Fig. 7-5a).

Local environmental factors determine which particular species of mosquito transmits malaria in a given area; therefore, local epidemiological surveys are used to assay the prevalent transmitters. Precipitin tests of ingested blood from infected mosquitoes reveal whether the vectors have zoophilic or anthropophilic feeding preferences.

Statistical computation of the average number of bites per person per night yields the **critical density**. A continuously declining critical density indicates that malaria in a survey area is waning and may eventually disappear. An accurate critical density assessment must include not only the number of mosquitoes and their feeding preferences, but also the frequency of feeding and the life expectancy of the mosquito species.

Critical density is influenced by environmental factors that affect breeding and/or sporogony. These functions require temperatures between 16 and 34°C and a relative humidity in excess of 60%. Water dependency for breeding varies greatly; some species of *Anopheles* favor small bodies of water, others require large bodies of water such as ponds and even lakes, and still others have intermediate requirements. Females' feeding habits also vary, even as to whether an indoor (**endophilic**) or outdoor (**exophilic**) locale is preferred. Mosquito populations in areas of low critical density produce a pattern of **stable malaria**, a universal low-grade infection with few, if any, disease symptoms. The immunity level in the human population is unaffected by environmental and climatic changes. On the other hand, mosquito populations displaying a high critical density are associated with **unstable malaria**. The disease pattern in such areas is noticeably affected by drastic environmental or climatic changes. Incidence is usually transient, and periods of high mortality alternate with periods of declining mortality as optimal conditions subside. Because there is insufficient time for immunity to become established under such circumstances, a pattern of recurring epidemics develops.

Although the areas affected by malaria have diminished over the past 50 years, control is becoming progressively more difficult, and earlier gains are being eroded. Under the auspices of the World Health Organization (WHO), malaria was either under control or drastically diminished in many parts of the world by the 1960s due primarily to the availability of antimalarial drugs, the use of screens on houses to keep out mosquitoes, the proper use of insecticides, the elimination of mosquito breeding sites, mosquito eradication, and other environmental measures. However, there has been a marked resurgence in the disease since the 1970s. Several elements have contributed to this resurgence, most important of which are the development of widespread resistance by anopheline mosquitoes to insecticides and the evolution of chloroquine-resistant *P. falciparum*. Another contributing element is the reduction in the number of personnel trained to maintain the WHO-established standards for control. Increased prevalence of malaria is also linked to activities such as road-building, mining, logging, and the introduction of new agricultural and irrigation projects in many third world countries. Wars, which have caused disintegration of health services and mass

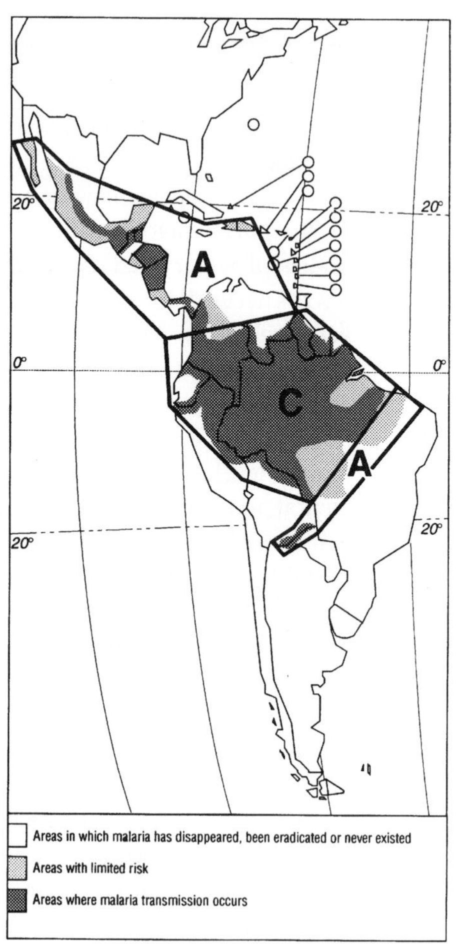

FIGURE 7-5
Malaria: global distribution suggested prophylaxis.

movements of refugees from malarial zones, have also contributed to the upsurge.

RELAPSE AND RECRUDESCENCE

It has long been known that victims of vivax or ovale malarias may suffer relapse after apparent recovery. Originally, such relapse was thought to be due to populations of cryptozoites entering the exoerythrocytic cycle. While one population progressed to the usual erythrocytic phase, underwent schizogony, and released merozoites into the circulating blood causing malaria, the other population was thought to maintain an ongoing exoery-

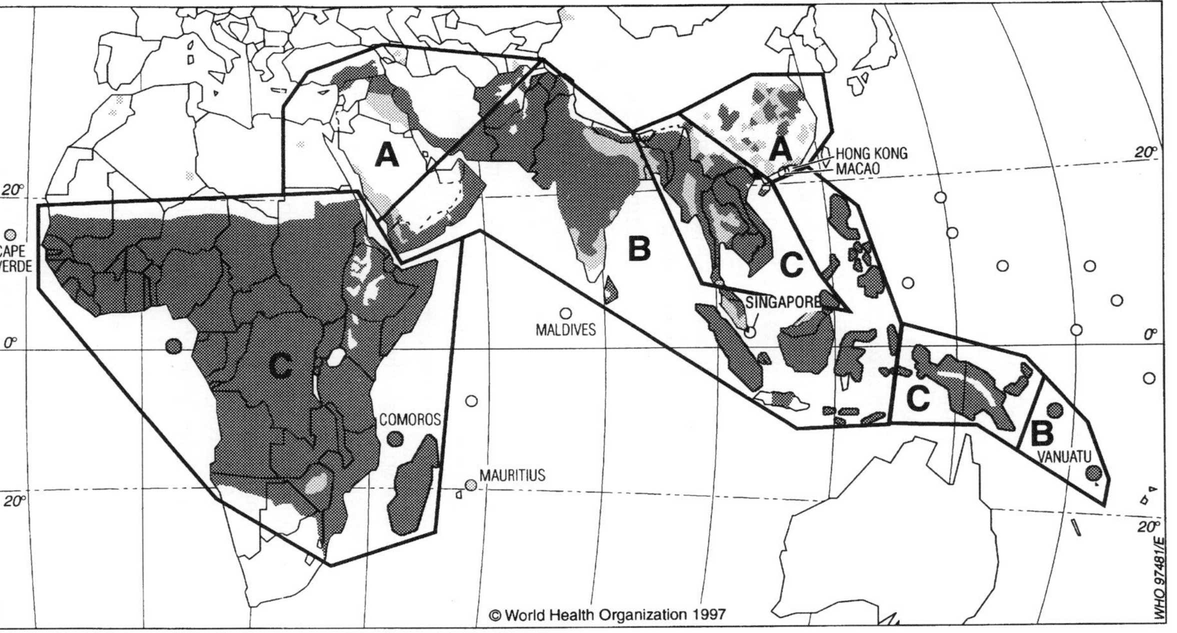

Zone	Characteristics (for details by country, see yellow pages)	Recommendations concerning prophylaxis (see Table 2 for dosages/regimens; see Table 3 for contraindications; see Box 5.3 for prophylaxis of pregnant women; see Tables 4 and 5 for stand-by emergency treatment)	
A	Risk generally low and seasonal; no risk in many areas (for example urban areas). *P. falciparum* absent or sensitive to chloroquine.	**prophylaxis:** chloroquine *or:* (in case of very low risk) no prophylaxis	Protection from mosquito bites should be the rule in all situations, even when prophylaxis is taken
B	Low risk in most areas. Chloroquine alone will protect against *P. vivax*. Chloroquine with proguanil will give some protection against *P. falciparum* and may alleviate the disease if it occurs despite prophylaxis.	**prophylaxis:** chloroquine + proguanil *or:* (in case of very low risk) no prophylaxis	
C	Risk high in most areas of this zone in Africa, except in some high-altitude areas. Risk low in most areas of this zone in Asia and America, but high in parts of the Amazon basin (colonization and mining areas). Resistance to sulfadoxine-pyrimethamine common in zone C in Asia, variable in zone C in Africa and America.	**prophylaxis:** first choice – mefloquine second choice – chloroquine + proguanil border areas Cambodia/Myanmar/Thailand – doxycycline } for details, see yellow pages *or:* (in case of very low risk) no prophylaxis	

FIGURE 7-5
Continued.

throcytic cycle known as a para-erythrocytic cycle. It was believed that parasites in the hepatic stages of the cycle remained protected from host antibodies until activated by some physiological change within the host that allowed them to erupt from the hepatocytes, precipitating another bout of malaria.

Now, it is recognized that there are two different populations of sporozoites. **Short prepatent sporozoites** (**SPP**s), upon entering the human host, undergo the usual exoerythrocytic phases of development and cause malaria. **Long prepatent sporozoites** (**LPP**s) or **hypnozoites**, remain dormant in the hepatocytes for an indefinite period. When a stimulus, such as the physiological fluctuation cited previously, activates hypnozoites into the exoerythrocytic and erythrocytic cycles, relapse occurs. The ratio of LPPs to SPPs in *P. vivax* infections in a given human population appears to vary according to strain. For instance, in a North Korean strain found in temperate zones, LPP sporozoites are far more numerous than SPP sporozoites. On the other hand, in strains common to tropical regions, the relative proportions are equal or sometimes reversed.

The recurrence of malaria among victims infected by *P. malariae* many years after apparent cure fostered an enduring belief that this species produced relapses like those produced by *P. vivax* and *P. ovale*. However, it has been shown that the periodic increase in numbers of parasites results from a residual population persisting at very low levels in the blood after inadequate or incomplete treatment of the initial infection. The number of parasites is usually so small that infected individuals remain symptomless. This situation has been known to persist for as long as 53 years before something, such as splenic dysfunction, triggers a parasite population explosion with accompanying disease manifestations, a phenomenon termed **recrudescence**. The difference, therefore, between relapse and recrudescence is that the former results from the activation of hypnozoites into exoerythrocytic stages in the liver, while the latter is due to a sudden increase in what was a persistent, low-level parasite population in the blood.

SYMPTOMATOLOGY AND DIAGNOSIS

Pathology in human malaria is generally manifested in two basic forms: host inflammatory reactions and anemia. Of the four species of *Plasmodium* responsible for human malaria, *P. falciparum* is the most virulent and causes by far the highest mortality.

The initial symptoms of malaria, such as nausea, fatigue, a

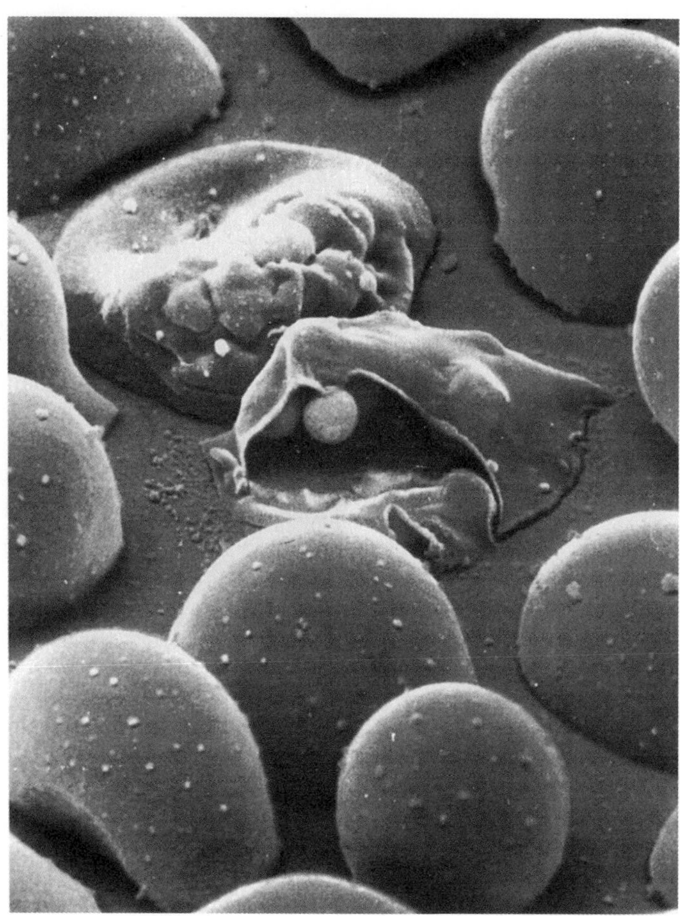

FIGURE 7-6
Scanning electron micrograph of *Plasmodium*-infected red blood cells.
One cell has burst open, releasing merozoites.

slight rise in temperature, mild diarrhea, and muscular pains, are often mistaken for influenza or gastrointestinal infection. Host inflammatory reactions are triggered by the periodic rupture of infected erythrocytes, which releases hemozoin and other malarial pigments, cellular debris, and parasite metabolic wastes into the circulatory system (Fig. 7-6). These ruptures are accompanied by fever paroxysms that are usually synchronous except during the primary attack. As explained earlier, the interval between paroxysms is species-specific. Synchrony may not be evident during the primary attack, however, since the infection may arise from several populations of liver merozoites at different stages of development. The mechanism by which the synchronous pattern gradually emerges remains unexplained, but *P. falciparum* tends to be the most persistently erratic. Macrophages, particularly those in the liver, bone marrow, and spleen, phagocytose released

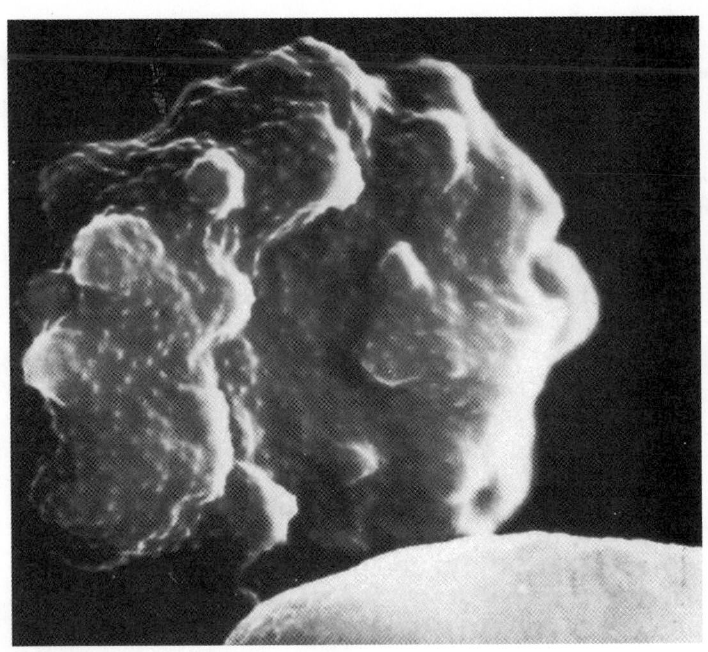

FIGURE 7-7
Erythrocyte, parasitized by *Plasmodium falciparum*, showing surface knobs.

pigment. In extreme cases of falciparum malaria, the amount of pigment is so great that it imparts a dark, reddish-brown hue to visceral organs such as the liver, spleen, and brain. With increased erythrocyte destruction, accompanied by the body's inability to recycle iron bound in the insoluble hemozoin, anemia develops.

One pathological element unique to *P. falciparum* infection is vascular obstruction. Plasma membranes of erythrocytes infected with schizonts, the more mature stages of the organism, develop electron-dense "knobs" by which they adhere to the endothelium of capillaries in visceral organs (Fig. 7-7). Engorged with hordes of infected erythrocytes, the capillaries become obstructed, causing the affected organs to become anoxic. In terminal cases, capillary blockage (**ischemia**) in the brain causes the brain to become swollen and congested.

A condition known as **blackwater fever** often accompanies falciparum malaria infections. Characterized by massive lysis of erythrocytes, it produces abnormally high levels of hemoglobin in urine and blood. Fever, vomiting with blood, and jaundice also occur, and there is a 20–50% mortality rate usually due to renal failure. The exact cause of this condition is uncertain; it may be a reaction to quinine, or it may result from an autoimmune phenomenon in which hemolytic antibodies are produced.

Diagnosis of malaria usually consists of microscopical demonstration of the parasites in stained thick and thin smears of peripheral blood. Even though synchrony is obvious, diagnostic blood samples can be drawn almost anytime, since a few "stragglers" from the previous episode always remain in the blood. Smears, however, should be made at regular intervals over a period of several days, especially if one smear fails to show parasites. Serological tests are of little clinical value, since they make no distinction between present and past infections.

CHEMOTHERAPY

Malaria control requires effective treatment of the disease in humans and continuous efforts to control mosquito populations. The first known effective antimalarial drug was quinine, an extract from the bark of the cinchona tree of South America and other tropical areas. The tree was named by Linnaeus in the seventeenth century in honor of the wife of the Peruvian envoy, Countess del Chinchón, who was treated for malaria with the bark. The drug destroys the schizogonic stages of the parasite, but has little or no effect on exoerythrocytic stages or gametocytes. During World War II, when the Japanese occupied the cinchona plantations in Indonesia, it became essential that researchers develop alternative drugs for the Allied forces. A synthetic drug, Atabrine dihydrochloride (quinacrine hydrochloride), developed in Germany in 1936, proved effective against the erythrocytic stages of all species of *Plasmodium* and in suppressing clinical symptoms. Like quinine, Atabrine is ineffectual against exoerythrocytic stages; consequently, vivax and ovale malaria patients treated with this drug are susceptible to relapse. Also, Atrabrine produces a number of undesirable side effects, such as jaundice and gastrointestinal disturbances. Since World War II, research has yielded a number of other synthetic drugs, of which the most commonly used are chloroquine, amodiaquin, and primaquine. Each, however, has limited effect on *Plasmodium* and, for maximum benefit, should be administered in combination with one or more other drugs. For instance, while chloroquine and amodiaquin act to suppress clinical symptoms by destroying the erythrocytic stages, the slow-acting drug primaquine destroys the exoerythrocytic stages. Currently, the optimal chemotherapeutic regimen for treatment of malaria includes taking chloroquine for

3 days followed by a single dose of primaquine after leaving endemic areas.

The folic acid cycle provides a suitable metabolic pathway for chemotherapeutic management of malaria. This cycle is vital to the parasite in synthesizing bases for nucleic acid formation. The drug pyrimethamine, used in combination with sulfadoxine (Fansidar), inhibits portions of the cycle and is therefore lethal to the parasites. In 1984, a new antimalarial drug, mefloquine, was tested and approved for use by health authorities. This drug acts against blood schizonts. Currently, mefloquine is being added to the pyrimethamine–sulfadoxine combination in a one-step treatment for chloroquine-resistant falciparum malaria, and mefloquine is prescribed as a prophylactic drug for travelers to areas where chloroquine-resistant falciparum malaria has been reported. The combination of quinine and tetracycline is used in Southeast Asia as standard treatment for uncomplicated malaria, while quinine has been reestablished as an alternative drug for the treatment of chloroquine-resistant strains.

As noted earlier, an alarming phenomenon in the treatment of malaria is the increasing resistance of the parasites to chemotherapy (Fig. 7-5b), most likely the result of mutagenic changes in some strains of *P. falciparum*. Chloroquine-resistant strains of *P. falciparum* are now common throughout Africa, pyrimethamine-sulfadoxine-resistant strains are present in Southeast Asia and South America, and strains resistant to mefloquine have been reported in Thailand, Cambodia, and Myanmar. Thus, the development of antimalarial drugs must be a continuous process. Similarly, the use of insecticides to eradicate mosquitoes has led to the appearance of resistant mosquito strains in areas that have been sprayed extensively. In Greece, for example, only a few years after apparently successful efforts to control *Anopheles* with DDT, it was necessary to alternate DDT application with dieldrin in order to control the malaria-carrying species.

Ideally, the search for new antimalarial drugs and new insecticides should be directed toward development of compounds that block a critical metabolic pathway within the parasite or mosquito. Further, such new compounds need to be inexpensive, safe, and able to produce long-lasting effects. Such an approach, however, must be predicated upon a thorough understanding of the biochemical processes occurring within these parasites, knowledge requiring years of intensive research employing sophisticated techniques.

IMMUNITY

In addition to research in chemotherapy, development of a protective vaccine against malaria is being vigorously pursued. Indeed, the development of vaccines and immunodiagnostic tests are two of the major priorities of WHO. The basis for development of a successful vaccine is identifying those stages that stimulate protective immune responses in the vertebrate host. As many of the developmental stages of malarial parasites in the vertebrate host are intracellular and therefore protected from the host's immune mechanism, the extracellular forms (sporozoites and merozoites) become the targets for vaccine. The main types of vaccines currently being studied are **anti-sporozoite vaccines,** directed against the sporozoites when introduced by the mosquito to the vertebrate host; **anti-asexual blood stage vaccines**, directed against various blood-stage antigens, such as those attributed to merozoites as well as those introduced to the surface of infected erythrocytes; and **transmission-blocking vaccines**, aimed at arresting development of the parasite in the mosquito. A number of approaches using gene cloning, genetic engineering, and related technology are creating a degree of cautious optimism in the quest. Certain singular characteristics of the sporozoite surface coat already have been identified. The coat acts as as a renewable "decoy" to the vertebrate host's immune system, stimulating the production of antibodies. When the sporozoite is attacked and its "decoy" coat sloughs off, a replacement coat is synthesized, and the "decoy" effect continues. This system provides ideal protection for the sporozoite, which resides only briefly in the blood before it enters a liver cell, where it is protected from circulating antibodies. It also suggests a brief window of opportunity for targeting a potential vulnerable developmental stage. Protection afforded the sporozoite by its surface coat in its brief transit through the host circulatory system contrasts with that in African trypanosomes (p. 118), which are exposed to the immune system for a long time throughout a lengthy residence in the blood. The surface antigens of African trypanosomes, it will be recalled, undergo continual change, each dominant population keeping one step ahead of the vertebrate host's immune system.

In endemic areas, premunition (p. 33) is the basis for protective immunity as long as low-level infection persists. With complete cure, however, the victim regains susceptibility. While nursing infants in endemic areas are protected through antibodies in the mother's milk, at the time of weaning the children are at greatest risk, and the highest mortality rate in such regions is among children. Also, *P. falciparum* has been reported to cross the placenta and cause infection of the fetus.

Factors other than immunological ones may also influence susceptibility among humans. Several genetic conditions affect the malarial organism. Susceptibility conferred by the presence of Duffy antigens has already been discussed. Genetic deficiency in glucose-6-phosphate dehydrogenase in erythrocytes (**favism**) creates an inhospitable environment for the parasites. This enzyme is rate-limiting in one of the erythrocyte's metabolic pathways that, among other functions, provides reducing potential to protect the erythrocyte's plasma membrane against toxic by-products, such as those produced by the parasite. The lack of protection causes excessive leakage of potassium from the infected cell. Since the malarial parasite may require a higher level of potassium than is available, it dies. Humans heterozygous for **sickle cell anemia** possess a selective advantage over individuals with normal hemoglobin in regions where *P. falciparum* is endemic. The tendency to "sickle" is accelerated when affected erythrocytes are subjected to low oxygen tensions. One explanation for such a selective advantage is that *P. falciparum*-infected erythrocytes sickle when trapped in visceral capillaries, damaging the erythrocyte membrane, which causes excessive leakage of potassium from the cells. In a heterozygous host, up to 40% of the cells are of this type and are, therefore, unsuitable for the parasite's development, thus accounting for the resistance to the disease among such persons. Ironically, the severe pathological effects of falciparum malaria have resulted in the maintenance of this highly deleterious mutation in the human population. The requirement of malarial organisms for intracellular potassium has been questioned. *In vitro* experiments have indicated that the parasite may grow normally in erythrocytes with high sodium and low potassium content. An alternative explanation for the advantage of sickle cell anemia is that it enhances the possibility of detection and removal of infected cells by host phagocytic cells.

PHYSIOLOGY

Metabolic characteristics of *Plasmodium* provide targets for drug action and immunological control. Unfortunately, many gaps remain in our understanding of several metabolic aspects of the intracellular stages in the life cycle, due in part to the fact that there was no culture technique for reproducing these stages *in vitro* until recently. For example, glucose is the chief carbohydrate required by the parasite, which appears to derive most of its energy from glycolysis. However, while some intermediates of the Krebs cycle have been demonstrated, there is no evidence of functional mitochondria in the erythrocytic stages, although the mosquito stages do possess these organelles. In the erythrocytic stages, the parasites are facultative anaerobes; i.e., they use oxygen when it is available, primarily during the synthesis of nucleic acids.

The end-products of carbohydrate metabolism are lactic acid, formic acid, and a limited amount of acetic acid. The parasite does fix carbon dioxide, and the enzymes that catalyze this process are believed to be vulnerable to quinine and chloroquine.

Hemoglobin is essential for the parasite's development, although it is uncertain precisely which components are required. The parasite digests hemoglobin intracellularly, producing an insoluble by-product, hemozoin. In addition to its possible disruption of carbon dioxide fixation, chloroquine appears to interfere with the intracellular digestive processes of the parasite. Chloroquine and quinine are both weak bases that raise the pH of the lysosomal compartment, reducing the ability of the parasite to digest host hemoglobin efficiently.

Although the malarial parasite depends on host erythrocytes for many essential molecules, it does have the ability to synthesize folic acid, a key compound in pyrimidine synthesis, from basic molecules. Host cells, on the other hand, require outside sources of folic acid. Therefore, drugs that block the synthesis of folic acid (**antifols**) by the parasite possess immense chemotherapeutic potential.

SELECTED READINGS

Desowitz, R. S. 1976. How the wise men brought malaria to Africa. *Natural History* **85**, 36–44.

Friedman, M. J., and Trager, W. 1981. The biochemistry of resistance to malaria. *Scientific American* **244**, 154–165.

Galinski, M. R., and Barnwell, J. W. 1996. *Plasmodium vivax*: Merozoites, invasion of reticulocytes and considerations for malaria vaccine development. *Parasitology Today* **12**, 20–29.

Godson, G. N. 1985. Molecular approaches to malaria vaccines. *Scientific American* **248**, 52–59.

Hermentin, P. 1987. Malaria invasion of human erythrocytes. *Parasitology Today* **3**, 52–55.

Knell, A. J. (Ed.). 1991. *Malaria.* Oxford University Press, Oxford, England (A publication of the Tropical Programme of the Wellcome Trust).

Leete, T. H., and Rubin, H. 1996. Malaria and the cell cycle. *Parasitology Today* **12**, 442–444.

Meis, J. F. G. M., and Verhave, J. P. 1988. Exoerythrocytic development of malarial parasites. *Advances in Parasitology* **27**, 1–61.

Chapter Eight

BLOOD AND TISSUE PROTOZOA III: OTHER APICOMPLEXANS

BABESIA

Infections of humans by *Babesia* spp. have been known since 1957; in recent years, however, human babesiosis has become sufficiently common on Nantucket Island and Martha's Vineyard in Massachusetts, at Shelter Island on Long Island, New York, and in Wisconsin to warrant the attention of medical parasitologists. In each of these locales, the causative agent has been identified as *Babesia microti*, a natural parasite of the meadow vole and other rodents, with the vector in all instances being the tick, *Ixodes dammini*. *Ixodes dammini* may also serve as the vector for Lyme disease among humans (see p. 435). Humans acquire the infection when an infected tick feeds on a human host. Splenectomized persons seem especially vulnerable to babesiosis; indeed, such individuals appear to be susceptible to more than one species of *Babesia*, and most of the recorded fatalities have occurred in splenectomized individuals.

Life Cycle

Infection in the vertebrate host is initiated when **vermicles** (sporozoites) are introduced through the bite of an infected tick (Fig. 8-1). The vermicle is approximately 2 μm long and varies in shape from pyriform to spiral. The vermicle enters a host erythrocyte, where it develops into a trophozoite that rapidly increases in size and undergoes binary fission, producing numerous merozoites. The merozoites erupt from the infected erythrocyte and enter other erythrocytes, where the cycle of growth, division, and reentry continues, resulting in an extremely large intraerythro-

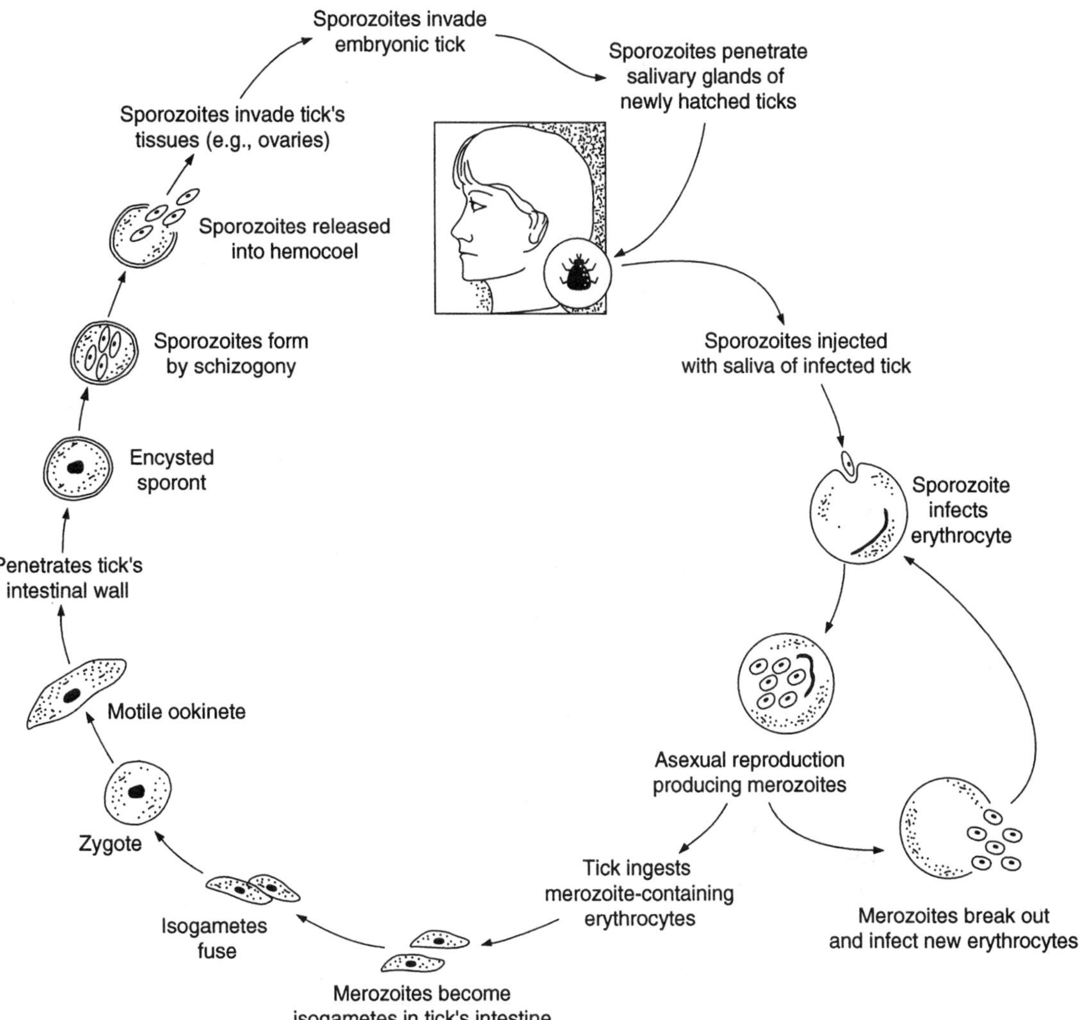

FIGURE 8-1
Life cycle of *Babesia microti.*

cytic population in a short time. There is neither an exoerythrocytic nor a sexual phase in the vertebrate portion of the life cycle.

The tick acquires the infection by ingesting infected vertebrate blood. Parasites are released into the tick's intestine and immediately transform into motile, polymorphic isogametes. Gametic fusion to form zygotes occurs within 24 hours after the blood meal. The zygotes transform into cigar-shaped ookinetes, 8–10 μm long, which penetrate the tick's intestine and become encysted sporonts, each of which grows to about 16 μm in diameter within 2 days. Each sporont nucleus then undergoes schizogony, and the resulting vermicles, each 9–13 μm long, migrate into the hemocoel, whence they invade various tissues of the tick, particularly ovarian tissues. In the ovaries, the vermicles undergo several more divisions and invasions within embryonic ticks. Final generations of vermicles eventually migrate to the salivary glands of the newly hatched tick and are injected into the vertebrate host when the young tick takes a blood meal. The passage of *Babesia* from a tick to its progeny in this manner is known as **transovarian transmission.**

Symptomatology and Diagnosis

Human babesiosis can be fatal in immunologically compromised individuals. The disease mimics mild malaria, and unless there is reason to suspect babesiosis, the erythrocytic stages in blood smears are often mistaken for malarial organisms. The usual manifestation of the infection is basically hemolytic anemia.

Treatment

Since babesiosis can be mistaken for malaria, it is sometimes treated with chloroquine. In spite of some claims of success, there is no real evidence that the drug is effective against babesiosis. Because most individuals recover spontaneously, treatment of symptoms may be the best way to manage the disease. For patients in whom the number of parasites becomes life-threatening, exchange transfusion is a viable option.

TOXOPLASMA GONDII

Human toxoplasmosis is caused by a coccidian, *Toxoplasma gondii*, originally discovered in 1908 in a desert rodent. This potentially perilous parasite is estimated to infect 50% of the population of the United States. Fortunately, most of the infections are asymptomatic, with clinical toxoplasmosis affecting only a limited number of individuals. Occasionally, however, minor epidemics do occur. The principal means of acquiring the infection is either by ingestion of inadequately cooked meat, primarily beef, pork, and lamb, or by contact with feral or domestic cats. Any cat, no matter how well cared for, may carry and pass the infective stage of *Toxoplasma*. Congenital toxoplasmosis is a very serious disease, and for this reason pregnant women should avoid contact with litter box filler used by cats. Flies and cockroaches have also been implicated as carriers of the infective stages from cat feces to food. At least five different strains of *T. gondii* have been identified and studied. They differ primarily in life cycle duration and the number and morphology of merozoites produced.

Life Cycle

Toxoplasma can attack a wide variety of tissue cells but seems to favor muscle, lymph nodes, and intestinal epithelium. Infection of intestinal epithelial cells occurs only in felines, probably the "normal" hosts, and this developmental pathway is termed the **enteric** or **enteroepithelial phase** (Fig. 8-2). It is during this phase that the formation of sporozoite-containing oocysts, the primary source of human infection, occurs. In other hosts, including many species of carnivores, insectivores, and primates, there is only the **extraintestinal** or **tissue phase**. Ingestion of a sporulated oocyst is the precursor for either developmental phase. Each oocyst, measuring 10–13 μm by 9–11 μm, contains two sporocysts, and each sporocyst contains four sporozoites. The sporozoites are released from the oocyst in the lumen of the host's small intestine. In cats, some sporozoites penetrate intestinal epithelial cells to begin the enteric phase, while others penetrate the mucosa and develop in cells of underlying tissues, including lymph nodes and leukocytes.

In the enteric phase, the sporozoites enter the host cell, are enclosed in a parasitophorous vacuole, become trophozoites, and reproduce by endodyogeny and/or endopolyogeny. The number of asexual cycles varies according to the physiological condition of the feline host, but about 2–40 merozoites (Fig. 8-3) arise from

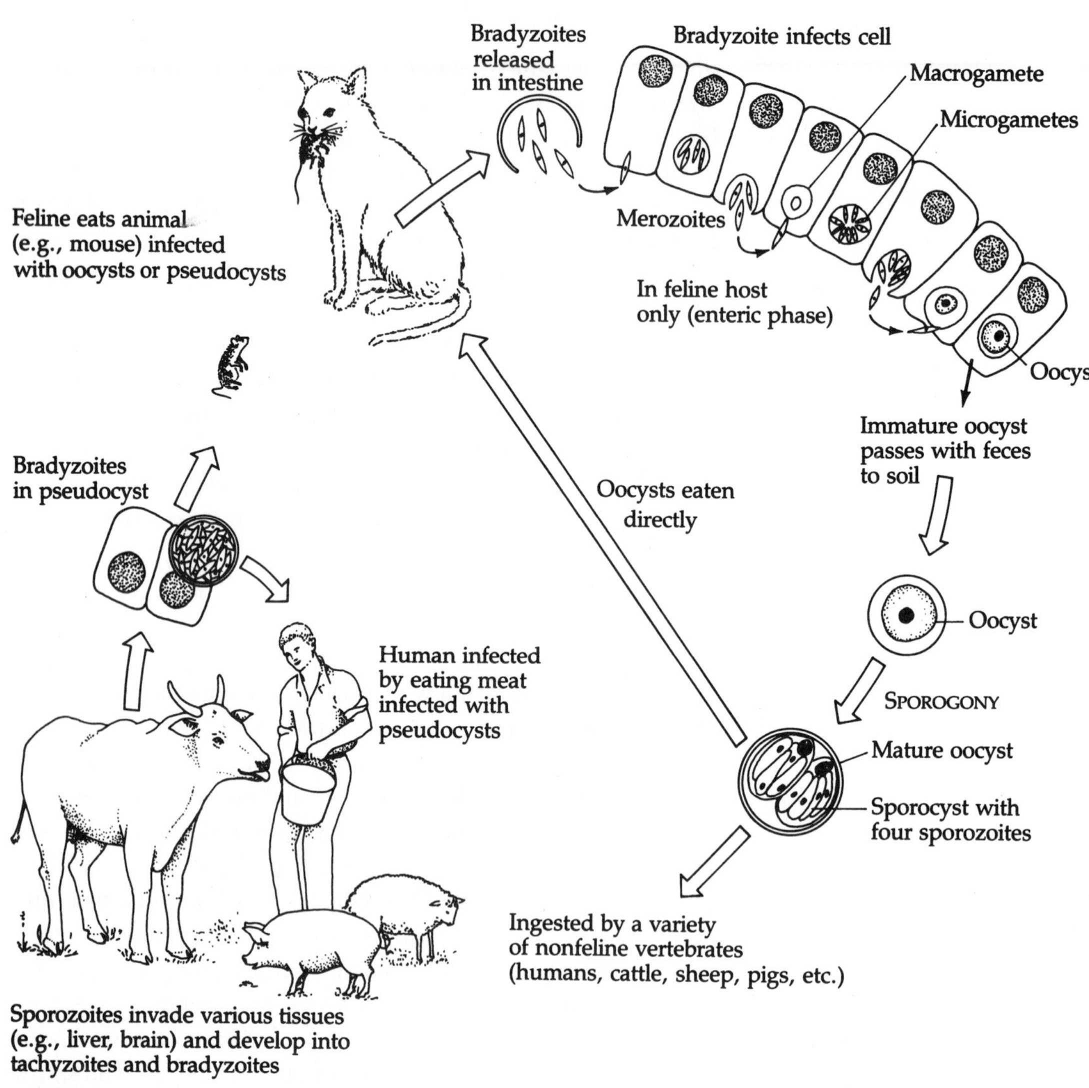

FIGURE 8-2
Life cycle of *Toxoplasma gondii*.

each trophozoite. Three to 15 days after infection, some of the merozoites enter new host cells and develop into either microgametocytes (males) or macrogametocytes (females). About 2–4% of the gametocytic population is microgametocytes, and each produces about 12 microgametes. Fertilization is intracellular, the microgametes bursting from their host cell to invade other

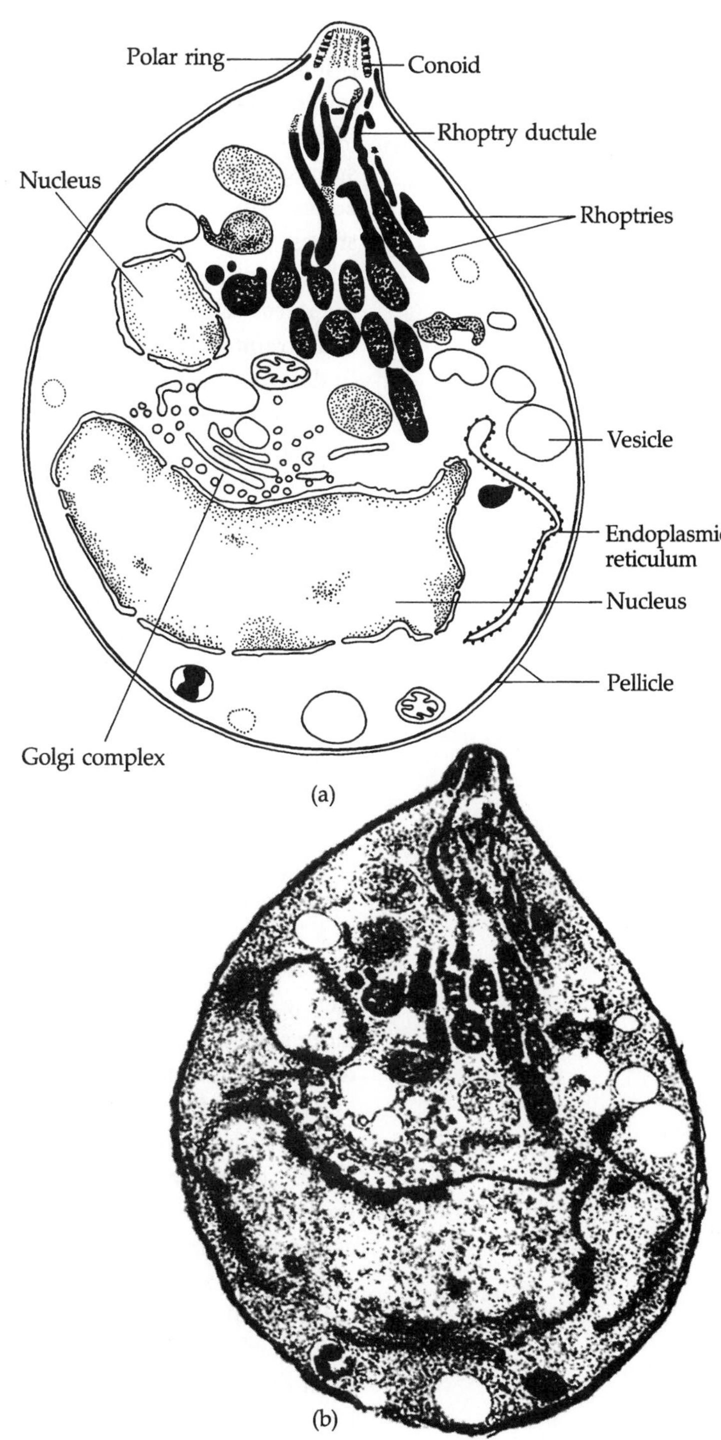

FIGURE 8-3
Apical complex.
(a) Drawing of merozoite of *Toxoplasma gondii* showing some constituents of the apical complex. (b) Transmission electron micrograph from which (a) was drawn.

host cells containing macrogametes. Following fertilization, the resulting zygote develops into an oocyst that breaks out of the cell into the lumen of the feline intestine to be passed out with feces. Within 2–5 days, in the presence of oxygen, the oocyst undergoes sporogony, forming two sporocysts, each containing four sporozoites. The feline enteric phase, then, proceeds through three stages: asexual reproduction producing merozoites, gamogony producing gametes, and sporogony producing oocysts containing the infective sporozoites.

Extraintestinal and enteric development, which follow entirely different patterns, can occur simultaneously in the cat. Only the extraintestinal phase occurs in mammals other than cats, including humans.

In extraintestinal development, there are two avenues for infection: infective oocysts may be ingested, in which case sporozoites invade cells other than those of the intestinal epithelium; or tissue infected with pseudocysts may be ingested, whereupon liberated bradyzoites can invade cells. In either case, the intestinal wall is penetrated and the parasites are engulfed by macrophages and transported throughout the body. Protected from the lysosomal activity of the macrophage, the parasites form rapidly dividing merozoites called **tachyzoites**, which measure 7 μm by 2 μm. In acute infections, 8–16 tachyzoites are produced within a parasitophorous vacuole in the host cell, eventually causing the cell to disintegrate, probably by pressure, releasing the parasites to invade new cells. An accumulation of tachyzoites in a host cell is known as a **group**. Many types of cells are vulnerable to infection. As the disease becomes chronic, parasites infecting cells of the brain, heart, and skeletal muscles reproduce more slowly than during the acute phase. At this time, they are designated as **bradyzoites** and accumulate in large numbers within an infected cell. Gradually, thick walls develop around the masses of bradyzoites to form **pseudocysts** that may persist for months or even years, especially in nerve tissue. Therefore, all animals except cats can be considered paratenic hosts, since the parasite never completes its sexual phases in those creatures.

Pseudocyst formation coincides with the development of immunity in the host. This immunity, involving both humoral and cellular reactions, is usually permanent and precludes establishment of a new infection. If immunity wanes, it is restored by release of bradyzoites from cysts, restimulating the host's immune system.

Epidemiology

Toxoplasma gondii is cosmopolitan in distribution. All mammals, including humans, are capable of transmitting toxoplasmosis transplacentally. Sporulated oocysts, tachyzoites, and bradyzoites all serve as infective agents. Sources of infection range from direct contamination, as from handling cat litter, to ingestion of inadequately cooked meat or raw milk.

Immunologic surveys reveal that humans throughout the world carry antibodies to *Toxoplasma*; as stated earlier, clinical toxoplasmosis is rare, and infections are generally asymptomatic. Although not all of the influential factors are presently known, it has been established that the following affect the level of pathology: (1) the age of the host, with older hosts being more resistant to the disease; (2) the virulence of the strain of *T. gondii* involved; (3) the natural susceptibility of the host; and (4) the degree of acquired immunity of the host.

Symptomatology and Diagnosis

Symptomatic, or clinical, toxoplasmosis may be classified as acute, subacute, chronic, or congenital. Acute toxoplasmosis in humans is characterized by parasitic invasion of the mesenteric lymph nodes and liver parenchyma. The most common symptom is the development of painful, swollen lymph glands in the inguinal, cervical, and subclavicular regions, frequently accompanied by fever, headache, anemia, and muscle pain, and sometimes by pulmonary complications. The tachyzoites proliferate in many tissues and tend to kill host cells rapidly. When cells from sites such as the retina or brain are involved, serious lesions often develop. Subacute toxoplasmosis is merely a prolongation of the acute stage.

Normally, the duration of the chronic stage is limited by the host's immune system. If immunity develops slowly, however, the course of clinical toxoplasmosis can be protracted. During this period, tachyzoites continue to destroy cells, producing extensive lesions in the lungs, heart, liver, brain, and eyes. Damage is usually greater to the central nervous system than to non-nervous tissues because of lower immunocompetence in the former. Toxoplasmosis becomes chronic when immunity in the host, accompanied by the formation of pseudocysts, becomes sufficient to suppress tachyzoite proliferation. The pseudocysts may remain intact for years, producing no clinical symptoms. A pseudocyst wall may occasionally rupture, however, releasing bradyzoites. Most of them are destroyed by host responses, but some may penetrate cells and form new pseudocysts. Death of bradyzoites elicits a hypersensitive response. In the brain, nodules of glial cells gradually form at the sites of such reactions. In cases in which there are sufficient numbers of such nodules, the victim may develop symptoms of chronic encephalitis, sometimes accompanied by spastic paralysis. This is especially true of AIDS patients (see pp. 29–30), in whom *Toxoplasma* can cause severe brain damage. The presence and rupture of pseudocysts in the retina and choroid can lead to blindness. Chronic toxoplasmosis can also cause myocarditis, leading to permanent heart damage and pneumonia.

Congenital toxoplasmosis results from fetal transplacental infection. Such infection may result in stillbirth or a number of severe birth defects. Approximately 12% of infected infants born alive die shortly after birth, and fewer than 20% of those surviving are normal by age 4. Abnormalities occur in the central nervous system, eyes, and viscera with symptoms such as jaundice, microcephaly, and hydrocephaly appearing at birth or shortly thereafter.

Diagnosis is based primarily on serological tests using killed antigens. Demonstration of the parasite in mice following inoculation with suspected fluid or biopsied tissue (xenodiagnosis) constitutes positive diagnosis.

Treatment

Oral administration of pyrimethamine, usually accompanied by sulfadiazine, is the treatment of choice at this time. Because pyrimethamine is an antifol and thus can cause folic acid deficiency in the host, supplemental folic acid may be added to the regimen as a precautionary measure.

PNEUMOCYSTIS CARINII

There has been a dramatic upsurge in the incidence of *Pneumocystis carinii* pneumonia (PCP) coincident with the increasing incidence of AIDS (see p. 29). Of the opportunistic diseases associated with AIDS, PCP is the most common cause of death, affecting an estimated 60% of AIDS patients in the United States and Europe. In addition to its prevalence among AIDS patients, PCP is common in children and premature infants who are malnourished or debilitated or who suffer from primary immune deficiency disorders. The disease is also found in cancer and transplant patients being treated with immunosuppressive drugs.

A universally accepted taxonomic designation for *P. carinii* has yet to be agreed upon. A number of authorities place it provisionally in the kingdom Protista, phylum Apicomplexa. Others classify *Pneumocystis* as a protistan of independent systematic position. Still others place it in the kingdom Fungi. Not only is its systematics open to question, but its life cycle, natural reservoirs, and modes of transmission are obscure.

Life Cycle

Little of the life cycle of *P. carinii* has been established (Fig. 8-4). Existing data have been derived from morphological studies of forms collected from infected humans and other mammals. No information is available on forms existing outside these hosts. *P. carinii* is an extracellular parasite found in interstitial tissues of the lungs and their alveoli.

Three morphological stages, **trophic, precystic**, and **cystic,** have been identified. In the pleomorphic trophic stage (Fig. 8-5), the parasite measures 2–8 μm and is bounded by a thin pellicle 10–40 nm thick, consisting of a plasma membrane and an electron-dense outer layer. Associated with the pellicle are small, tubular expansions sometimes regarded as filopodia. The trophic stage form is usually uninucleate, although binucleate forms occasionally occur.

The precystic stage is a transitional link between the trophic and cystic stages. The precystic organism is oval and 3–5 μm long, with a clump of mitochondria in its cytoplasm. During this stage, the pellicle thickens to 40–120 nm and has few tubular expansions, and the number of nuclei increases to eight.

The cyst measures 4–6 μm in diameter and has a thick pellicle (70–140 μm) consisting of three layers: plasma membrane, electron-lucent middle layer, and electron-dense outer layer. During sporogony, a rosette of eight **intracystic bodies**, or sporozoites, form meiotically within the cyst. Each intracystic body (Fig. 8-6)

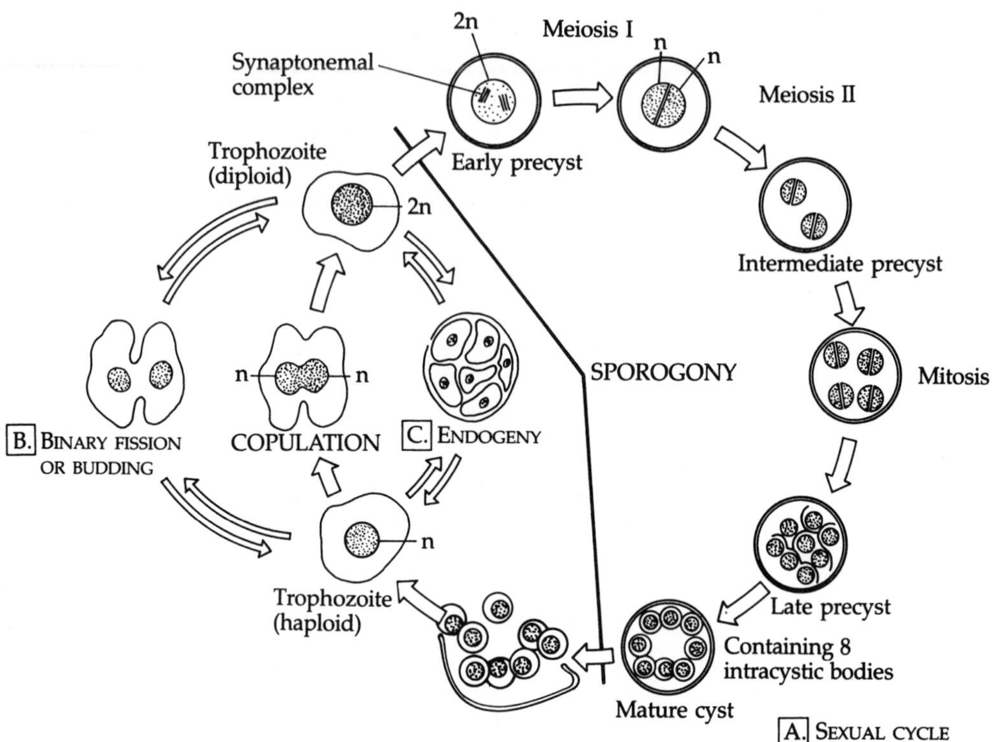

FIGURE 8-4
Life cycle of *Pneumocystis carinii*.
Only the intrapulmonary cycle is known. In the sexual cycle (trophozoite–cyst cycle, A), the diploid trophozoite meiotically divides through the precyst stages into a mature cyst with eight haploid intracystic bodies. The cyst ruptures, releasing the intracystic bodies, which develop into haploid trophozoites. This process is equivalent to sporogony. In addition to the sexual cycle, the trophozoites seem to have two modes of asexual division: binary fission or budding of the trophozoite (B) and endogeny (C). It is unknown which type of trophozoite (diploid or haploid) is involved in asexual development. All cycles occur extracellularly.

measures 1–1.5 μm and possesses a nucleus, a mitochondrion, and rough endoplasmic reticulum; intracystic bodies can be spherical, crescent-shaped, or amoeboid. After rupturing from the cyst, each intracystic body develops to the trophic stage. This activity occurs in the alveolar lining layer of the lung, and each new form selectively attaches to squamous (type I) alveolar epithelial cells (Fig. 8-7). While the mode of transmission from one human to another has not been established, the most plausible hypothesis, based on rat-to-rat transmission studies, suggests inhalation of cysts from the air.

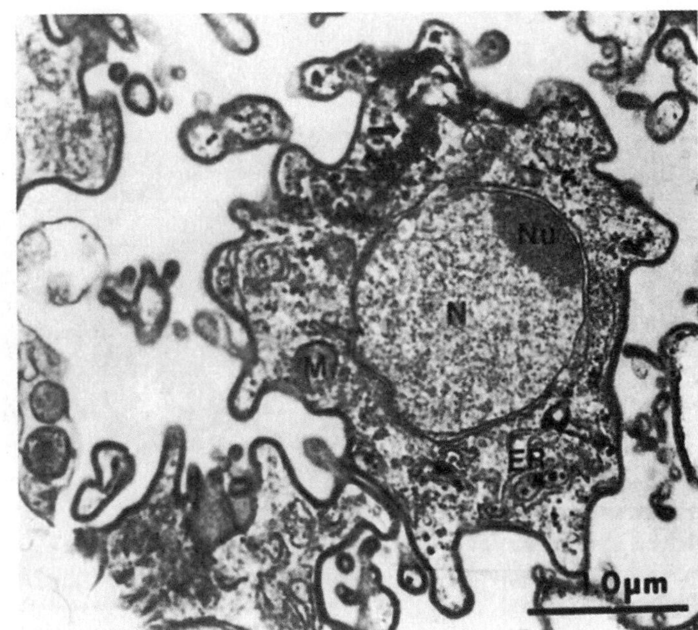

FIGURE 8-5
Trophozoite of *Pneumocystis carinii*.
Note the nucleus (N), nucleolus (Nu), mitochondrion (M), and sparse endoplasmic reticulum (ER).

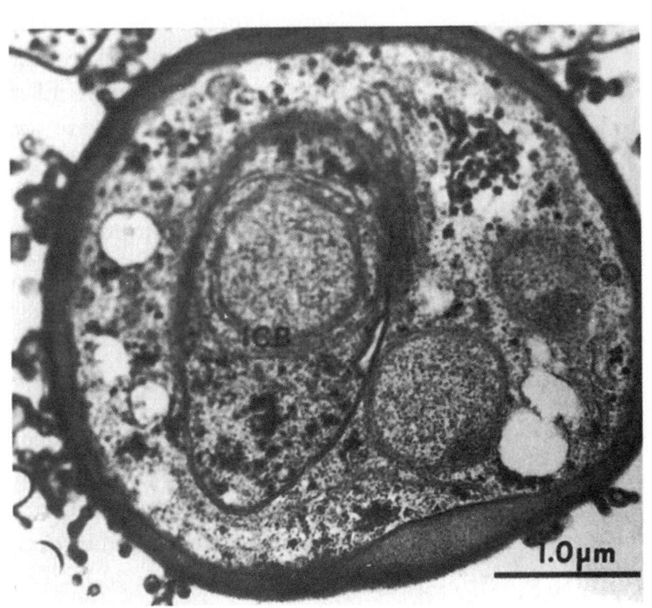

FIGURE 8-6
Cysts of *Pneumocystis carinii* with developing intracystic body (ICB).

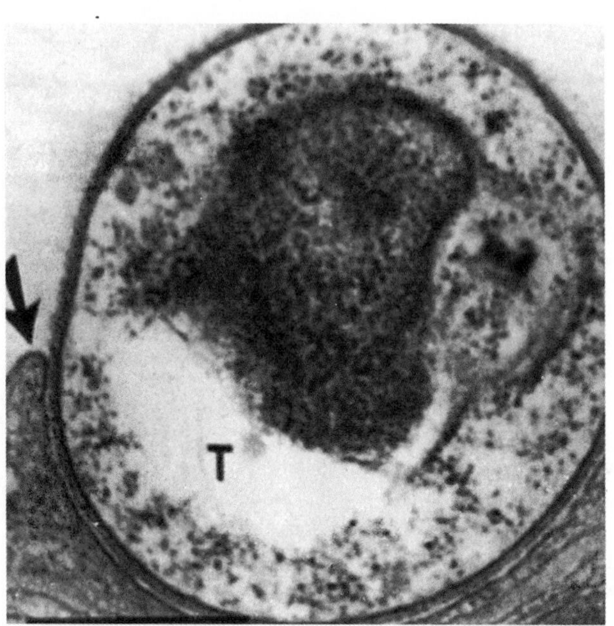

FIGURE 8-7
Trophozoite (T) of *Pneumocystis carinii* attached to an alveolar cell. Note the cytoplasmic projections of the host cell (arrow).

Symptomatology and Diagnosis

In immunologically normal individuals, *Pneumocystis* infection is asymptomatic, but immunosuppression can activate such latent infections into virulent ones. *Pneumocystis* is found in the lungs of the host, usually in the lumina of the alveoli. The alveolar septa thicken and are infiltrated by plasma cells, and the *Pneumocystis* organisms fill the alveoli. These events occur in rapid succession and are accompanied by fever, difficulty in breathing, coughing, and cyanosis. In untreated patients, death from pneumonia is the inevitable outcome. Diagnosis is confirmed by identification of the organism in lung biopsies and bronchial lavages.

Treatment

First-line chemotherapy is cotrimoxazole, which is also recommended for other opportunistic parasites. A potential hazard is that continued use of the drug may encourage the development of resistant forms. Other drug regimens that have proven successful in some cases are trimethoprim–sulfamethoxazole, pyrimethamine–sulfadoxine, and inhaled nebulized pentamidine.

CRYPTOSPORIDIUM PARVUM

Three other apicomplexans which hitherto caused only minor clinical symptoms in persons with competent immune systems have gained renewed attention from the medical profession by causing severe symptoms to immunodeficient patients. These are *Cryptosporidium parvum*, *Cyclospora cayentanensis*, and *Isospora belli.*

Cryptosporidiosis is a condition caused by the coccidian *Cryptosporidium parvum.* The organisms live in the brush border of the small intestine and respiratory epithelium of a number of mammals, including humans. Acquisition is by ingestion of the oocyst, usually in contaminated drinking water.

Life Cycle

The infective oocysts are oval, measuring 4–5 μm wide, and contain four slender sporozoites but no sporocysts (Fig. 8-8). Oocysts are expelled with the feces of a number of infected mammals. When ingested, the oocysts release sporozoites that excyst in the small intestine and attach to the epithelial surfaces of the ileum and colon (Fig. 8-9). Once enclosed in a parasitophorous vacuole formed from the convergence of microvilli of infected cells, each sporozoite becomes a trophozoite (Fig. 8-10), which undergoes schizogony to produce eight first-generation merozoites. The merozoites erupt from the infected cells and enter the intestinal lumen. The following sequence of events then transpires: (1) attachment of each first-generation merozoite to an uninfected epithelial cell surface, (2) envelopment of the merozoite by microvilli, (3) transformation of the merozoite to a trophozoite, (4) schizogony to form a second generation of four merozoites, (5) eruption of second-generation merozoites from the infected cell, and (6) incorporation of these merozoites to the surface of still other uninfected epithelial cells. The second-gen-

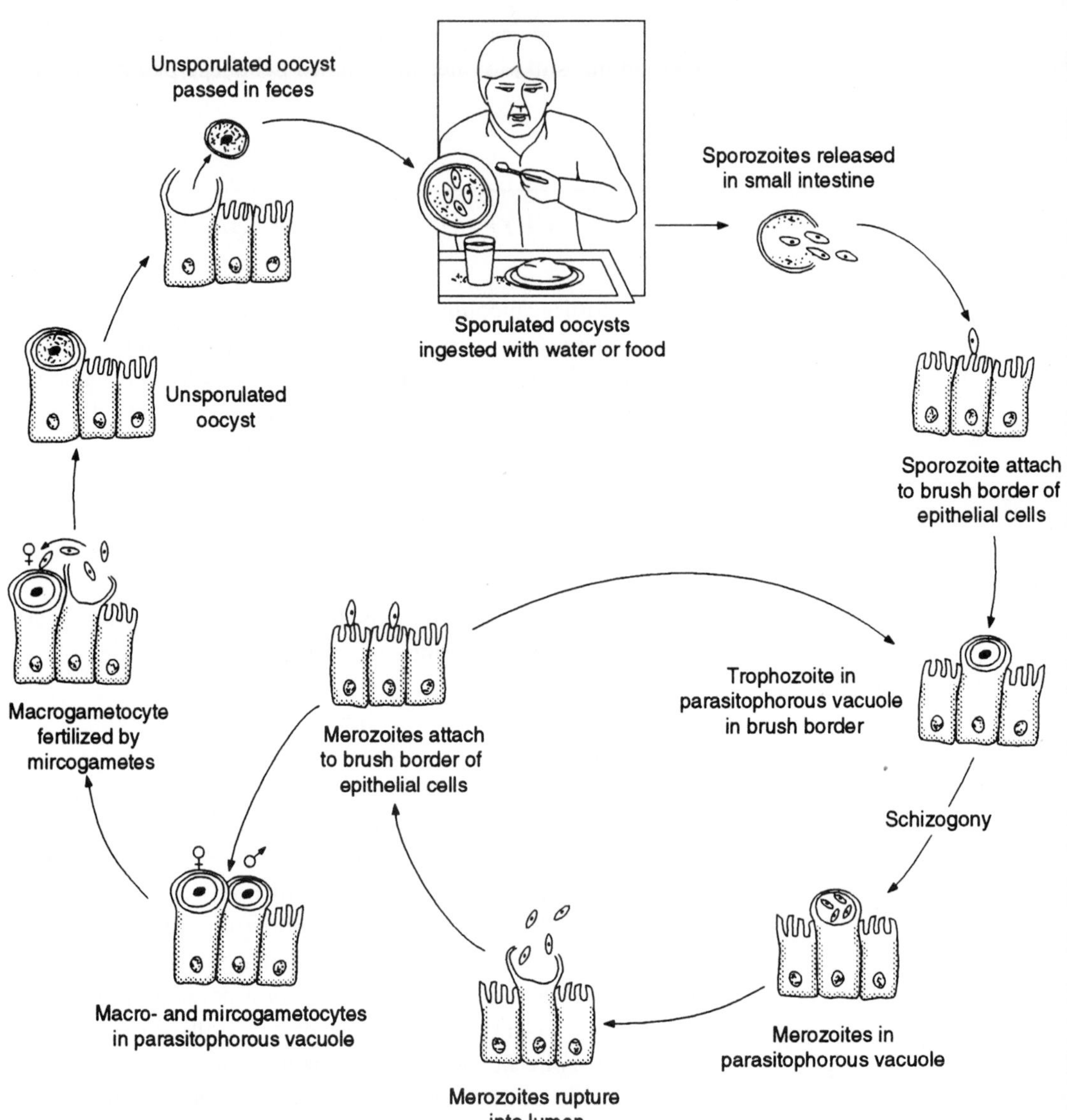

FIGURE 8-8
Life cycle of *Cryptosporidium parvum*.

eration merozoites differentiate into microgametocytes and macrogametocytes. The former undergo several divisions to produce numerous microgametes, while the latter transform into macrogametes, usually one per parasitophorous vacuole. The microgametes burst from the infected cell and enter cells containing

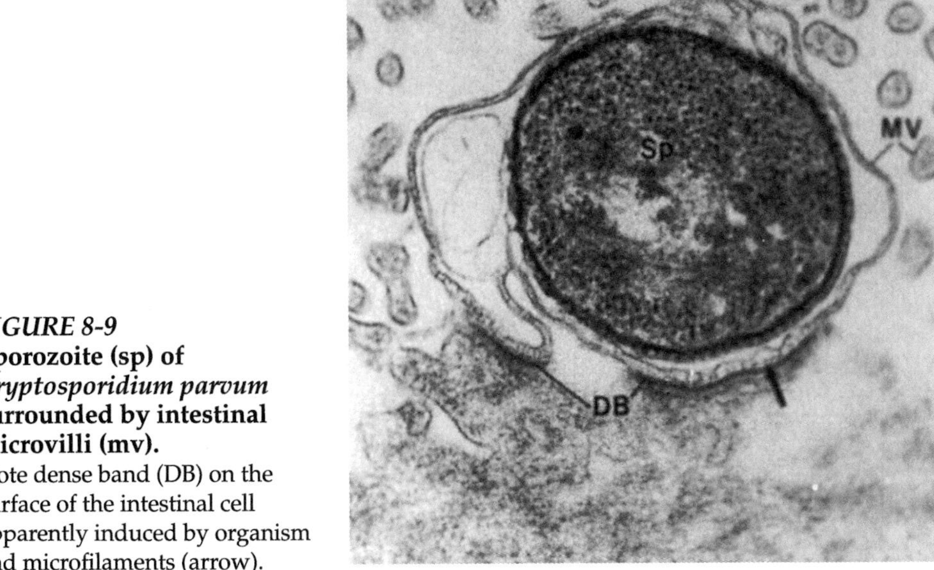

FIGURE 8-9
Sporozoite (sp) of *Cryptosporidium parvum* surrounded by intestinal microvilli (mv).
Note dense band (DB) on the surface of the intestinal cell apparently induced by organism and microfilaments (arrow).

macrogametes. Following fertilization, the resulting zygote differentiates into an unsporulated oocyst, which frees itself from the superficial parasitophorous vacuole and is shed with the feces of the host. The oocyst is infectious upon shedding. Each oocyst sporulates in the soil or when swallowed by a new host.

Epidemiology

Cryptosporidium occurs in a wide variety of hosts, including humans and other primates, cattle, sheep, rodents, and birds. Although several distinct species of *Cryptosporidium* have been described, studies have shown a surprisingly high degree of cross-infectivity of *Cryptosporidium* recovered from different hosts, with C. *parvum* being the most dominant species in nature. Therefore, a large number of hosts can act as reservoirs. Outbreaks of cryptosporidiosis were reported in 1993 in Milwaukee, Wisconsin, and in Washington, DC. Spring flood water laden with infective oocysts, ostensibly washed downstream in cattle manure, were blamed for overloading the cities' water purification systems. In Washington, drinking water was brought in from

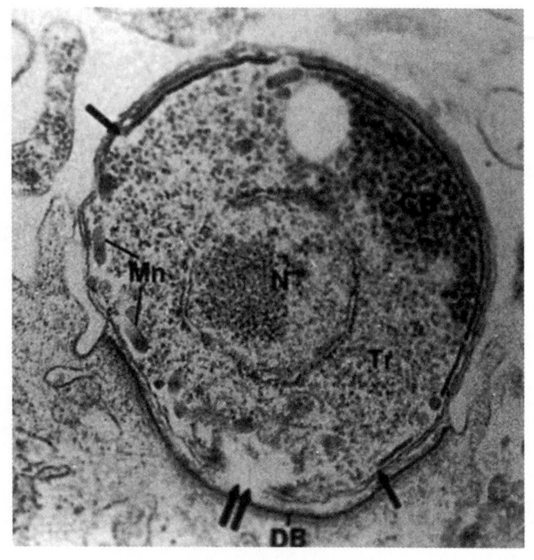

FIGURE 8-10
Early trophozoite (Tr) of *Cryptosporidium parvum.* Note the micronemes (Mn), nucleus (N), crystalloid bodies (CB), and dense band (DB) of the trophozoite. Arrows point to the parasite's plasma membrane.

Charlottesville, Virginia, for use by athletes participating in a weekend football game to protect them from infection. Lesser outbreaks have been reported in other cities. None of the purification chemicals used in municipal water treatment plants is effective against the oocysts. Filtration is the best means of reducing the number of oocysts in public drinking water. The number of asymptomatic individuals who pass oocysts has been found to be higher than previously thought, and outbreaks attributed to person-to-person transmission, especially in daycare centers and nursing homes, have been reported.

Symptomatology and Diagnosis

Morphological alterations of the intestinal epithelium of infected individuals include villous atrophy, mitochondrial changes, and increased lysosomal activity in infected cells. Symptoms range from none, through mild diarrhea, to diarrhea with severe cramping, anorexia, nausea, and vomiting. In immunologically competent individuals, the infection is self-limiting and lasts from several days in most patients to several weeks. In immunologically compromised individuals, however, cryptosporidiosis is a chronic disease lasting months or even years. In extreme cases, e.g., AIDS patients, the disease can be extremely severe, and patients can lose as much as three liters of fluid daily. Mortality in such instances may reach 50%, and there are often secondary extraintestinal complications, such as biliary disease and pneumonitis from respiratory tree infection. Diagnosis depends upon identification of oocysts in the stool. Histological sections from biopsy of intestinal epithelium showing any of the stages of the organism also constitute positive identification.

Treatment

No treatment is recommended in immunocompetent patients, because the infection is self-limiting. For immunosuppressed patients, no chemotherapeutic agents have yet proven effective, but the antibiotic agent Azithromycin has been used successfully to treat severe diarrhea in immunosuppressed children. Octreotide also has no effect on the organism but has been used to control diarrhea. Paromomycin has been used with some success to control the organism.

CYCLOSPORA CAYENTANENSIS

Cyclospora cayentanensis is a relatively new addition to the realm of organisms dangerous to human health. It is now considered an emerging pathogen. Although the organism has been known since 1979, it was first isolated from patients from Peru in 1985. The first outbreak of cyclosporidiosis in the United States was recorded in 1990 in Chicago, Illinois. Subsequently, at least 1,000 cases of the disease have been reported in the United States, and numerous incidents have been confirmed from Central and South America, the Caribbean, Asia, and Eastern Europe. In Kathmandu, Nepal, for example, *Cyclospora* has been identified in 11% of individuals with gastrointestinal symptoms. Most infections have been traced to drinking water contaminated with sporulated oocysts. However, an outbreak of cyclosporidiosis in Charleston, South Carolina, in 1996 was traced initially to contaminated strawberries and later to contaminated Guatemalan raspberries. The infective stage is a sporulated oocyst measuring 8–10 μm in diameter. In the laboratory, sporulation requires 7–13 days at 25–32°C, with each sporulated oocyst enclosing two sporocysts, each of which contains two sporozoites. Sporozoites measure 1.2 μm wide by 9 μm long. The complete life cycle and epidemiological features of *Cyclospora* are still largely unknown.

Symptomatology and Diagnosis

Clinical symptoms of cyclosporidiosis resemble those of cryptosporidiosis: nausea, vomiting, anorexia, weight loss, and explosive watery diarrhea lasting 1–7 weeks. Diagnosis is difficult, because *Cyclospora* oocysts recovered from the feces of infected humans are often mistaken for those of *Cryptosporidium.* It is strongly recommended that precise measurements of the oocysts' dimensions be made to differentiate between *Cyclospora* oocysts and those of *Cryptosporidium.*

Treatment

As in any diarrheic incident, it is important to correct and maintain hydration. *Cyclospora* can be treated successfully in children and adults with Trimethoprim–sulfamethoxazole.

ISOSPORA BELLI

Isospora belli, the causative agent of isosporiasis in humans, is endemic in South America, the Caribbean, Africa, and Southeast Asia. The infective stage is the sporulated oocyst containing two sporocysts, each with four sporozoites. This apicomplexan attacks the columnar epithelium of the small intestine, causing diarrhea that is usually mild in healthy patients. In immunologically compromised individuals, however, the infection can be life-threatening, causing high fever and persistent, severe diarrhea. In Haiti, there is a 15% prevalence among AIDS patients. A second species, *I. hominis*, has been implicated in some human cases of isosporiasis. Trimethoprim–sulfamethoxazole is an effective treatment.

SELECTED READINGS

Clark, D. P., and Sears, C. L. 1996. The pathogenesis of cryptosporidiosis. *Parasitology Today* **12,** 221–225.

Coop. R. L., Wright, S. E., and Casemore, D. P. 1998. Cryptosporidiosis. In *Zoonoses* (Palmer, S. R., Soulsby, E. J. L., and Simpson, D. I. H., Eds.), pp. 563–578. Oxford University Press, Oxford, England.

Dubey, J. P. 1998. Toxoplasmosis, sarcocystosis, isosporosis, and cyclosporosis. In *Zoonoses* (Palmer, S. R., Soulsby, E. J. L., and Simpson, D. I. H., Eds.), pp. 579–597. Oxford University Press, Oxford, England.

Hughes, H. P. A. 1985. Toxoplasmosis—A neglected disease. *Parasitology Today* **1,** 41–44.

Jackson, M. H., and Hutchison, W. M. 1989. The prevalence and source of *Toxoplasma* infection in the environment. *Advances in Parasitology* **28,** 55–105.

Lindsay, D. S., and Blagburn, B. L. 1994. Biology of mammalian *Isospora. Parasitology Today* **10,** 214–220.

Matsumoto, Y., and Yoshida, Y. 1986. Advances in pneumocystis biology. *Parasitology Today* **2,** 137–142.

Perkins, M. E. 1992. Rhoptry organelles of apicomplexan parasites. *Parasitology Today* **8,** 28–32.

Spielman, A. 1988. Lyme disease and human babesiosis: Evidence incriminating vector and reservoir hosts. In *The Biology of Parasitism* (Englund, P. T., and Sher, A., Eds.), pp. 147–165. Wiley-Liss, New York.

Ynes R., Ortega, M. S., Sterling, C. R., Gilman, R. H., Cama, V. A., and Diaz, F. 1993. *Cyclospora* species—A new protozoan pathogen of humans. *New England Journal of Medicine* **328,** 1308–1312.

Zipori, T. 1988. Cryptosporidiosis in perspective. *Advances in Parasitology* **27,** 63–129.

PART TWO

THE TREMATODA

Chapter Nine

GENERAL CHARACTERISTICS OF THE TREMATODA

The phylum Platyhelminthes includes various dorsoventrally flattened animals commonly known as flatworms (Fig. 9-1). All members are typically bilaterally symmetrical and lack a body cavity. The digestive tract, if present, is incomplete; i.e., the caeca end blindly. Therefore, the only opening to the exterior, the mouth, serves for both ingestion and egestion. Skeletal, circulatory, and respiratory systems are usually lacking. The space between the body wall and the internal organs contains connective tissue fibers, muscle, and unattached and fixed cells of various types. The intercellular spaces are filled with body fluids. The fibers, cells, and spaces between them are referred to collectively as the **parenchyma.**

Four classes make up the phylum. Two of these, Trematoda and Cestoidea, contain flatworms parasitic to humans. One evolutionary scheme for the trematodes proposes that they arose from a stock of free-living flatworms (progenitors of present-day rhabdocoel turbellarians), became intimately associated with molluscs, and ultimately developed into parasitic forms. Evolutionary divergence within this endoparasitic population gave rise to two groups, designated as subclasses Digenea and Aspidogastrea. The ancestral digeneans proliferated asexually in the mollusc; later adult forms parasitized evolving vertebrates. The ancestral, nonproliferative, aspidogastrean forms, on the other hand, remained within their molluscan hosts through adulthood. All trematodes parasitic to humans belong to the subclass Digenea. Digenetic trematodes constitute one of the largest groups of platyhelminths, parasitizing a wide range of invertebrate and vertebrate hosts. Within human hosts, these worms are found in numerous organs, including the intestine, lungs, liver, and vascular system.

STRUCTURE OF THE ADULT

Despite superficial differences, the morphology of the various groups of digenetic trematodes is basically uniform. The following description represents a hypothetical composite exemplifying the various anatomical features (Fig 9-1).

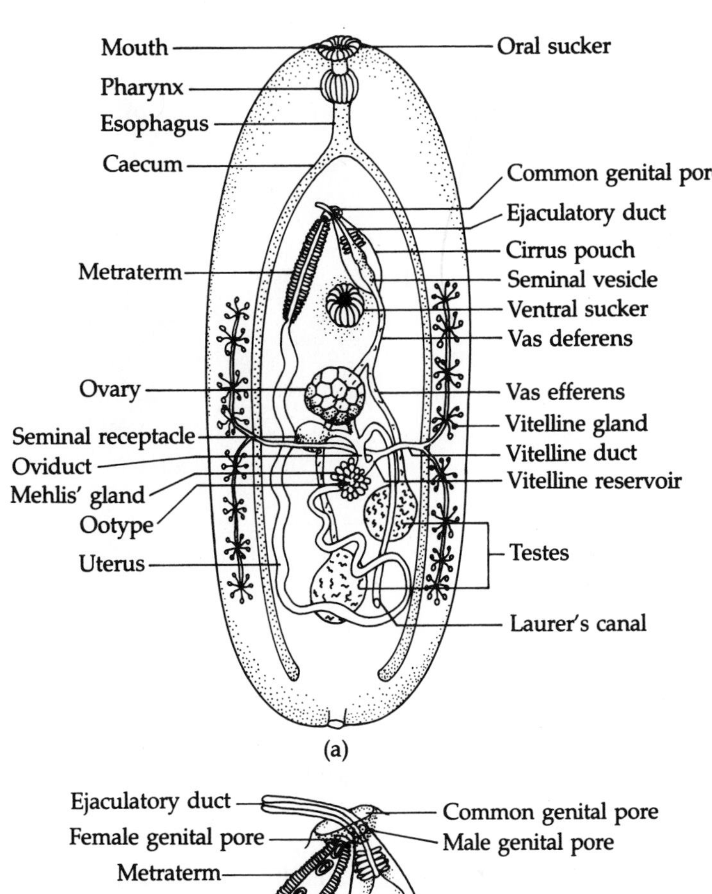

FIGURE 9-1
Generalized digenetic trematode.
(a) Diagram of entire organism. (b) Detailed diagram of male (right) and female (left) genitalia.

TEGUMENT

Once considered a nonliving, protective "cuticle," the tegument is now recognized as a dynamic, cellular structure. Under light microscopy, it appears as a generally homogeneous layer about 7–16 μm thick (Fig. 9-2). The tegument is a **syncytium,** i.e.,

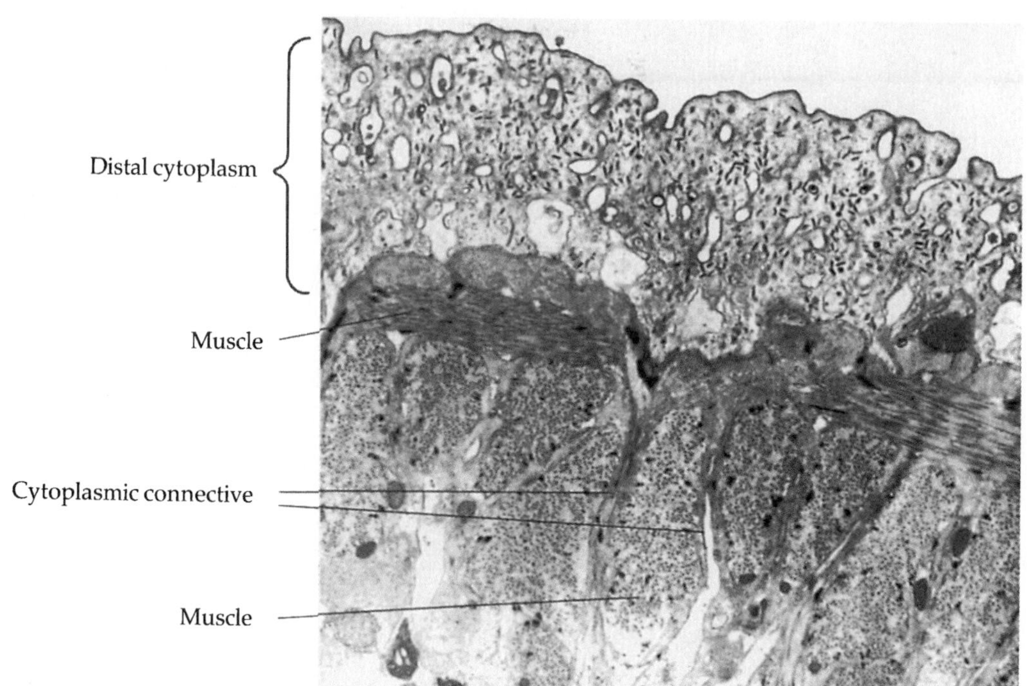

FIGURE 9-2
Transmission electron micrograph of the tegument of a digenetic trematode.

a multinucleated tissue with no cell boundaries (Fig. 9-3). The outer zone of this syncytium, the **distal cytoplasm,** is delineated at its surface by a plasma membrane measuring about 10 nm thick. Associated with the plasma membrane is a surface coat, or **glycocalyx,** that varies in thickness according to species. Surface invaginations, the number and extent of which also vary according to species, serve to increase tegumental surface area, much like microvilli on the surface of human intestinal cells. The ability of the tegument to absorb exogenous molecules is generally proportional to the number and extent of invaginations and the number of mitochondria in the distal cytoplasm. Hydrolytic enzymatic activity in the glycocalyx facilitates the uptake of certain molecules from the environment. The glycocalyx is also a protective structure, shielding the worm from such hostile environmental influences as antibodies and host digestive enzymes. For example, the presence of acid mucopolysaccharides in the glycocalyx is of particular significance, as such molecules are known to inhibit a number of digestive enzymes. Their presence on the

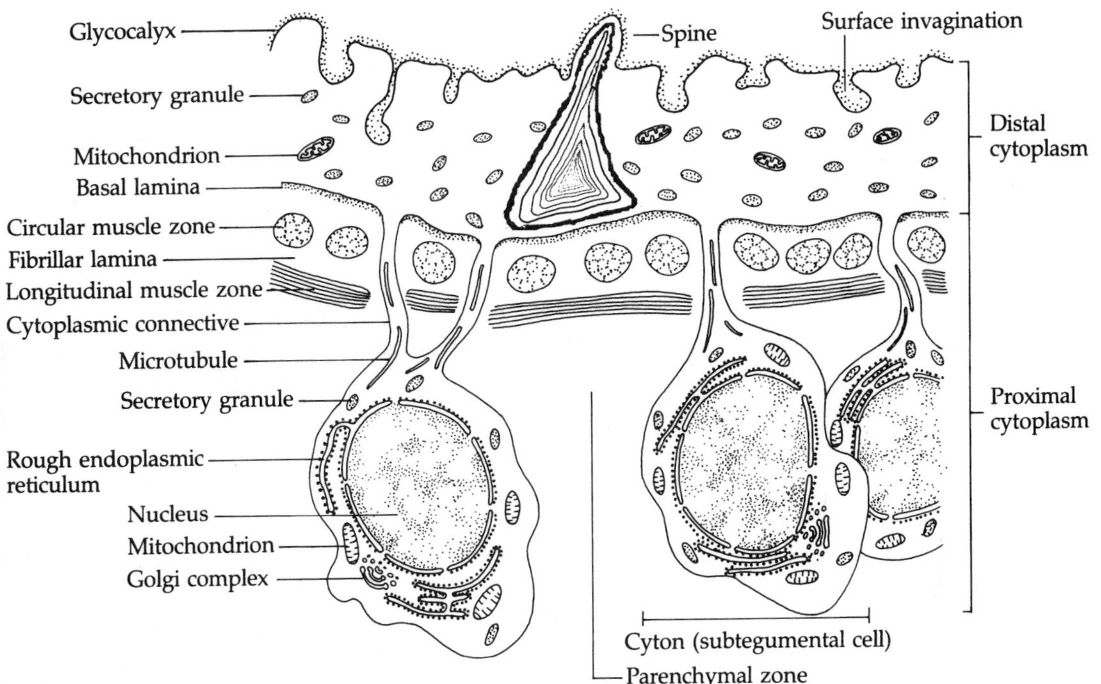

FIGURE 9-3
Tegument of a digenetic trematode.

body surface may account for the ability of intestinal trematodes to resist host digestive enzymes.

Embedded in the distal cytoplasm of some species are tegumental spines, with bases lying just above the basal plasma membrane of the distal cytoplasm and tips projecting outward but still covered by the surface membrane. Although the function of these spines has not been firmly established, it is speculated that they may serve as ancillary holdfast mechanisms and/or storage sites for certain essential molecules. The matrix of the distal cytoplasm also contains one or two types of secretory vesicles.

The distal cytoplasm is connected to the inner, **proximal cytoplasm** (**cyton region**) by cytoplasmic bridges. The proximal cytoplasm contains nuclei, endoplasmic reticulum, Golgi complexes, glycogen deposits, mitochondria, and various types of vesicles. This region of the tegument is the site where materials for the repair and maintenance of the distal cytoplasm are synthesized. The vesicles in the distal cytoplasm are packets of substances produced in the proximal cytoplasm that continually maintain the outer plasma membrane and its glycocalyx and assist in the maintenance of the matrix and spines. The translocation of these vesicles from proximal to distal cytoplasm is facilitated by microtubules in the cyton region and in the cytoplasmic bridges.

DIGESTIVE TRACT

Digenetic trematodes possess an incomplete digestive tract (Fig. 9-1). The anterior mouth, surrounded by a muscular oral sucker, leads into a bulbous, muscular pharynx, in many species via a short prepharynx. The esophagus connects the pharynx and the alimentary tract, the latter bifurcating into two **caeca**. The mouth, pharynx, and esophagus make up the foregut, analogous to that of more complex animals. The lining of the foregut is morphologically similar to the general tegument; i.e., it is a syncytium consisting of distal and proximal cytoplasmic zones. There are, however, no spines associated with this lining. The foregut is the site of ingestion and assimilation of food, and the ability to accomplish these functions is enhanced by specific modifications of the foregut in these organisms. In many forms, for instance, the proximal cytoplasm produces enzymes that are released into the lumen of the foregut, where they partially degrade ingested food. In addition, heavily muscularized regions of the foregut, such as the pharynx or, in some species, the esophagus, mechanically break food into smaller particles.

The transition from the tegument-like structure of the foregut to the simple epithelium, or **gastrodermis**, of the two caeca is abrupt and marked by a prominent cell junction (Fig. 9-4). The gastrodermis may be syncytial or may consist of cells with distinct lateral cell boundaries. There is no discernible physiological basis for this variation. The caeca are two longitudinal, blind tubes of variable length. In many species, they extend almost to the posterior tip of the body; in others, they may extend no farther than a third of the body length. In certain larger digeneans, the caeca exhibit extensive diverticulation.

The gastrodermal surface is bounded by a plasma membrane amplified in either fingerlike microvilli (Fig. 9-5a) or leaflike lamellae (Fig. 9-5b). Digestion and absorption of food occur in the caeca, and such amplifications increase the absorptive surface. The type of amplification is independent of the type of food ingested. Some blood-feeding digeneans, for example, exhibit a

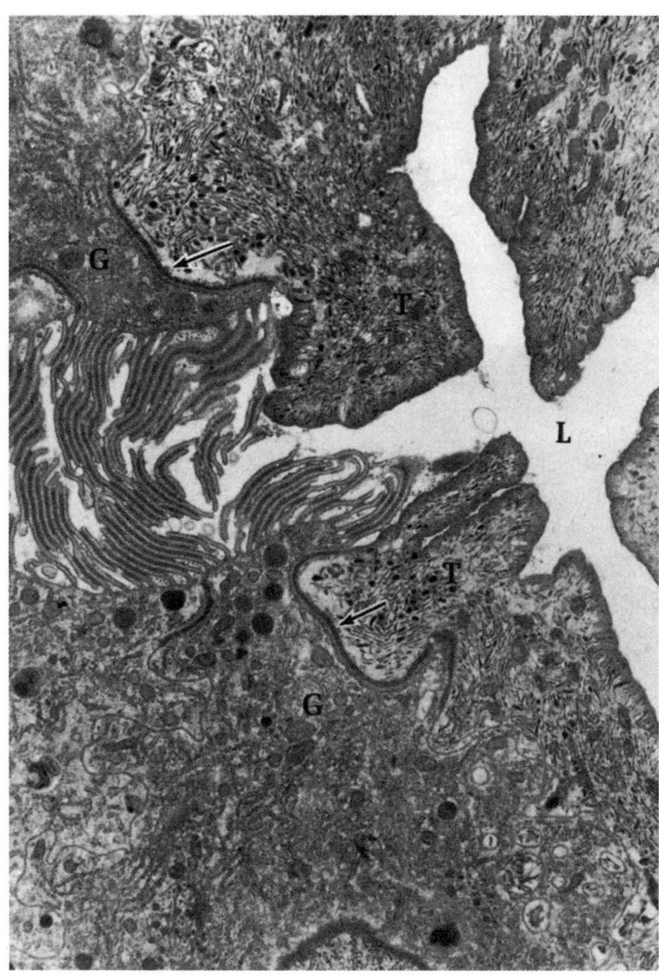

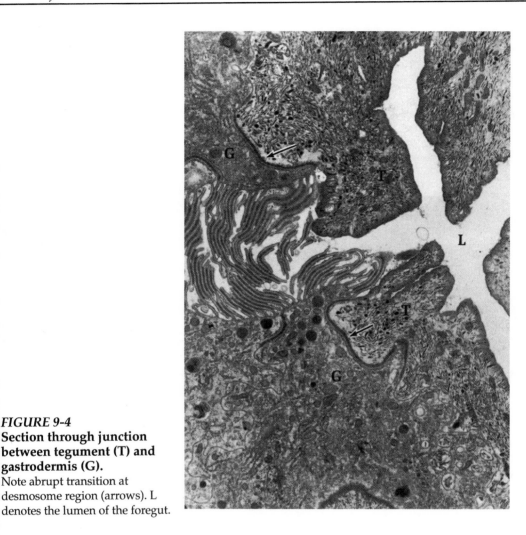

FIGURE 9-4
Section through junction between tegument (T) and gastrodermis (G).
Note abrupt transition at desmosome region (arrows). L denotes the lumen of the foregut.

microvillar type, while others display the lamellar type. Associated with the plasma membrane is a prominent glycocalyx that, like the tegumental glycocalyx, appears to afford protection as well as aid in the uptake of certain molecules, the latter function abetted by its enzymatic activity. Digestion is typically extracellular, occurring in the gut lumen.

The gastrodermis is highly active in protein synthesis and secretion, for which it possesses abundant rough endoplasmic reticulum, Golgi complexes, mitochondria, and vesicles. Most of the vesicles originate from the Golgi complex and contain either material for maintaining the glycocalyx or hydrolytic enzymes that are released into the caecal lumen for the purpose of diges-

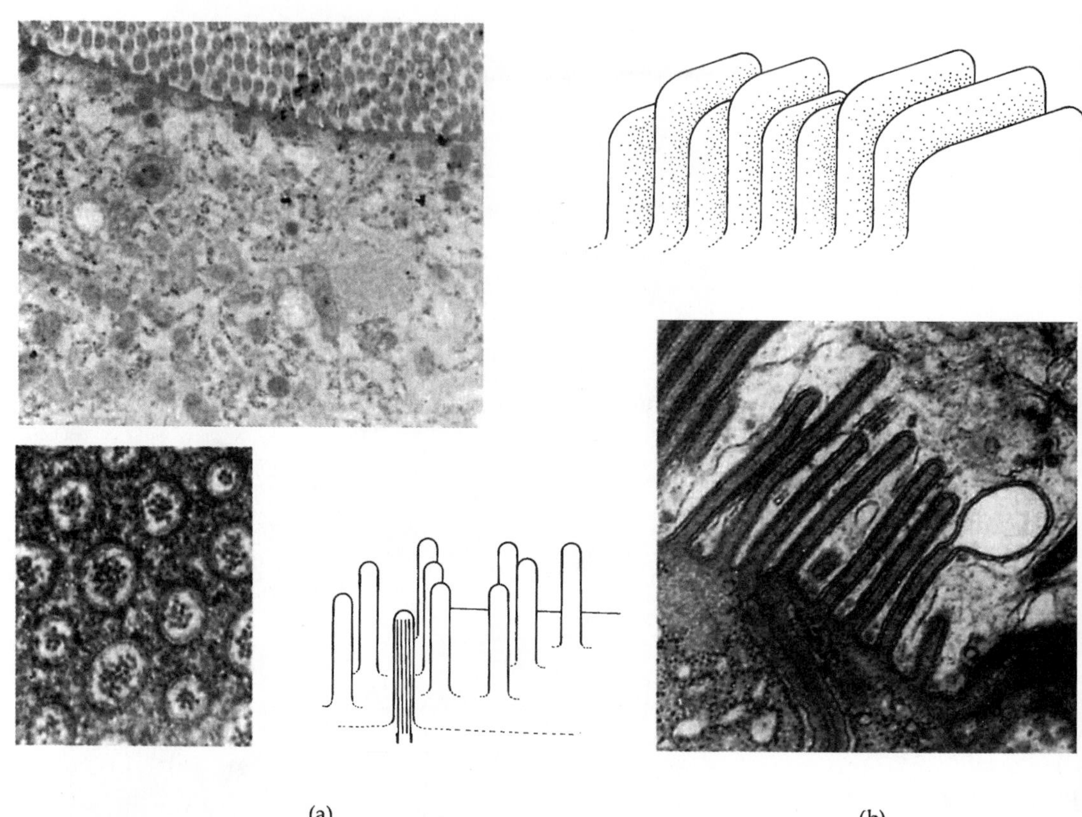

FIGURE 9-5
(a) Microvillar amplification of gastrodermis.
Bottom left is a cross section through microvilli.
(b) Lamellar amplifications of gastrodermis.

tion. The basal plasma membrane of the gastrodermis often contains extensive infoldings that seem to be associated with the organism's ability to transport ions. The basal plasma membrane rests on an extensive **basal lamina** in which are embedded two layers of muscles, one circular, the other longitudinal.

MUSCULAR AND NERVOUS SYSTEMS

There are two muscle zones in adult digenetic trematodes. Underlying the tegument is the **subtegumental zone,** which consists of three layers of muscle—longitudinal, circular, and diagonal.

Contractile activity by these muscles is usually minimal, although certain species exhibit more active subtegumental musculature. The muscle layers are typically more distinct in the anterior part of the body. The orientation of contractile fibers allows the organism to elongate, contract, and/or twist its body in almost any given plane. This zone of smooth muscles contains a nucleated region, or **myoblast**, connected to the bundles of myofibers. The second zone of musculature, the **gastrodermal zone**, described in the previous section, helps move food up and down the caecal lumen. Well-developed contractile fibers are also present in the oral and ventral suckers.

The nervous system of adult digeneans (Fig. 9-6) is of the "ladder" type. Three pairs of longitudinal nerve trunks—a prominent ventral pair, a lateral pair, and a dorsal pair—extend posteriorly and anteriorly from two connected dorsal ganglia (brain) near the pharynx; all three pairs of trunks are interconnected by transverse commissures. Smaller nerve branches, emanating from the brain and longitudinal trunks, supply motor and sensory innervation to the tegument, suckers, reproductive systems, and other organs.

Sensory organs are evident in some tissues of the digenean body, particularly the tegument and gastrodermis. These organs usually appear as modified cilia projecting from bulbous nerve endings, and they extend outward from the tegumental surface

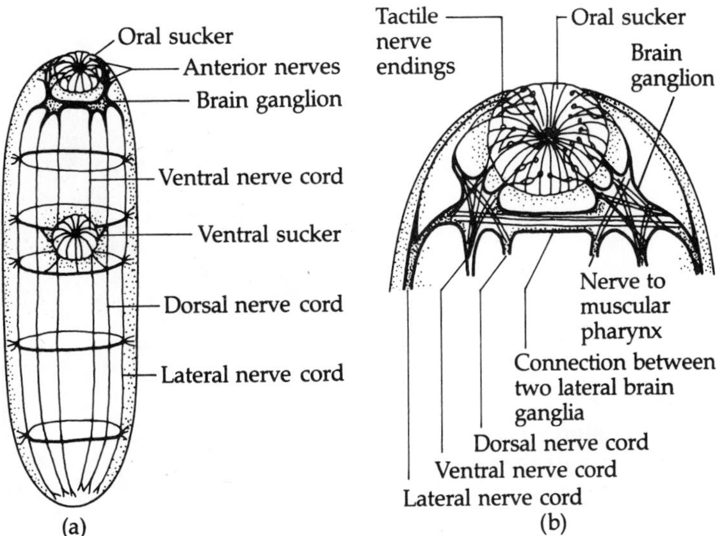

FIGURE 9-6
(a) Nervous system of a digenetic trematode. (b) Innervation of the anterior end and oral sucker of a digenetic trematode.

or from the gastrodermis into the lumen of the digestive tract. They may serve as pressure, touch, rheotactic, or chemical sensors. In larval stages, sensory organs may include papillae, pigmented eyespots, uniciliated organs, and organs containing up to six ciliary eyespots. Such diversity undoubtedly aids free-swimming larvae in locating hosts. Nerve end organs act as chemo-, mechano-, and photoreceptors.

OSMOREGULATORY SYSTEM

The osmoregulatory system of digenetic trematodes is of the typical protonephridial type, a tubular system closed at one end and open at the other. Currents are produced at the closed ends by **flame cells**, each of which is equipped with a tuft of fused, vigorously beating cilia (Fig. 9-7). The number and arrangement of such cells in digeneans are specific enough to serve as taxonomic indicators of phylogenetic relationships. Each cell opens into a terminal tubule, several of which converge to form larger collecting ducts. The collecting ducts on each side of the body lead

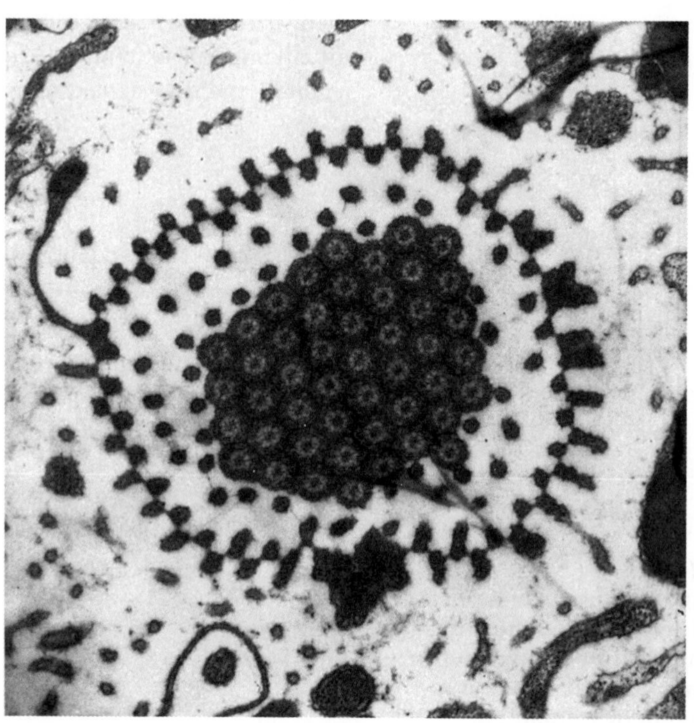

FIGURE 9-7
Transmission electron micrograph of the ciliary tuft of a trematode flame cell.

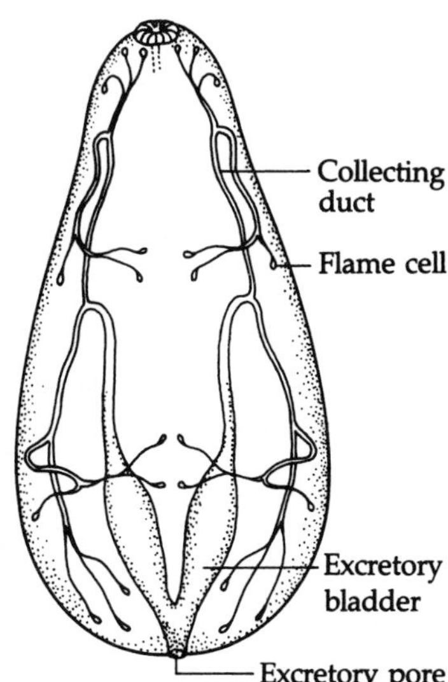

FIGURE 9-8
Excretory system of *Heterophyes heterophyes.*

posteriorly and empty into a common **excretory bladder** (Figs. 9-8, 9-9), the duct of which opens to the exterior through the excretory pore located at or near the posterior end of the body.

While it seems likely that this system serves in both osmoregulation and/or excretion, not all details of these functions are clearly defined. In some forms, structural and biochemical features suggest reabsorptive functions. For instance, microvilli and alkaline phosphatase activity, both characteristic of absorptive epithelium, occur in the walls of the collecting ducts in such forms.

The major nitrogenous waste product in digeneans is ammonia, although urea and other soluble compounds also occur. It is not entirely clear how much of each of these compounds is eliminated through the tegument, digestive tract, or excretory system.

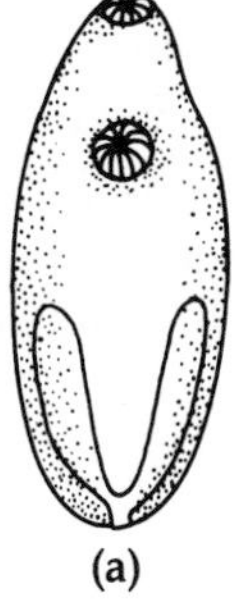

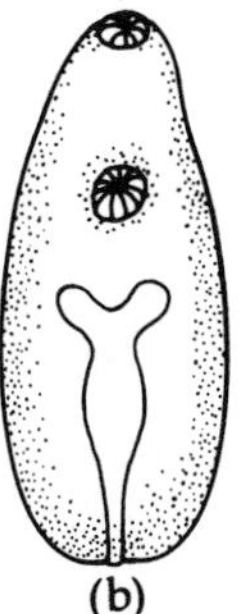

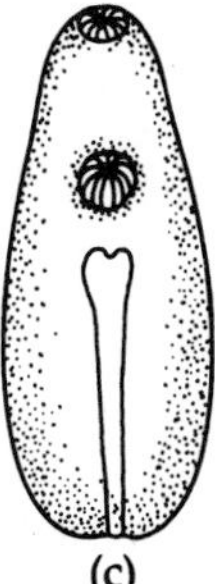

FIGURE 9-9
Shapes of excretory bladders of digenetic trematodes.
(a) V-shaped. (b) Y-shaped. (c) I-shaped.

In a number of forms, uric acid forms in the excretory bladder and tubules and is eliminated as insoluble crystals via the excretory pore.

REPRODUCTIVE SYSTEMS

With the exception of schistosomes, digenetic trematodes are hermaphroditic. The male reproductive system may mature prior to the female system, reducing the likelihood of self-fertilization.

Male System

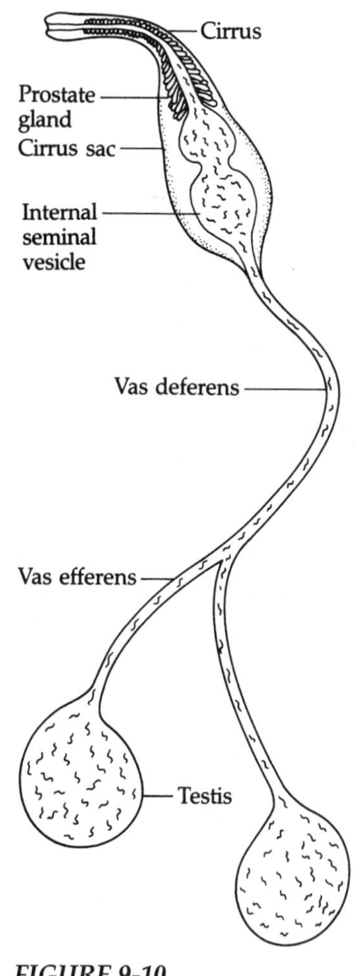

FIGURE 9-10
Male reproductive system of a digenetic trematode.

The male reproductive system (Fig. 9-10) generally includes two testes, although schistosomes are multitesticular. The position of the testes in the parenchyma varies according to species, as do the shape and orientation of the testes to each other. For instance, testes can be located anywhere from the middle to the posterior portion of the body. They can be ovoid, round, smooth, branched, or lobed. They can be tandem, side by side, or diagonal to each other. Such characteristics are useful in the identification of species. Spermatogenesis in the testes produces biflagellated sperm (Fig. 9-11).

Leading from each testis is a **vas efferens**, each of which unites with the others anteriorly to form the common **vas deferens.** Distally, this duct forms the male copulatory organ, or **cirrus.** The cirrus may be surrounded by a **cirrus sac** into which it can invaginate when not everted. Also enclosed by the cirrus sac are the sperm-storing **seminal vesicle** and the **prostate gland.** The eversible cirrus can be protruded to the exterior through a genital pore on the ventral surface of the organism.

Among digeneans, there are certain variations in the components of the vas deferens and their relative positions. One or more of these components may be missing (e.g., the prostate gland, the cirrus sac, and/or a protrusable cirrus), and the seminal vesicle often varies in size and position. The seminal vesicle is usually enclosed within the cirrus sac but is sometimes located outside the sac, in which case it is called an **external seminal vesicle.**

Female System

The female reproductive system consists of a single ovary embedded in the parenchyma anterior to, posterior to, or between

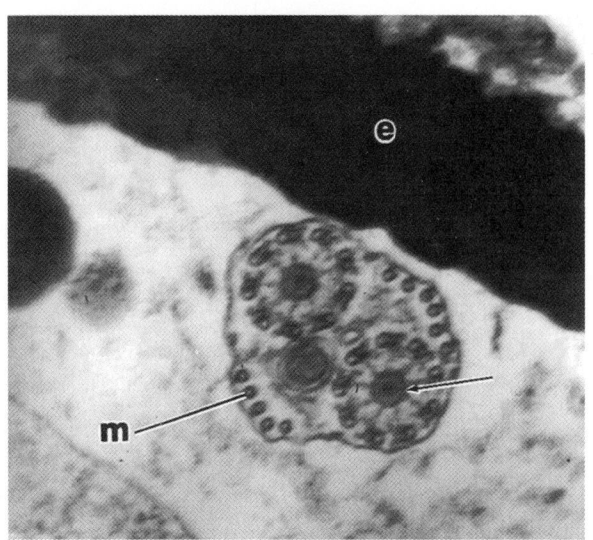

FIGURE 9-11
Cross section through a sperm of a digenetic trematode.
Note the pattern of nine outer doublets and a single, central microtubule (arrow) in each axoneme of the biflagellated sperm. m, Cortical microtubule; e, eggshell.

the testes, depending upon the species. **Ova** (actually secondary oocytes), are formed in the ovary and released via a short **oviduct.** They undergo a sequence of events analogous to an assembly line (Fig. 9-12). After leaving the ovary, each ovum passes down the oviduct to a minute chamber, the **ootype.** In this vicinity, the oviduct is joined by the duct of the seminal receptacle, in which sperm deposited earlier are stored. Fertilization occurs at this point, whereupon oogenesis is completed and cleavage begins. The ootype is surrounded by **Mehlis' gland,** which consists of two groups of unicellular glands: one group secretes a membranous body, and the other secretes a dense body. Among several functions suggested for these secretions, the most likely is that the membranous body provides a template for the deposition of shell material (Fig. 9-13), while the dense body lubricates the passage for the shelled egg. Other functions postulated for these secretions include activation of sperm, activation of vitelline glands to release shell material, and enhancement of eggshell hardening. Other glands that empty into the ootype are the **vitelline glands** (Fig. 9-14). In digeneans, these glands are composed of numerous multicellular clusters. Each cell synthesizes globules, which are then stored in its cytoplasm. When a cell attains a certain level of maturity, it detaches and enters a vitelline ductule. Groups of glands are usually situated bilaterally, although their distribution may vary according to species. The smaller vitelline ductules converge to form right and left **vitelline ducts** which, in turn, merge to form the **common vitelline duct,** which opens into the

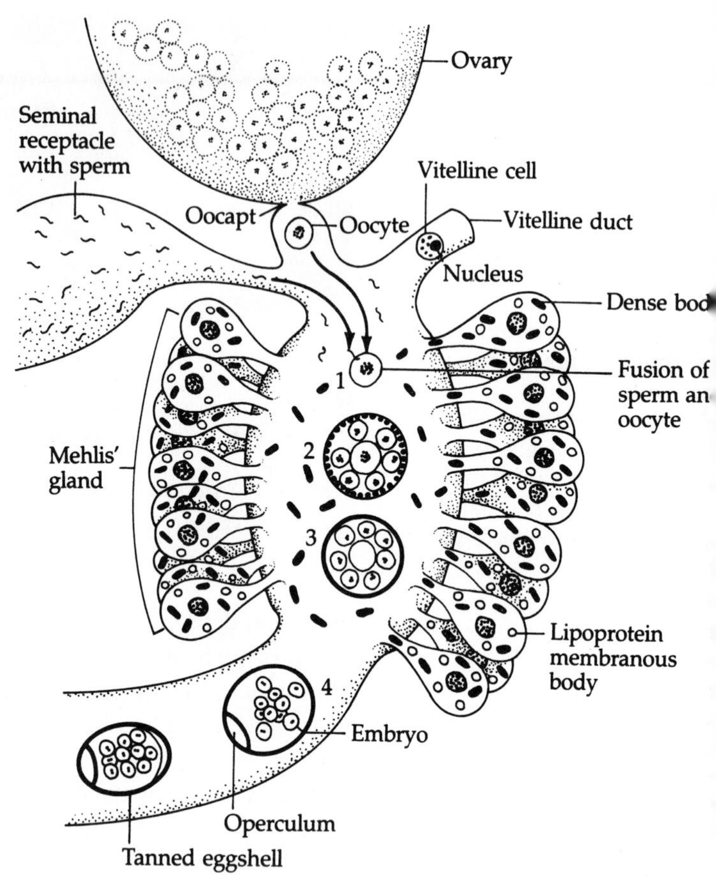

FIGURE 9-12
Sites of formation of constituents of a digenetic trematode egg (see text for description).

ootype. In some digeneans, the right and left vitelline ducts merge into a common chamber, the **vitelline reservoir**, which is connected to the ootype by a short duct.

The vitelline gland cells are essential to eggshell formation. The globules they release into the ootype become aligned against the membranous template derived from Mehlis' gland. These globules coalesce and eventually toughen to form the shell. This toughening process is accomplished by enzymatic cross-linking of proteins in the coalesced globules. In some species, tyrosine residues of the proteins are oxidized to "tan" the eggshell. This type of shell is rather hard and brown. In other forms, disulfide links are formed, producing an eggshell more elastic than the tanned form. The cytoplasm of vitelline cells provides nourishment for the developing embryo. According to some authorities, the uterine lining in some digeneans may also supply essential elements for eggshell formation.

The uterus is a long, often convoluted tube through which

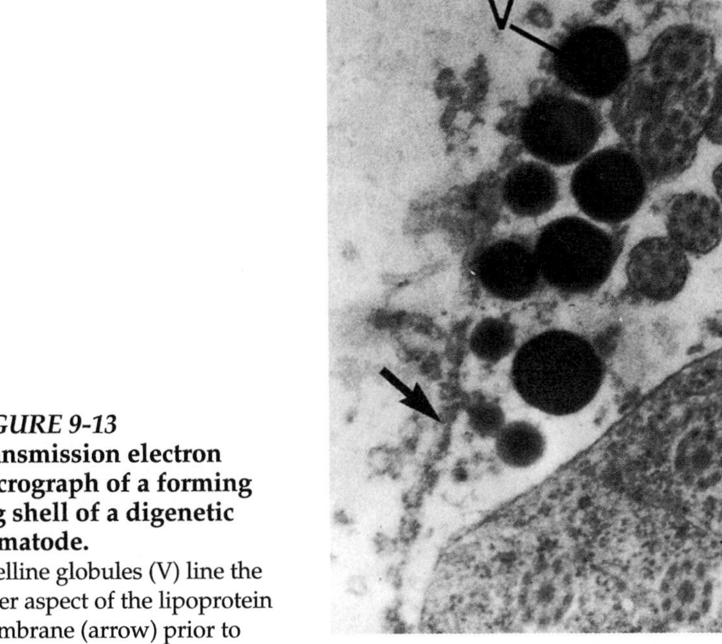

FIGURE 9-13
Transmission electron micrograph of a forming egg shell of a digenetic trematode.
Vitelline globules (V) line the inner aspect of the lipoprotein membrane (arrow) prior to fusion.

shelled eggs are transported to the exterior via the genital pore. In some species, a muscular, distal portion of the uterus, the **metraterm**, helps propel the eggs out of the uterus and aids in copulation. In addition to transporting eggs to the exterior, the uterus also permits sperm to move in the opposite direction, to the seminal receptacle. During copulation, the cirrus is inserted into the distal end of the uterus; sperm, ejaculated into the metraterm of the uterus, then swim to the seminal receptacle, where they are stored. In some species, a **Laurer's canal**, originating on the surface of the ootype, passes to the dorsal surface, where it may or may not open to the exterior. This canal may represent a vestigial vagina, or it may serve as an outlet for excess sperm and extraneous matter produced during egg formation.

The Egg

The ovoid, shelled egg contains vitelline substance, the embryo, ancillary membranes, and other materials (Fig. 9-15). The typical eggshell is equipped at one end with a lidlike structure, the **operculum**, which allows the larva to hatch. The eggshells of human

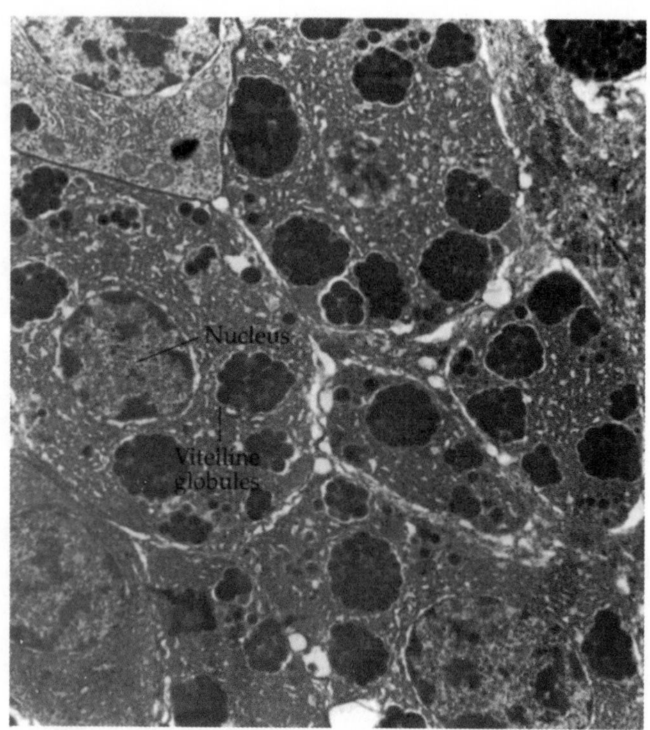

FIGURE 9-14
Transmission electron micrograph through the vitelline gland of a digenetic trematode.

a
Operculum
Viscous cushion
Developing miracidium
Vitelline membrane
Shell

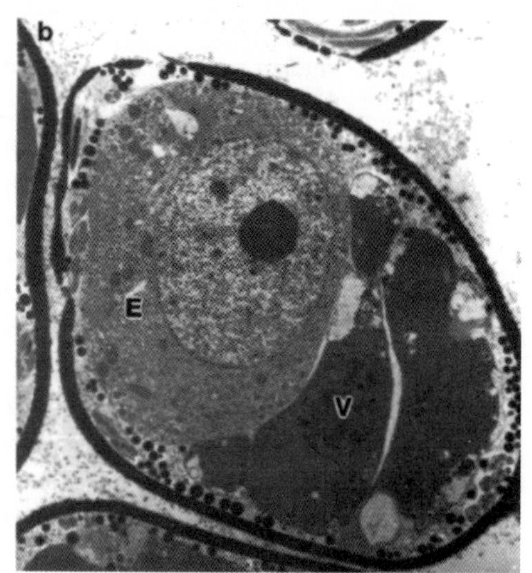

FIGURE 9-15
(a) Typical digenetic trematode egg. (b)Section through a digenetic trematode egg *in utero*. The embryo (E) is surrounded by a forming eggshell. Two vitelline cells (V) can be seen, with their expelled globules under the eggshell surface.

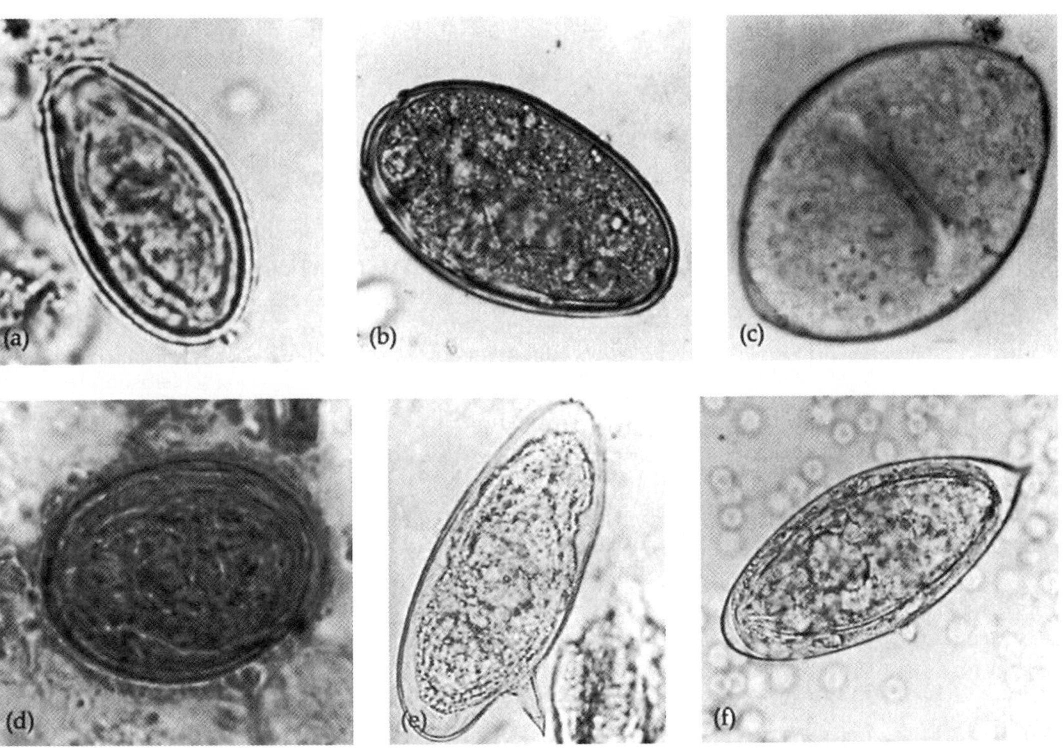

FIGURE 9-16
Eggs of some digenetic trematodes parasitic in humans.
(a) *Clonorchis sinensis*, 27–35 μm by 12–20 μm, urn-shaped, operculum at narrow end. (b) *Paragonimus westermani*, 80–118 μm by 48–60 μm, oval, operculum at flattened end. (c) *Fasciolopsis buski*, 130–140 μm by 80–85 μm, ellipsoidal, inconspicuous operculum. (d) *Schistosoma japonicum*, 7–100 μm by 50–65 μm, round to oval, inconspicuous lateral spine, no operculum. (e) *Schistosoma mansoni*, 114–175 μm by 45–68 μm, elongate oval, longer lateral spine, no operculum. (f) *Schistosoma haematobium*, 112–170 μm by 40–70 μm, spindle-shaped, posterior terminal spine, no operculum.

blood flukes possessing no operculum rupture longitudinally when those larvae hatch. Hatching occurs only under precise conditions of temperature, osmolarity, and light. For instance, in schistosomes that infect humans, hatching of embryonated eggs is inhibited by an osmolarity equivalent to 0.85% saline and a temperature of 37°C, thereby reducing the likelihood that the egg will hatch prematurely within the host's body. Most digenean eggs are unembryonated when they pass out of the human host and are unable to hatch without further development. Specific size and structural characteristics of trematode eggs, especially those of medically important species, are useful in diagnosis (Fig. 9-16).

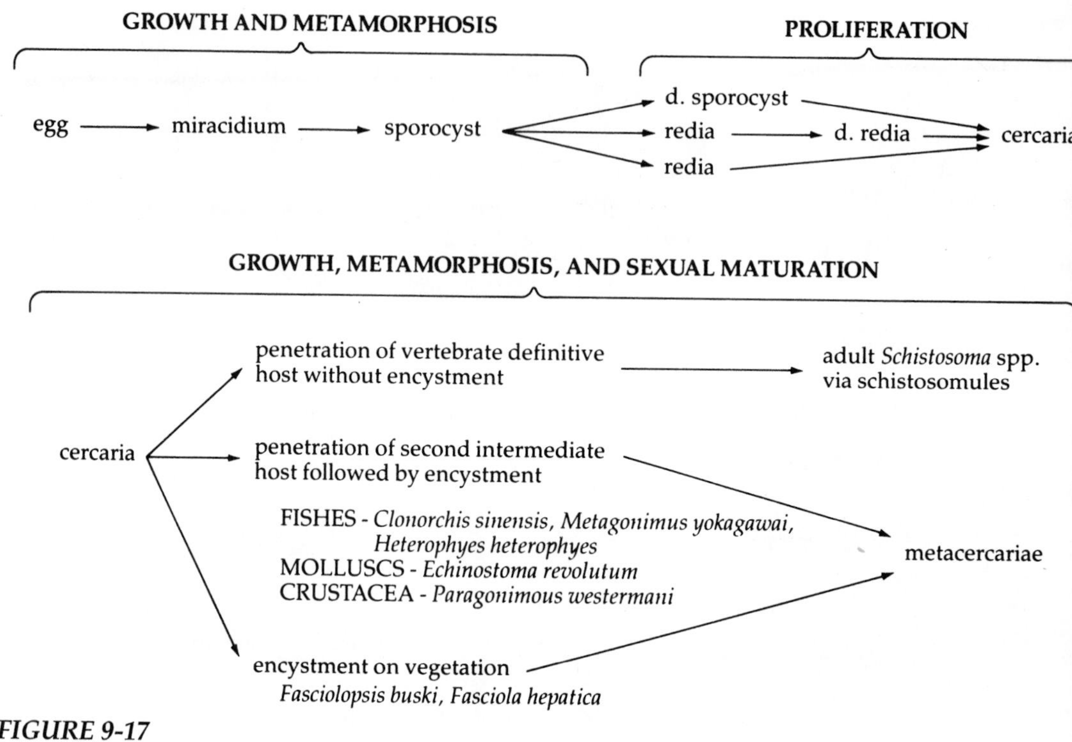

FIGURE 9-17
Flowchart showing life cycles of trematodes that infect humans.

GENERALIZED LIFE CYCLE PATTERNS

The following brief overview of the life cycles of digeneans that infect humans will illustrate the various larval stages and the relationship of each to the succeeding one (Fig. 9-17).

Eggs are usually released into the lumen of the host's organ housing the adult worm (gut, lungs, urinary bladder, etc.) and pass to the exterior through feces, sputum, or urine. If the egg is deposited in water, it completes its development, and a free-swimming **miracidium** (Fig. 9-18) hatches. Within 24 hours, the miracidium must find and penetrate the integument of a suitable freshwater snail host (the first intermediate host), shedding its ciliated epidermis in the process and metamorphosing into a **primary sporocyst** (Fig. 9-19), which may produce numerous secondary sporocysts or **primary rediae** asexually (Fig. 9-20). In

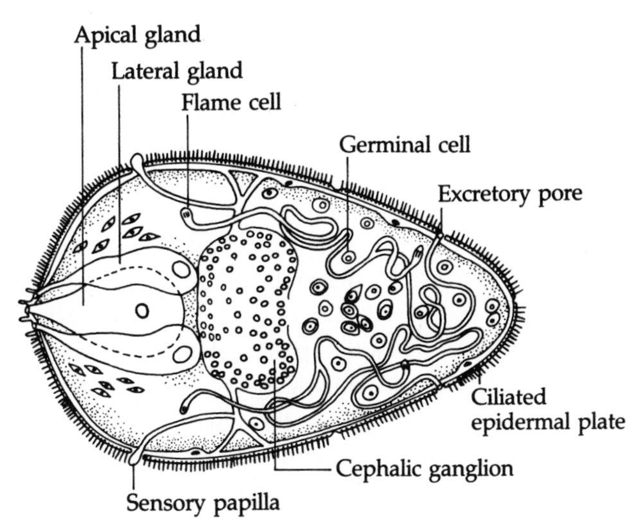

FIGURE 9-18
Miracidium of *Schistosoma*.

some forms, the egg must be ingested by the snail (particularly if the snail is terrestrial) before the miracidium hatches.

While the digestive gland of the snail is a common site for further development, other organs, including the gonad, the mantle, and the lymph spaces surrounding the intestine may also serve for such development. Once established in a suitable location, the sporocyst or redia grows, matures, and continues to proliferate.

Sporocysts are commonly elongate and hollow and contain germ cells, formed in the miracidium, that multiply by mitosis and develop into **germ balls.** Unlike a sporocyst, a redia possesses a functional, saclike gut and a pharynx.

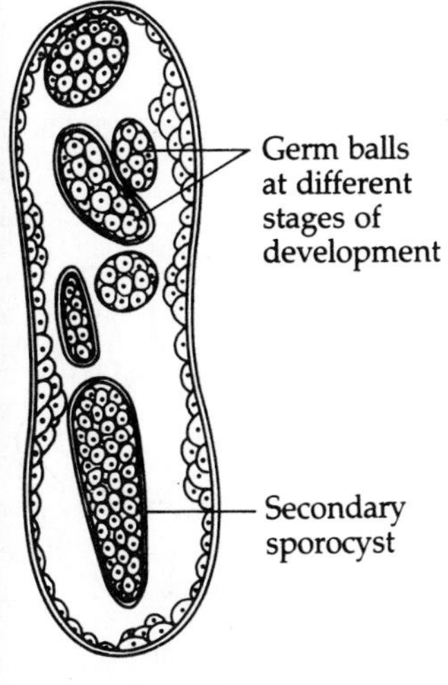

FIGURE 9-19
Primary sporocyst.

The redia or secondary sporocyst (depending on species) eventually gives rise to a tailed larva called a **cercaria** (Fig. 9-21). Cercariae that escape from the molluscan host experience only a brief (several-hour) free-swimming existence, because they do not feed outside the host. In some species, the cercariae may actively penetrate or attach to the surface of a second intermediate host or attach to vegetation; they lose their tails, encyst, and are then known as **metacercariae** (Fig. 9-22). Upon ingestion by a vertebrate definitive host, the encysted metacercaria excysts in the host's small intestine, migrates to the definitive site, and gradually matures into the adult stage. In schistosomes, cercariae penetrate the definitive host directly, thereby foregoing an encysted metacercarial stage.

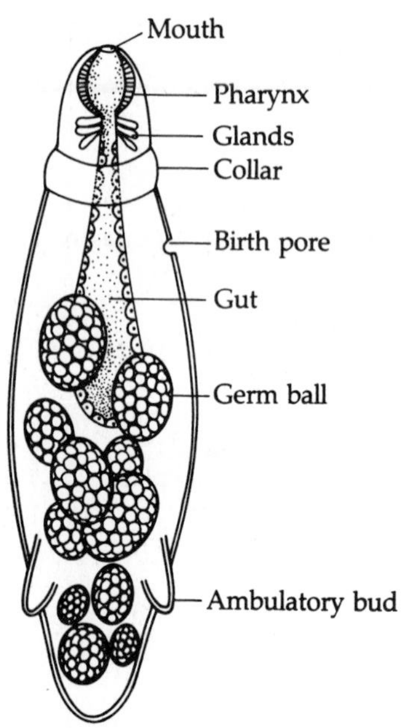

FIGURE 9-20
Redia of *Fasciola hepatica*.

THE MIRACIDIUM

The miracidium is a ciliated, nonfeeding larva (Fig. 9-18). Under favorable conditions, it escapes from the eggshell, usually through the operculum, and enters the environment. The miracidium is elongated and covered with flattened, ciliated epidermal plates. At the junctures of adjacent epidermal plates are **cytoplasmic ridges,** which play a prominent role during the miracidium's metamorphosis into the next larval stage. Beneath the epidermal plates are well-developed circular and longitudinal muscles.

At the anterior tip of the miracidium is a flexible **apical papilla** with sensory organs and three secretory glands—the apical gland and two lateral glands—that release materials at the tip of the papilla during host penetration (Fig. 9-23). During penetration, the papilla becomes partially invaginated, and secretions from the glands are captured in the depression. The papilla thus acts as a suction cup, holding the miracidium to the site of penetration and allowing the secretions to exert both adhesive and lytic actions.

In addition to the sensory structures in the papilla, there may be two to three anterior **eyespots** as well as **lateral papillae** on each side of the body. The "brain" of the miracidium lies in the parenchyma behind the apical region, from which nerve fibers innervate various tissues and organs of the body. The miracidium also has a simple, protonephridial excretory system. Waste-containing body fluids are collected by two or three pairs of flame cells and excreted through two lateral excretory pores.

During differentiation of the miracidium, germ cells grow and

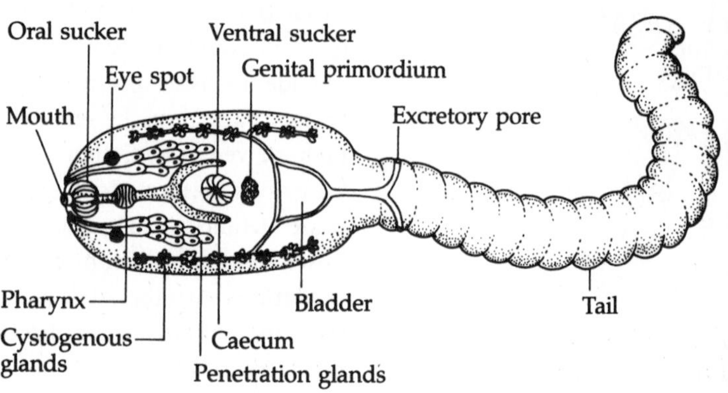

FIGURE 9-21
Cercaria of *Clonorchis sinensis*.

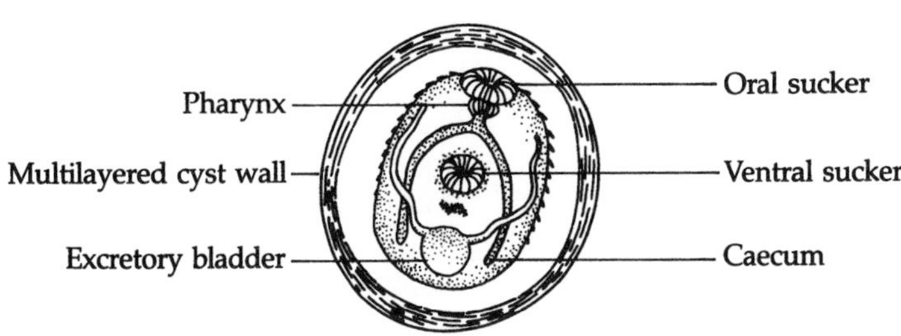

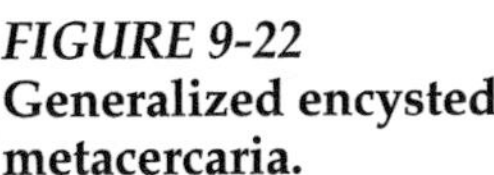

FIGURE 9-22
Generalized encysted metacercaria.

divide to form germ balls. Each germ ball eventually develops into a distinct, membrane-enclosed entity that is the next larval generation.

THE SPOROCYST

First-generation sporocysts, having differentiated from miracidia, usually accumulate near the site of penetration (mantle and head-foot), but occasionally they may reach the hemocoel in the digestive gland of the molluscan host. Less often, they may congregate along the digestive tract in certain species. The sporo-

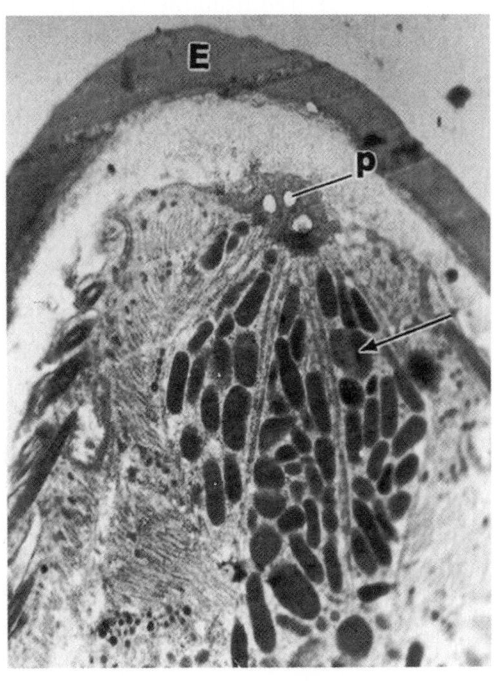

FIGURE 9-23
Section through a miradicium enclosed by an eggshell (E).
Note the gland openings in the apical papilla (p). The arrow points to gland contents.

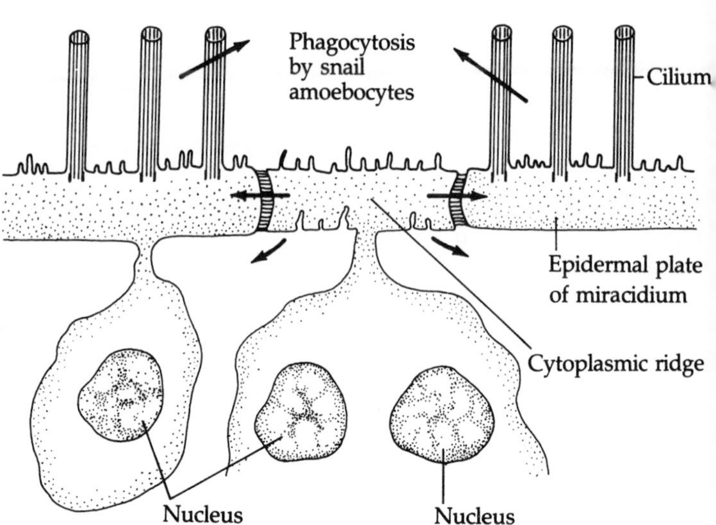

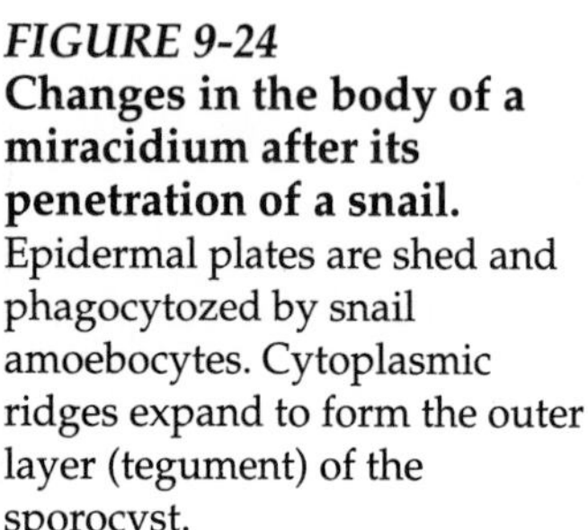
FIGURE 9-24
Changes in the body of a miracidium after its penetration of a snail. Epidermal plates are shed and phagocytozed by snail amoebocytes. Cytoplasmic ridges expand to form the outer layer (tegument) of the sporocyst.

cyst varies in shape from ovoid to elongate to tubular and may even be extensively branched (Fig. 9-19).

Seen in cross section, the thickness of the sporocyst wall varies according to age and species. As in all subsequent stages in the life cycle of digeneans, its outermost layer is a syncytial tegument derived from the cytoplasmic ridges of the miracidium. Prior to completing penetration of the first intermediate host, or shortly thereafter, the miracidial epidermal plates are shed; as the miracidium transforms into a sporocyst, the cytoplasmic ridges spread to form the tegument (Fig. 9-24). In most sporocysts, microvilli produce extensive amplification of the tegumental surface.

Beneath the tegument lies a thin basal lamina in which is embedded a layer of circular muscles. A thin layer of parenchyma underlies this area. These layers form the lining of the fluid-filled **brood chamber,** a cavity containing the germ balls. Sporocysts possess no digestive tract, and essential nutrients must diffuse across the absorptive tegument. Carbohydrates derived from body fluids of the infected mollusc are the chief source of energy for this stage. Definitive nervous and reproductive systems are also lacking, although flame cells are generally present.

In some species, germ balls in the brood chamber of mother (or primary) sporocysts differentiate to form daughter (or secondary) sporocysts. In other species, the germ balls differentiate into rediae or directly into cercariae. Daughter sporocysts usually are morphologically similar to primary sporocysts but can be distinguished by their larger size and their common occurrence in deeper body organs of the molluscan host, such as the digestive gland and gonads.

THE REDIA

Rediae, if present, develop from germ balls in the brood chamber of the primary sporocyst. They eventually escape from the sporocyst and migrate through the molluscan tissue to the digestive gland.

Each redia is elongate and normally possesses two or four budlike, antero- and posterolateral projections, the **ambulatory buds (procruscula)** (Fig. 9-20). As their name implies, the ambulatory buds facilitate movement of the larva through the tissues of the molluscan host. This movement is abetted by contractions of the redial body. Unlike the sporocyst, the redia possesses a digestive tract with an anterior mouth, a muscular pharynx, and an unbranched caecum. As the redia moves through the host's tissues, it actively ingests host cells, digesting them in the lumen of the caecum. Some rediae augment these intestinal feedings by secreting hydrolytic enzymes to the exterior and lysing surrounding host cells. The resulting molecules are then absorbed through the tegument, which is morphologically similar to that of the sporocyst. The physical effect of rediae upon the molluscan host is considerably more deleterious than that produced by sporocysts.

On each side of the pharynx is a cephalic ganglion from which nerve fibers radiate. Flame cells occur in most rediae, terminating at the bladder(s) in either single or multiple excretory pores.

Near the mouth of the redia there is usually a birth pore leading from the brood chamber. Within the brood chamber, germ balls differentiate into either secondary (daughter) rediae or the next larval stage, the cercaria.

THE CERCARIA

Cercariae differentiate from the germ balls in the brood chambers of secondary, tertiary, or subsequent generations of sporocysts or rediae, depending upon the life cycle of the particular digenean. A cercaria is usually equipped with a tail that enables it to swim (Fig. 9-25); a few species, such as the human lung fluke, have minute tails, limiting the cercaria to crawl on a substrate

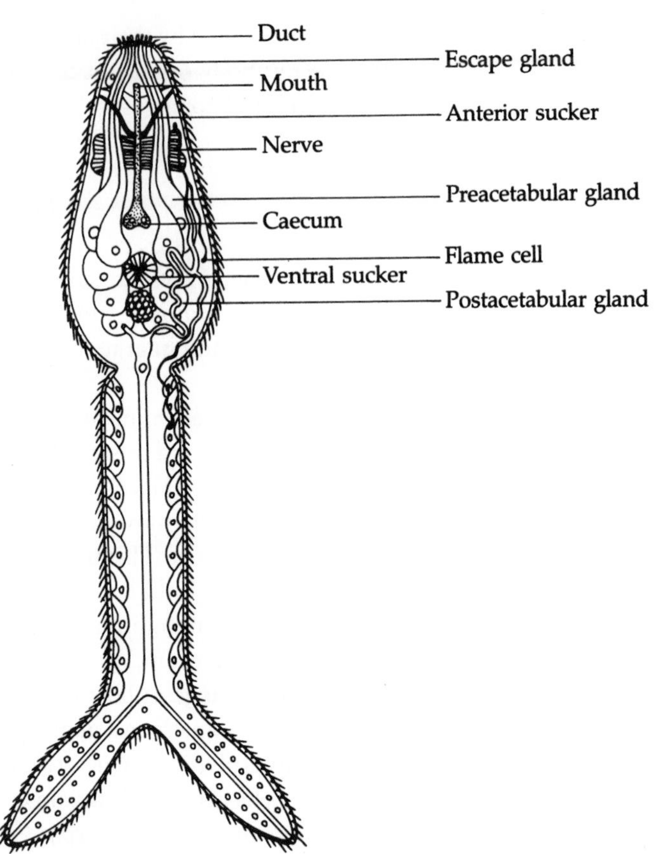

FIGURE 9-25
Fork-tailed cercaria of *Schistosoma* spp.

rather than swim. After escaping from the brood chamber through the birth pore, cercariae leave the molluscan host and actively seek the next host or suitable vegetation.

Regardless of species, the distribution of internal organs in all cercariae usually resembles that of the adult worm (Fig. 9-21). The mouth, situated at the anterior end of the body and surrounded by the oral sucker, leads into the foregut and paired caeca. There is a variably positioned ventral sucker whose location remains constant through adulthood. In many cercariae, several types of glands open anteriorly. The name of a gland indicates its assumed function. For example, in schistosome cercariae, a pair of **escape glands** lies near the mouth. The contents of these glands are secreted during the cercaria's emergence from the sporocyst in which it had developed as well as during its exit from the snail host. In liver fluke cercariae, **cystogenous glands** secrete substances to form a cyst wall. Other glands, such as **penetration glands** and **mucoid glands,** may play a role in host penetration, which may be further augmented by cuticular stylets capable of puncturing chitin-covered arthropods.

Embedded in the parenchyma, near the ventral sucker, is a genital primordium, a mass of germinal cells that eventually forms the male and female reproductive systems of the adult.

Cercariae also have protonephridial (flame cell) excretory systems. But, unlike sporocysts and rediae, cercariae have two lateral collecting tubules that empty into a common, posterior, excretory bladder from which a tube may extend posteriorly into the tail. The arrangment of flame cells in cercariae is similar to the arrangement in the adult. Thus, if the flame cell pattern in a cercaria is known, it can be used to correlate the larval form with its adult stage.

THE METACERCARIA

The next larval stage of most digeneans is the metacercaria (Fig. 9-22). When the free-swimming (or crawling) cercaria locates a suitable substrate or penetrates a second intermediate host, it sheds its tail and encysts. Within the cyst wall, the metacercaria may grow and develop into a more mature juvenile preadult, or its genital primordium may differentiate into a complete reproductive system that usually is nonfunctional. Many cercarial features, including certain glands and sensory structures, disappear.

Very little is known about the metabolism of metacercariae. It is generally assumed that they subsist primarily if not exclusively on stored nutrients. However, while many metacercariae appear metabolically quiescent, some encysted in animal tissues grow and, in fact, may exert a dynamic effect upon their host's metabolism. They commonly induce the host's cellular defenses, whereby they are encapsulated in fibrous connective tissue. All metacercariae, however, undergo one common developmental change: they become infective to their definitive hosts.

GERM CELL CYCLE

Reproduction in the miracidium–sporocyst–redia–cercaria progression is asexual, with the progeny arising through differentiation of germinal cells passed from one generation to the next. This phenomenon is known as the **germ cell cycle.** Only in the adult does sexual reproduction occur. Currently, the most widely accepted concept of intramolluscan reproduction among digeneans is that of **sequential polyembryony,** the production of multiple embryos from the same zygote with no intervening gamete production. There is some evidence of parthenogenesis in sporocysts of several digeneans as well as polyembryonic proliferation.

Of particular importance to those interested in gene expression is the observation that all stages in the digenean life cycle carry identical sets of genes. Yet the expression of these genes differs among the several stages. It is apparent, then, that certain genes are activated while others are suppressed at various times during the sequence of larval development. For example, genes responsible for the development of an intramolluscan larva into a redia are suppressed in circumstances in which development into a sporocyst is indicated, and vice versa. What triggers this activation–suppression cycle has yet to be established.

Although the life cycle in a given species almost always follows the same pattern, the sequential pattern can be altered in some digeneans by environmental factors, such as temperature changes, and by experimental manipulations, such as transplanting the parasite from one mollusc to another. These alterations consist primarily of variations in the number and type of intramolluscan generations of larvae.

PHYSIOLOGY

During the past two decades, considerable information has been compiled concerning the biochemistry and physiology of digenetic trematodes. Much of this information has been derived from studies of the adult sheep liver fluke *Fasciola hepatica*. A number of factors are responsible for this emphasis: the adult worms are large and easy to work with, the life cycle can be easily maintained in the laboratory, and the economic and medical importance of this species attracts interest and funding for experimentation. The physiology of human blood flukes, or schistosomes, has also been studied intensively for similar reasons. Unfortunately, physiological and biochemical information on other genera and on larval forms is meager. Much of the following overview of the physiology of digeneans is derived from studies of the genera *Fasciola* and *Schistosoma*.

Substrate-level phosphorylation, via glycolysis, is the main source of energy for these adult digeneans, with glycogen and glucose as the principal metabolized carbohydrates. Even in the presence of oxygen, as occurs in the blood vessels, for example, glycolysis provides the primary energy supply. In *Fasciola*, oxygen is used when available, but its contribution toward satisfying the organism's overall energy requirements is difficult to assess. It is debatable whether a functional Krebs cycle exists in *Fasciola* or in the schistosomes. If such a cycle does function, its overall role in energy production is probably minimal. Some enzymes usually involved in the Krebs cycle may actually serve in other metabolic pathways in some instances.

The dependence of adult digeneans on glycolysis for energy has been useful in the search for effective drugs to treat patients infected with these parasites. For example, the efficacy of trivalent antimony compounds in treating schistosomiasis derives from their ability to inhibit phosphofructokinase, an important enzyme in the glycolytic pathway. A requisite for any effective drug is that the equivalent host enzyme must not be affected by the same concentration of drug that affects the parasite.

The miracidia and cercariae of all species studied to date are obligate aerobes, relying on oxidative phosphorylation for energy. Intramolluscan stages, on the other hand, resemble more the adult forms in their dependency upon substrate-level phosphorylation to supply energy-rich compounds.

The limited information available on the synthetic abilities of *Fasciola* and the schistosomes shows that these parasites depend upon their hosts for a number of essential compounds, including pyrimidines, arginine, and lipids such as sterols and saturated and unsaturated fatty acids. The worms can probably synthesize complex lipids, provided they are supplied with fatty acids and other basic essential molecules.

TREATMENT

The most effective chemotherapeutic regimen against the majority of trematodes infecting humans is the oral administration of the drug praziquantel. While the mode of action of this drug is still being investigated, it is known that its primary target is the tegument. It produces vacuolization and, by affecting calcium ion permeability, causes rapid diffusion of calcium ions, resulting in rapid muscle paralysis in the parasite. However, praziquantel is not effective against *Fasciola hepatica*. Apparently, at the dosage used for treatment, the tegument of *F. hepatica* is more resistant to the drug than those of other flukes. Whether this increased resistance is due to differences in the permeability of the tegument or to differences in the susceptibility of the worm's tissues is not known. However, the amount of the drug required to produce muscle tetany is 100 times greater for *F. hepatica* than for other worms.

SELECTED READINGS

Bogitsh, B. J. 1986. An overview of surface specializations in the digenetic trematodes. *Hydrobiologia* **132,** 305–310.

Fried, B., and Haseeb, M. A. 1991. Platyhelminthes: Aspidogastrea, monogenea, and digenea. In *Microscopic Anatomy of the Invertebrates* (Harrison, F. W., and Bogitsh, B. J., Eds.), Vol. 3, pp. 141–209, Wiley-Liss, New York.

Llewellyn, J. 1965. The evolution of parasitic platyhelminths. In *Evolution of Parasites* (Taylor, A., Ed.). Blackwell Scientific, Oxford, England.

Smyth, J. D. 1995. Rare, new and emerging helminth zoonoses. *Advances in Parasitology* **36,** 1–45.

Smyth, J. D., and Halton, D. W. 1983. *The Physiology of Trematodes,* 2nd ed. Cambridge University, New York.

Whitfield, P. J., and Evans, N. A. 1983. Parthenogenesis and asexual multiplication among parasitic platyhelminths. *Parasitology* **86,** 121–160.

CLASSIFICATION OF THE TREMATODA*

PHYLUM PLATYHELMINTHES

CLASS TURBELLARIA

Mostly free-living worms in terrestrial, freshwater, and marine environments; some are commensals or parasites of invertebrates, especially of echinoderms and molluscs.

*Only those taxa that include parasitic species discussed in this text are defined.

CLASS MONOGENEA

All parasitic, mainly on the skin or gills of fish; although most are ectoparasites, a few live within the stomadaeum, proctodaeum, or their diverticula.

CLASS TREMATODA

All parasitic, mainly in the digestive tracts of all classes of vertebrates; three subclasses.

Subclass Aspidogastrea

Most have only one host, a mollusc; a few mature in marine turtles or fishes and have a mollusc or lobster as intermediate host.

Subclass Digenea

At least two hosts in life cycle, the first almost always a mollusc; perhaps most diversification in marine bony fishes, although many species in all other groups of vertebrates.

SUPERFAMILY SCHISTOSOMATOIDEA

Dioecious adults in vascular system of definitive host; pharynx absent; no second intermediate host in life cycle; cercaria furcocercous with relatively short rami; oral sucker of cercaria replaced by protractile penetration organ; cercarial eyespots either pigmented or not; parasites of fishes, reptiles, birds, and mammals. (Genus mentioned in text: *Schistosoma*.)

SUPERFAMILY ECHINOSTOMATOIDEA

Adult and cercaria usually with circumoral collar, commonly armed with spines; parasites of reptiles, birds, and mammals. (Genera mentioned in text: *Fasciola, Fasciolopsis, Echinostoma*)

SUPERORDER EPITHELIOCYSTIDIA

Wall of embryonic excretory vesicle (bladder) replaced by epithelial cells of mesodermal origin; cercaria with simple, straight tail; cercarial oral stylet commonly present.

SUPERFAMILY ALLOCREADIOIDEA

Adult one of several morphologic types; with or without eyespots; oral sucker usually simple, some with appendages; acetabulum in anterior half of body; testes in posterior half of body; ovary pretesticular; cercaria one of several morphologic types; cercaria usually with eyespots; parasites of fish, amphibians, reptiles, and mammals. (Genus mentioned in text: *Paragonimus*)

SUPERFAMILY OPISTHORCHIOIDEA

Cercaria with well-developed penetration glands; cercarial oral sucker protractile; cercarial ventral sucker rudimentary; cercarial tail one of several types; parasites of fish, amphibians, reptiles, birds, and mammals. (Genera mentioned in text: *Opisthorchis, Clonorchis, Heterophyes, Metagonimus*)

Chapter Ten

VISCERAL FLUKES

Species belonging to eight genera in five families commonly infect various visceral organs of humans. Members of the genera *Fasciola, Clonorchis*, and *Opisthorchis* reside in the liver; those of *Fasciolopsis*, *Heterophyes*, *Metagonimus*, and *Echinostoma* inhabit the small intestine; and several members of the genus *Paragonimus*, notably *P. westermani*, live in the lungs. For the sake of convenience, discussion of the organisms is organized according to the site of infection rather than phylogenetic relationships. The classification system at the end of Chapter 9 summarizes phylogenetic affinities.

LIVER FLUKES

FASCIOLA HEPATICA

Fasciola hepatica, the sheep liver fluke, is one of the largest digeneans parasitizing humans, measuring 30 mm long by 13 mm wide (Fig. 10-1a). In addition to its size, *F. hepatica* can be distinguished from other digeneans by its highly branched testes and intestinal caeca; the short, convoluted uterus; oral and ventral suckers of equal size, the former situated on an anterior prominence called the **cephalic cone**; and vitellaria that extend along the lateral edges of the body to the posterior end. Adult worms live in the bile ducts, gallbladder, and liver tissue of their mammalian hosts.

Life Cycle

Fasciola hepatica occupies a prominent place in parasitology because its life cycle (Fig. 10-2) was the first among digenetic trematodes to be completely elucidated, and that achievement has been the impetus for all subsequent investigations on life histories.

The ovoid eggs are relatively large (130–150 μm by 63–

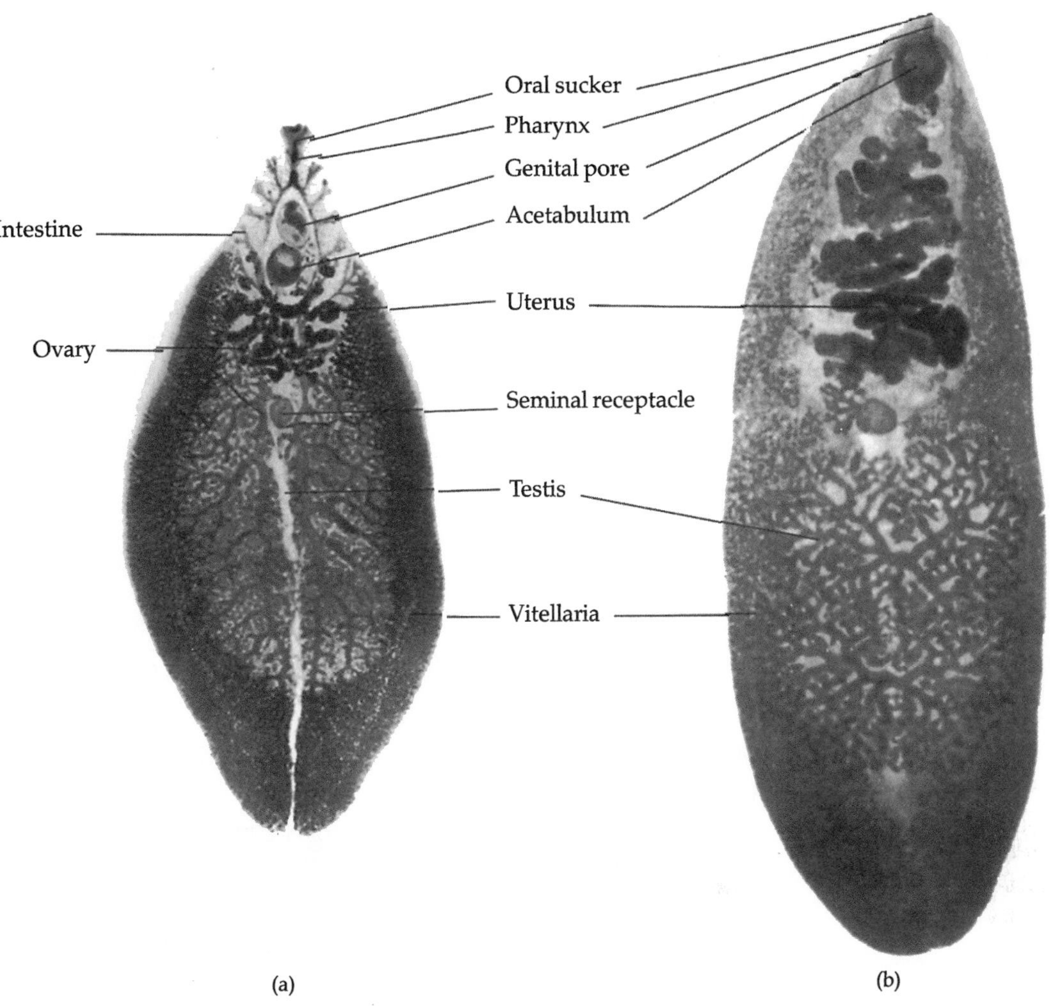

FIGURE 10-1
Two fasciolid flukes.
(a) *Fasciola hepatica*, the sheep liver fluke. (b) *Fasciolopsis buski*.

90 μm), operculate, and yellowish-brown in color. Expelled before the miracidium is fully developed, they pass into the host's alimentary tract via the common bile duct and eventually reach the exterior with feces, at which time they must encounter fresh water if the cycle is to continue.

After 4–15 days in water at approximately 22°C, the completely developed miracidium escapes when the operculum opens. The miracidium has eyespots and is positively phototaxic.

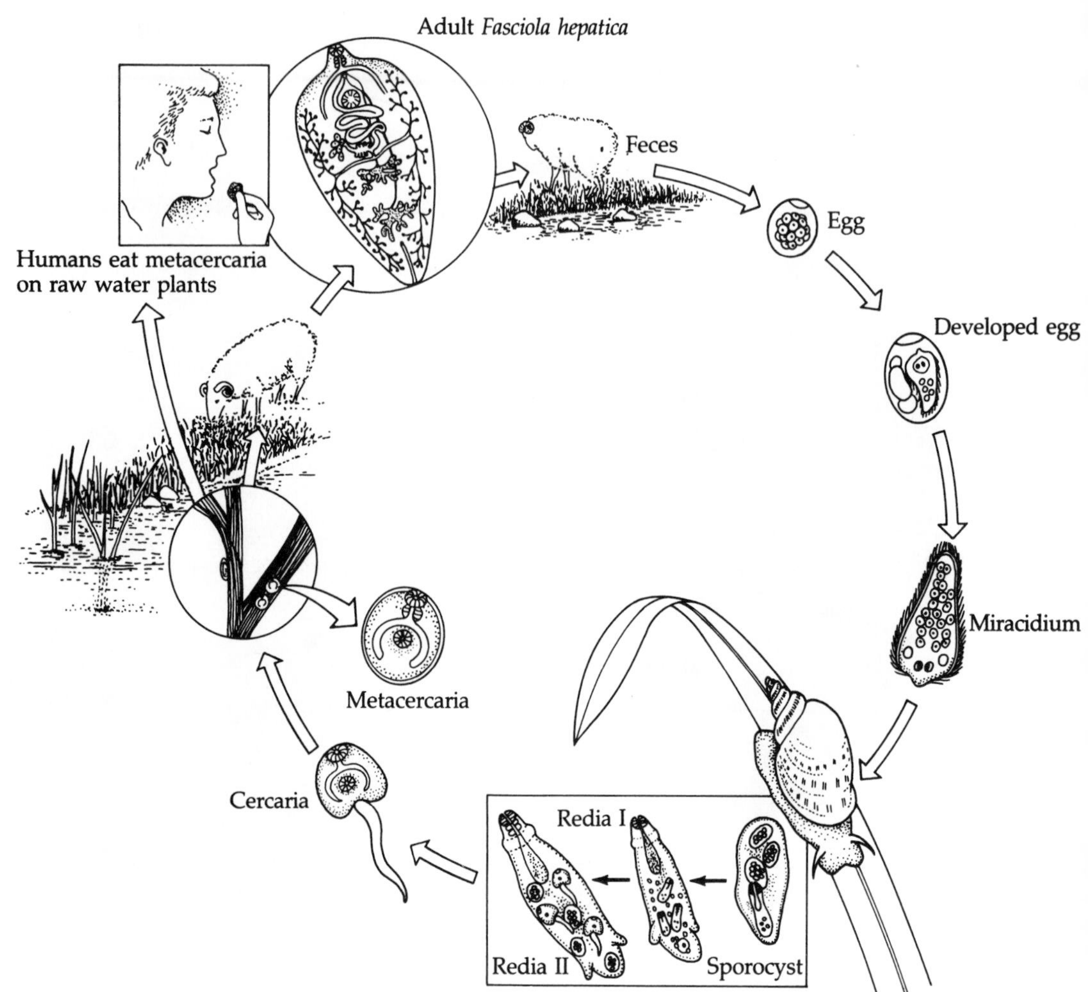

FIGURE 10-2
Life cycle of *Fasciola hepatica*.

Its survival depends upon its success in locating and penetrating a suitable snail host within 8 hours after hatching. Members of the amphibious snail genera *Lymnaea*, *Succinea*, *Fossaria*, and *Practicolella* serve as first intermediate hosts. Upon penetration, each miracidium metamorphoses into a sporocyst that gives rise to mother rediae which, in turn, produce daughter rediae. Germ balls in the brood chamber of daughter rediae develop into cercariae, which emerge from the snail and become free swimming. Upon reaching aquatic, emergent vegetation (e.g., grass) or even submerged bark, the cercariae shed their tails and encyst as metacercariae on plants upon which sheep and cattle commonly feed. Humans become infected by eating contaminated watercress and other vegetation.

Metacercariae swallowed by the definitive host excyst in the duodenum, penetrate the intestinal wall, and enter the liver capsule via the body cavity. Migration through the liver parenchyma allows them to consume liver cells and blood before they reach the bile ducts, where they attain sexual maturity in approximately 12 weeks. Adult *F. hepatica* can live up to 11 years.

Epidemiology

Human infection by *F. hepatica* occurs throughout the world and is of increasing importance in some Caribbean islands and South America, as well as southern France, Great Britain, and Algeria. Ecologically, human infection occurs most frequently in sheep- and cattle-raising regions. Livestock infections can result in heavy economic losses in wool, milk, and meat production. In one abattoir, annual economic losses from infected beef liver were estimated to be in the thousands of dollars.

Symptomatology and Diagnosis

F. hepatica infection in humans, or fascioliasis, is characterized by extensive destruction of liver tissue and bile ducts, hemorrhage, atrophy of portal vessels, and secondary, potentially lethal, pathological conditions. In addition to mechanical damage, the worms may evoke inflammatory reactions when the host becomes sensitized to the worms' metabolic products. Juvenile worms may get lost in the body cavity, encyst in ectopic tissues, and eventually become calcified.

Initial symptoms frequently include severe headache, backache, chills, and fever. An enlarged, tender, or cirrhotic liver, accompanied by diarrhea and anemia, indicates advanced infection.

Laboratory diagnosis is based on identification of the characteristic eggs (see Fig. 9-15) in patients' feces. Computer tomography (CT) scans are also diagnostically useful, and an enzyme-linked immunosorbent assay (ELISA) is especially effective in diagnosis of extrahepatic infections.

It is of interest that, when eaten by humans in the Middle East, raw bovine liver harboring *Fasciola hepatica* produces pain, irritation, hoarseness, and coughing due to the attachment of young worms to buccal or pharyngeal membranes. This condition, known as **halzoun,** is more commonly caused by pentastomids (tongue worms) and leeches acquired in a similar manner.

Treatment

Praziquantel, a drug that has proven successful in treating a wide variety of trematode infections, is ineffective against *Fasciola*. The current recommended treatment for fascioliasis is oral administration of Bithinol.

CLONORCHIS SINENSIS

Clonorchis sinensis, the Chinese or Oriental liver fluke, is distributed widely in Korea, Japan, China, Taiwan, and Vietnam and has been estimated to infect at least 19 million persons. A distinctive feature of these members of the family Opisthorchiidae is their small suckers. The flukes infect the biliary system of reptiles, birds, and mammals. Prosobranch snails serve as the molluscan hosts, and freshwater fishes, such as carp, serve as second intermediate hosts.

Life Cycle

The adult worm resides in the bile ducts of the human host (Fig. 10-3) and varies in size from 12–20 mm long and from 3–5 mm wide. The body is tapered anteriorly, while the posterior end is somewhat blunt (Fig. 10-4). The poorly developed ventral sucker lies about one-fourth the body length from the anterior end, just behind the common genital pore. The caeca extend to the posterior region of the body. A centrally located ovary lies just anterior to the branched, tandemly arranged testes. The vitellaria are lateral, and a loosely coiled, gravid uterus extends from the region of the ovary to the genital pore. The tanned eggs, which measure 29 μm by 16 μm, are operculated, with a ridge or collar at the base of the operculum, giving them an unusual urn shape (see Fig. 9-15). There is also a characteristic knob at the abopercular end of the shell.

Eggs containing partially developed embryos are deposited in the biliary ducts and pass out of the host's body with feces. Although the egg contains a fully developed miracidium by the time it reaches fresh water, it does not hatch immediately. Instead,

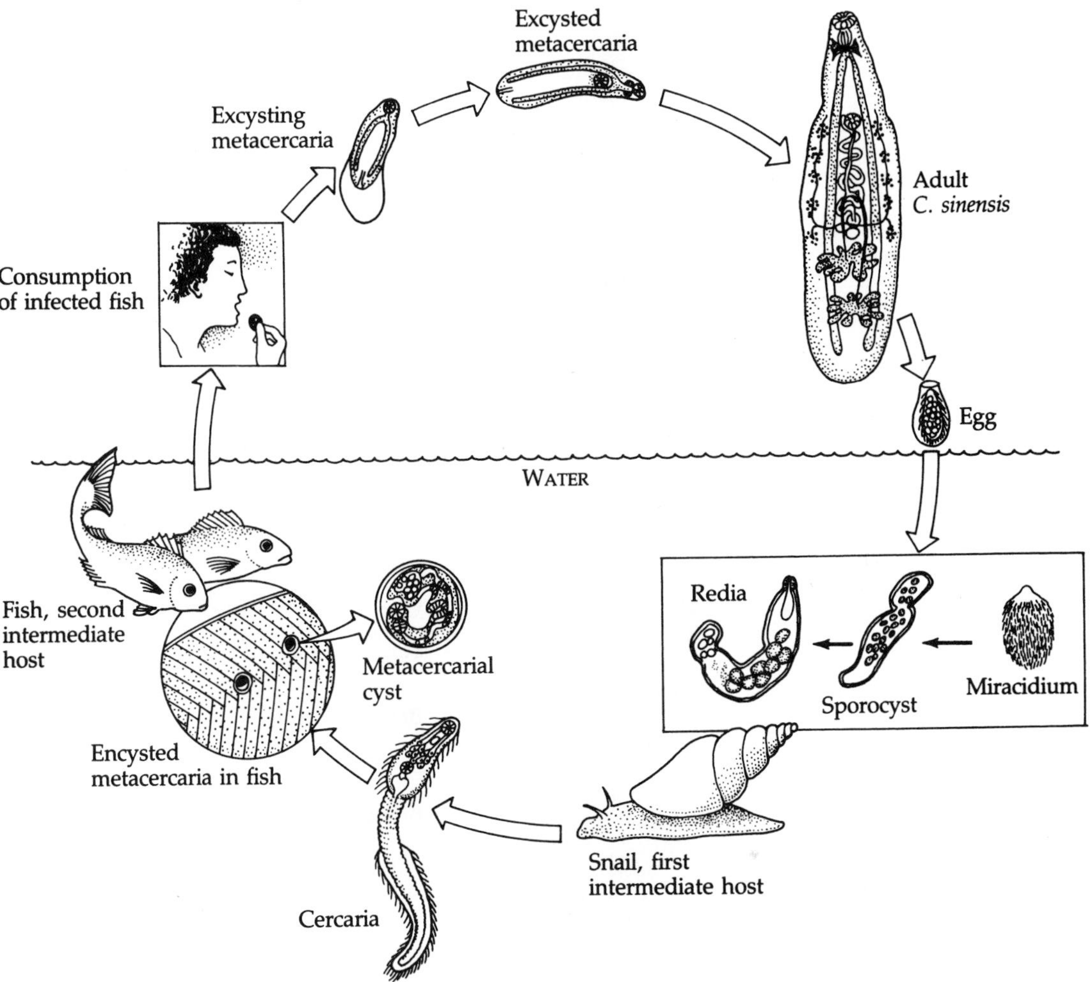

FIGURE 10-3
Life cycle of *Clonorchis sinensis*.

hatching is delayed until the egg reaches the digestive tract of a suitable snail intermediate host, one belonging to any of the genera *Parafossarulus*, *Bulimus*, *Semisulcospira*, *Alocinma*, and *Melanoides*. The released miracidium penetrates the intestinal wall of the snail and moves through the hemocoel to the digestive gland, where it metamorphoses into a sporocyst. The sporocyst gives rise to rediae, which erupt from the sporocyst and, in turn, produce cercariae. In order to survive, the free-swimming cercariae that emerge from the snail must penetrate the skin, gills,

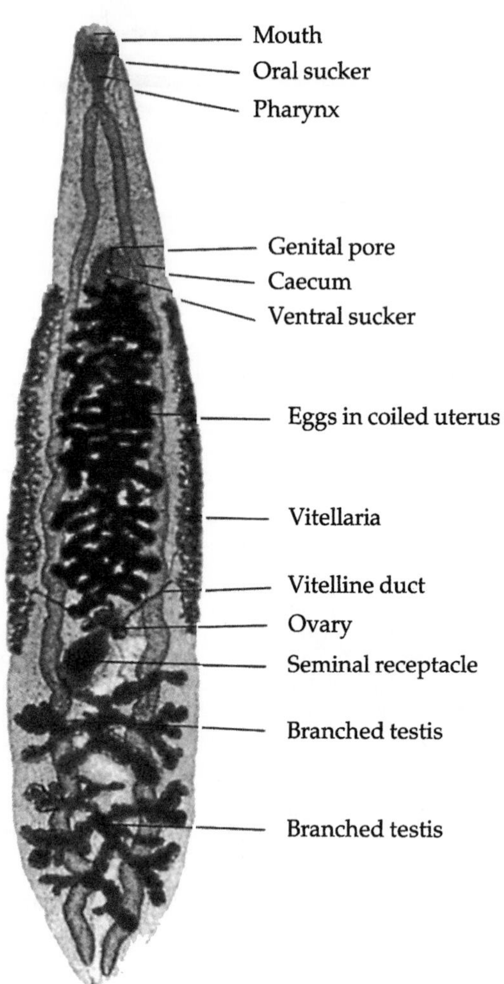

FIGURE 10-4
The digenetic trematode *Clonorchis sinensis*, the Chinese liver fluke.

fins, or muscles of a freshwater fish host within 24–48 hours. Each cercaria burrows into one of these tissues, loses its tail, and encysts as a metacercaria. A wide variety of fish species belonging to the family Cyprinidae serve as second intermediate hosts. Humans become infected by eating raw or poorly cooked fish (including steamed, smoked, or pickled fish). The metacercaria excysts in the duodenum and migrates up the common bile duct to the biliary ducts, feeding continually on the contents of the ducts. The worm reaches sexual maturity about a month after excystation and has been known to live up to 25 years in the human host.

Epidemiology

Reservoir hosts, including cats, dogs, tigers, foxes, badgers, and mink, play a significant role in maintaining Oriental fluke populations in endemic areas. The high incidence of mammalian infection, the increase in freshwater fish farming in the Orient, and the practice of eating fish raw have made clonorchiasis a serious problem. Oriental aquaculture ponds are commonly fertilized with human excrement to enhance the growth of vegetation on which the fish feed. In Hong Kong, where fish farming is very common, the prevalence of human clonorchiasis is about 14%; in rural endemic areas, it may reach 80%.

Symptomatology and Diagnosis

Damage to human hosts is most severe in the bile ducts, as manifested by mechanical and toxic irritation. The extent of damage is proportional to the number of worms present; over 6000 adult worms have been recovered from a single patient at autopsy. In such extreme cases, liver enlargement, thickening of the bile ducts, fibrosis, and some destruction of liver parenchyma are evident. Unlike *Fasciola*, however, *Clonorchis* does not invade liver tissues and, therefore, does not cause extensive necrosis. Intestinal disturbances are also common, but clonorchiasis is rarely fatal except when lowered resistance leaves patients vulnerable to secondary infections.

Positive diagnosis depends on identification of eggs in either feces or biliary drainage. Eggs must be differentiated from those of heterophyids (see the following sections). Clinical examination is warranted whenever there is liver enlargement coupled with a history of residence in endemic areas.

Treatment

Praziquantel administered over a two-day period is the treatment of choice. In light infections, prognosis is good even without treatment because tissue invasion is not involved.

OPISTHORCHIS FELINEUS AND *OPISTHORCHIS VIVERRINI*

Opisthorchis felineus and *O. viverrini* are parasitic in the bile ducts of fish-eating mammals, including humans (Fig. 10-5).

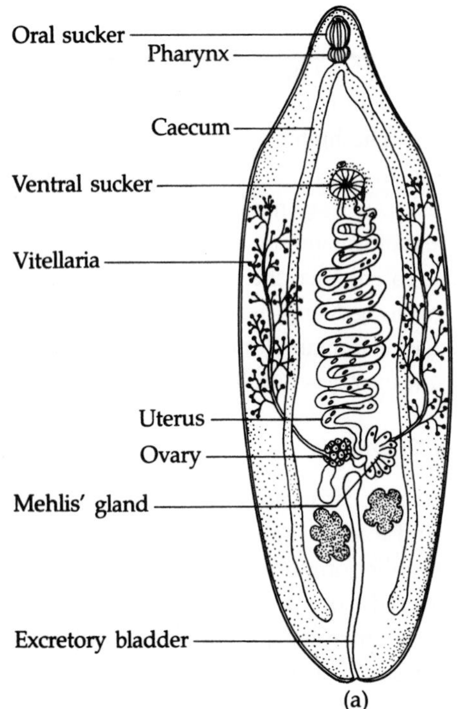

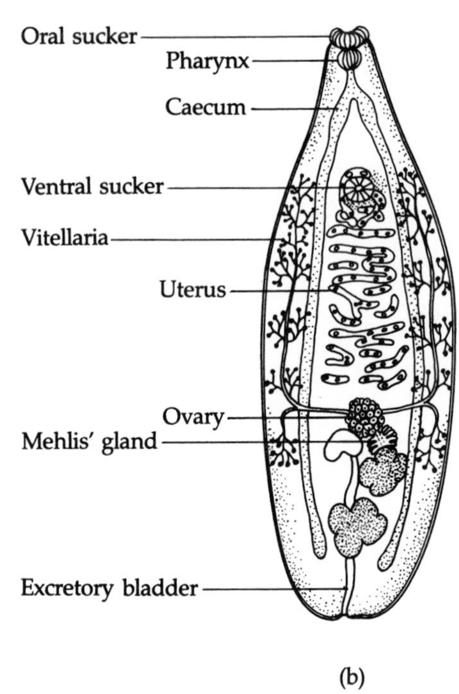

FIGURE 10-5
(a) *Opisthorchis felineus* adult. (b) *O. viverrini* adult.

Opisthorchis felineus is most commonly seen in southern, central, and eastern Europe, Turkey, the southern part of Russia, Vietnam, India, and Japan. It is also present in Puerto Rico and possibly other Caribbean islands. In Thailand, Laos, and southeast Asia, *O. viverrini* occurs in an estimated 1–3 million humans. Patients harboring these worms suffer from diarrhea and from thickening and eventual erosion of the bile duct wall.

The life cycles of *O. felineus* and *O. viverrini* are similar to that of *C. sinensis*, employing intermediate hosts of the snail genus *Bithynia* as well as cyprinid fishes, such as the chub or trench. Although infection by these worms is more common in animals, human infection results from eating raw or improperly cooked fish infected with encysted metacercariae. Felines are important reservoir hosts in endemic areas for both *O. felineus* and *O. viverrini.*

Opisthorchiasis is clinically indistinguishable from clonorchiasis, and treatment is similar to that for clonorchiasis.

INTESTINAL FLUKES

FASCIOLOPSIS BUSKI

Fasciolopsis buski is the largest digenean infecting humans, reaching a size of 75 mm by 20 mm. It is morphologically similar to *Fasciola hepatica* with a few notable differences (Fig. 10-1b). The most obvious of these are that, in *F. buski*, the caeca lack side branches, the ventral sucker is much larger than the oral sucker, and there is no cephalic cone. It differs further from all other members of the family Fasciolidae in that the definitive habitat is the small intestine of humans and pigs rather than the liver.

Life Cycle

Adult worms inhabit the duodenal and jejunal regions of the small intestine, either attached by their suckers to the mucosal epithelium or buried in the mucous secretions (Fig. 10-6). Each worm deposits about 25,000 eggs daily. The eggs, which are indistinguishable from those of *F. hepatica*, are expelled in feces and must reach fresh water in order to continue the cycle. In fresh water, miracidia develop and hatch in 3–7 weeks, depending on temperature. After locating and penetrating a planorbid snail of the genus *Segmentina* or *Hippeutis*, the miracidia metamorphose into sporocysts, which subsequently give rise to two sequential redial generations. Cercariae emerge from the daughter rediae 4–7 weeks after miracidial penetration of the snail, reenter the water, and encyst on freshwater vegetation, most commonly water chestnut, water caltrop, water bamboo, and lotus. Encysted metacercariae are ingested by humans when they eat contaminated raw plants or peel the pods or stalks with their teeth before eating, thereby freeing the encysted metacercaria, which are then swallowed. Metacercariae excyst in the small intestine, attach to the mucosa, and develop to sexual maturity in 25–30 days.

Epidemiology

Human infection by *F. buski* occurs throughout central and south China, Taiwan, Laos, Vietnam, Cambodia, India, Korea, and Indonesia. The infection is usually acquired by ingestion of encyst-

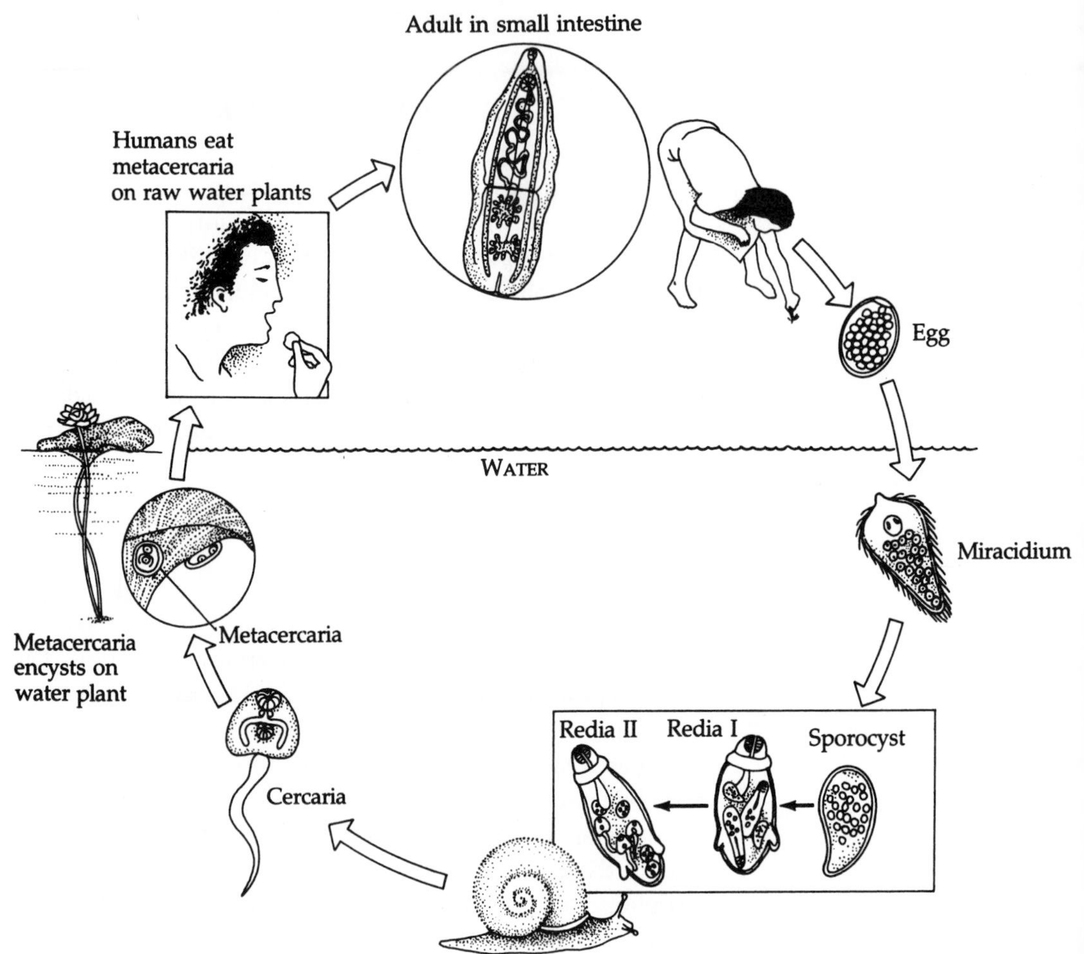

FIGURE 10-6
Life cycle of *Fasciolopsis buski.*

ed metacercariae from fresh plants grown in ponds fertilized with human or swine excrement. Drying or cooking the plants before eating kills the metacercariae. Hogs are the most important animal reservoirs for *F. buski.*

Symptomatology and Diagnosis

The worms feed actively not only on the host's intestinal contents but also on the superficial mucosa, causing inflammation, ulceration, and abscesses at sites of attachment. Diarrhea, nausea, and intestinal pain are common, especially in the morning hours. Intestinal edema occurs in heavier infections. Eating may relieve the abdominal distress unless the food happens to consist of infested aquatic plants, in which case symptoms will eventually be exacerbated. The large size of the worms may also lead to intestinal obstruction. Reaction to the worms' metabolites can produce such clinical symptoms as general leukocytosis, anemia, and eosinophilia. Patients purged of the worms usually recover completely, although advanced, heavy infections can be fatal.

When clinical symptoms appear in an endemic area, diagnosis must be confirmed by fecal examination for eggs or, occasionally, by retrieval of whole worms vomited or passed in feces.

Treatment

Praziquantel is the drug of choice.

ECHINOSTOMA TRIVOLVIS

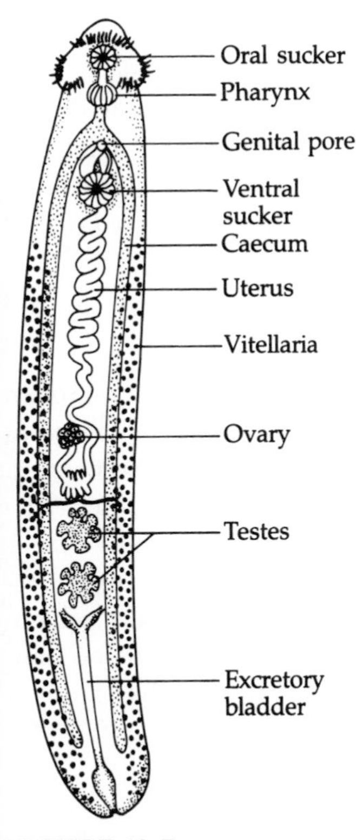

***FIGURE 10-7* *Echinostoma revolutum* adult.**

Several members of the genus *Echinostoma* and related genera occasionally infect humans as well as other mammals. Adult echinostomes, while varying greatly in size, are easily identified by the collar of spines along the dorsal and lateral sides of the head. In general appearance (Fig. 10-7), the adult worm is elongated, with a relatively large ventral sucker situated immediately behind the anterior end. The testes lie in tandem in the posterior portion of the body; the ovary is anterior to the testes, and the short uterus consists only of an ascending limb that terminates at the genital pore, anterior to the ventral sucker. Large, operculate eggs measure 90–126 μm long by 54–71 μm wide, with only a few in the uterus at any given time. *Echinostoma trivolvis* is the prototype for echinostome species that infect humans; essential differences between it and other species in its genus consist primarily of the number and arrangement of collar spines.

Life Cycle

The life cycle of *E. trivolvis* is typical of most echinostomes. Operculated eggs are passed from the definitive host with feces and must reach fresh water for the cycle to continue. The enclosed miracidium is at a very early stage of development when the egg is deposited and requires 2–5 weeks to reach maturity, after which it hatches and penetrates a snail of the genus *Lymnaea*, *Physa*, or *Bithynia*. Various freshwater pelecypods and gastropods serve as hosts for other echinostomes. A single sporocyst generation and two redial generations develop in the molluscan host. Free-swimming cercariae escape from daughter rediae, enter the water, and penetrate and encyst either in a variety of aquatic animals including molluscs—some of which may serve as first intermediate hosts—or, at times, on aquatic vegetation. The life cycle is completed when the definitive host ingests encysted metacercariae, which excyst and develop to sexual maturity in the small intestine.

Epidemiology

While as many as 15 species of *Echinostoma* have been reported in humans, most are incidental parasites. *E. trivolvis* and *E. revolutum*, for instance, are commonly parasites of birds in the United States and mammals in Europe. Human infections of *E. ilocanum* are most frequently reported from Oriental countries such as the Philippines, China, Taiwan, and Indonesia. Infection occurs when the infected second intermediate host is eaten either raw or improperly cooked. Because of the variety and number of potential intermediate and definitive hosts, it is impossible to control the parasite, but human infections can be prevented if food is cooked adequately.

Symptomatology and Diagnosis

Echinostomiasis in humans is usually a minor affliction, often causing nothing more serious than diarrhea. In heavy infections, the spinose collar may cause ulceration of the intestinal mucosa. Children sometimes experience abdominal pain, diarrhea, anemia, and/or edema.

The principal diagnostic technique, identification of eggs in feces, is facilitated by a number of distinctive features of echinostome eggs, namely, their dark brownish color and the very immature larvae, even uncleaved zygotes, that are unlike those of other intestinal trematodes.

Treatment

As with most intestinal flukes, best results are achieved with praziquantel.

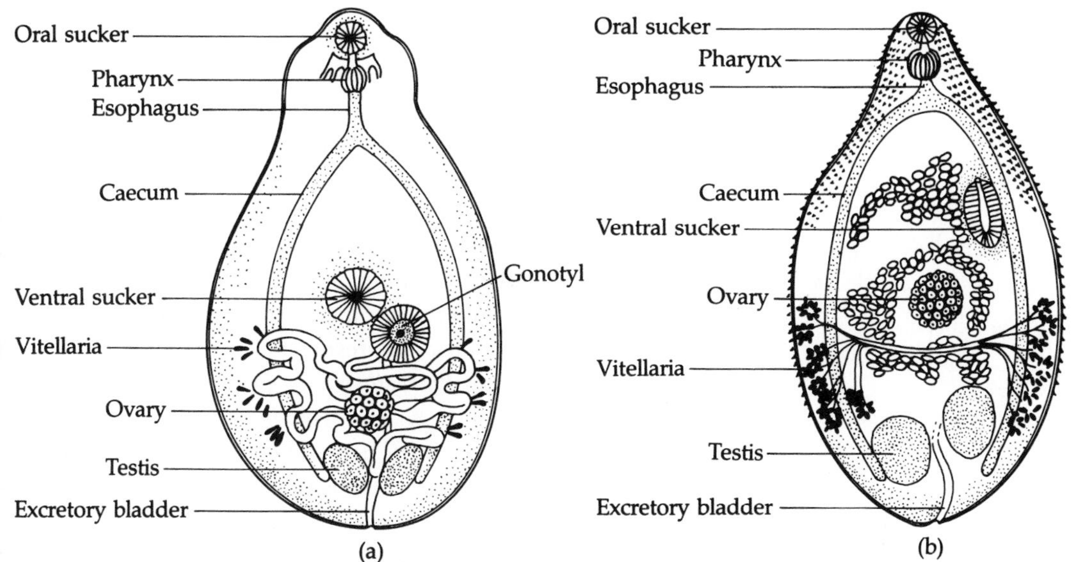

FIGURE 10-8
(a) *Heterophyes heterophyes* adult. (b) *Metagonimus yokogawai* adult.

HETEROPHYES HETEROPHYES AND *METAGONIMUS YOKOGAWAI*

Heterophyes heterophyes and *Metagonimus yokogawai* belong to the family Heterophyidae. Measuring 1.4 mm by 0.5 mm, they are among the smallest digeneans infecting humans (Fig. 10-8). The tegument of these pyriform flukes contains scalelike spines. In *H. heterophyes*, the genital pore, situated posterolateral to the prominent ventral sucker, is surrounded by a genital sucker or **gonotyl.** In *M. yokogawai*, the ventral sucker and gonotyl are fused, and the complex is displaced to the left side of the body. The reproductive system is located in the posterior half of the body, with the testes lying side by side; the ovary is medial, just anterior to the testes, and lateral, follicular vitelline glands are restricted to the posterior third of the body. The gravid uterus loops between the long intestinal caeca, terminating at the gonotyl. The eggs of both species resemble those of *Clonorchis sinensis* except for their indistinct opercular shoulders and the absence of an abopercular knob.

Life Cycle

Heterophyes heterophyes and *Metagonimus yokogawai* commonly inhabit the midregion of the small intestine, and their life cycles are almost identical. Human infection by *H. heterophyes* occurs in Asia, Egypt, and Hawaii, while *M. yokogawai* is the most common intestinal fluke of humans in the Far East, Spain, and the Balkan countries. Eggs containing fully developed miracidia pass out of the human host in feces and hatch only when ingested by a suitable molluscan first intermediate host. In *H. heterophyes*, this host is a freshwater or brackish water snail belonging to the genus *Pirenella* (in Egypt), *Cerithidia* (in Japan), or *Tarebia* (in Hawaii); *M. yokogawai* infects members of the snail genus *Semisulcospira*. The hatched miracidium penetrates the intestine of the snail and transforms into a sporocyst in the digestive gland. Two generations of rediae follow the sporocyst; daughter rediae give rise to cercariae that escape to the external environment, penetrate the musculature of any of a number of food fishes, and encyst as metacercariae. One of the principal fishes used by *H. heterophyes* as the second intermediate host is the mullet, *Mugil cephalus*, which can harbor several thousand metacercariae. Salmonoid fishes commonly serve as second intermediate hosts for *M. yokogawai* metacercariae. Human infection results from consumption of raw or improperly cooked fish. The metacercariae excyst in the duodenum, migrate to the jejunum, and attain sexual maturity in about a week.

Epidemiology

In addition to *Heterophyes heterophyes* and *Metagonimus yokogawai*, at least 14 other heterophyids have been reported in humans. There is an unusually high incidence of infection by *H. heterophyes* in Egypt, especially in parts of the lower Nile Valley. Poor sanitation practices by local fishermen, boatmen, and other residents continually pollute the water with eggs. One of the principal food fishes in the region is the mullet, and parasitic infection results from eating fresh mullet, either incompletely cooked or poorly pickled. Human infection with *H. heterophyes* is also common in Japan, central and south China, Korea, Taiwan, Greece, Israel, and Hawaii. Infection with *M. yokogawai* occurs when the infected second intermediate host, such as a salmonoid fish, is consumed raw or improperly processed. A variety of fish-eating mammals, including cats and dogs, serve as reservoirs for these parasites.

Symptomatology and Diagnosis

The pathology, symptomatology, and diagnosis in cases of infection by these two digeneans are very similar. Adult worms often produce little distress to the patient, but heavy infections may elicit inflammatory reactions at sites of contact as well as diarrhea and abdominal pain. Eosinophilia is also common but without anemia. Adult worms sometimes erode the mucosa and deposit eggs, which may infiltrate the lymphatics or venules. The eggs are then carried to various parts of the body, where they may cause granulomatous responses in organs such as the heart and brain. Heterophyid myocarditis sometimes precipitates fatal heart attacks, and neurological complications also have been reported.

Diagnosis depends on positive identification of eggs in feces. Because of the great degree of similarity, care must be exercised to differentiate the eggs from those of other heterophyids and of opisthorchids.

Treatment

Praziquantel is the treatment for both parasites.

LUNG FLUKES

PARAGONIMUS WESTERMANI

Paragonimus westermani, the Oriental lung fluke, belongs to the family Troglotrematidae and is one of several digeneans of the same genus that infect the human respiratory tract. The first report of human infection was from Taiwan during the latter part of the nineteenth century. Following that initial account, numerous other infections were quickly diagnosed in the Orient, where the condition remains prevalent today.

The thick-bodied, reddish-brown adult worm measures 7.5–12 mm by 4–6 mm (Fig. 10-9). The male reproductive system consists of two irregularly lobed testes situated side by side about two-thirds down the length of the body. The lobed ovary,

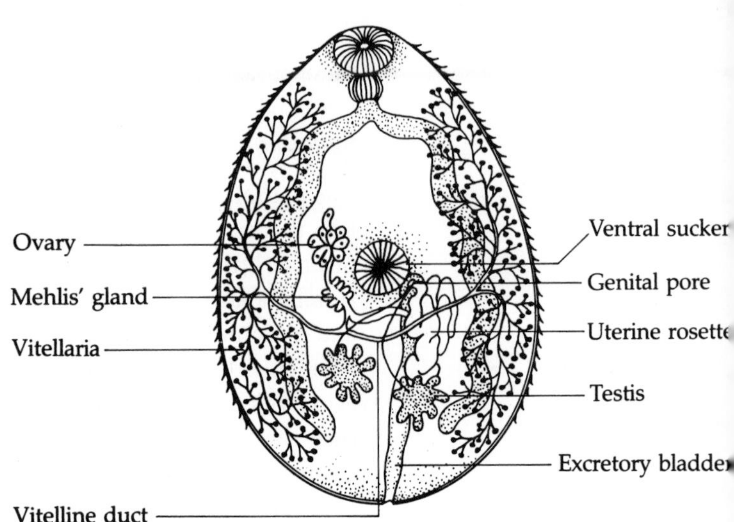

FIGURE 10-9
Paragonimus westermani
adult.

anterior to the right testis, is connected via the oviduct to the uterus, a tightly coiled rosette that lies anterior to the left testis at the same level as the ovary. Vitellaria extend bilaterally along the length of the body, lateral to and paralleling the caeca. A medially located ventral sucker lies between the ovary and the uterus. Brownish, operculated eggs (see Fig. 9-15), smaller than but similar to those of *Fasciola hepatica*, are released through the genital pore situated in the center of the uterine rosette.

Life Cycle

Paired adult *P. westermani* are usually found encapsulated in the bronchioles of the victim's lungs (Fig. 10-10). Commonly, eggs containing uncleaved embryos or zygotes are coughed up and expelled with sputum when the capsules enclosing the adult worms rupture. However, some eggs may be swallowed with sputum, pass through the digestive system, and be expelled with feces; others become trapped in the surrounding lung tissue and produce bronchial abscesses. Once the egg reaches water, several weeks are required for the miracidium to develop. Fully developed miracidia hatch spontaneously, and each must then locate and penetrate a suitable snail host of the genus *Semisulcospira*, *Tarebia*, or *Brotia* within 24 hours or perish. Following penetration of the snail host and metamorphosis into a sporocyst, two

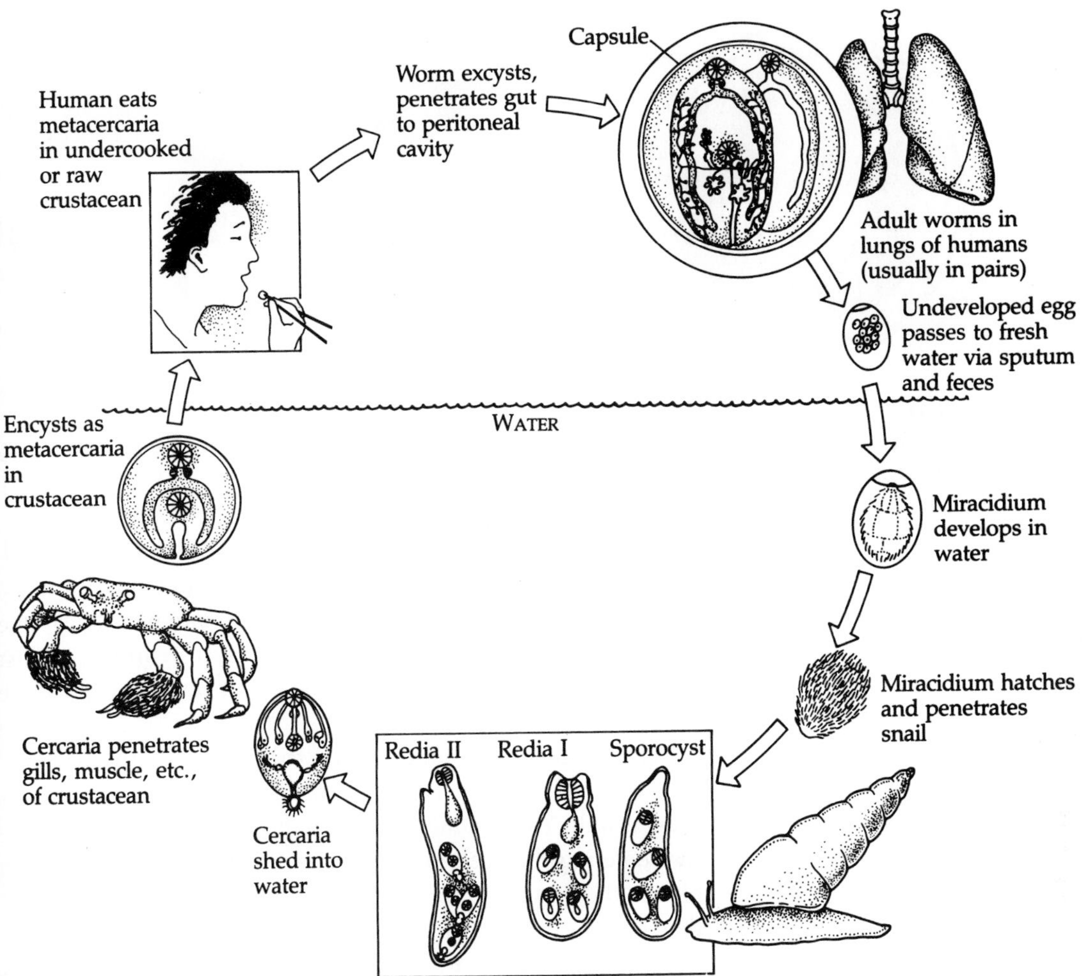

FIGURE 10-10
Life cycle of *Paragonimus westermani*.

redial generations are produced in the digestive gland. Cercariae, formed within the brood chambers of the daughter rediae, emerge from the snail tissue into the surrounding water approximately 11 weeks after the snail is infected. The cercariae possess knoblike tails useless for swimming; instead, the cercariae crawl over solid surfaces until they encounter suitable crustaceans, such as freshwater crabs and crayfish. Using a sharply pointed, cuticular stylet, they penetrate the crustacean's exoskeleton at various vulnerable sites. There is evidence that the crustacean second in-

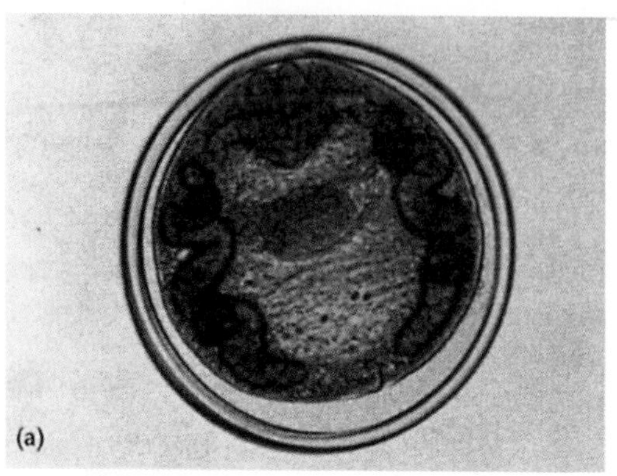

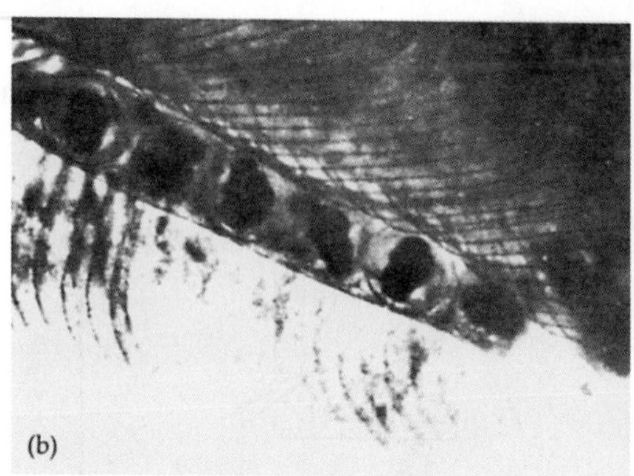

FIGURE 10-11
(a) Encysted metacercaria of *Paragonimus westermani*. (b) Several metacercariae encysted in gill filament of crab host.

termediate host may also acquire infection by eating infected snails. Once inside the host, the cercariae encyst in muscles, gills, and viscera (Fig. 10-11), where they develop into metacercariae. The encysted metacercaria is not folded over ventrally, as are most encysted metacercariae, but lies in an extended position within the cyst wall.

When a human consumes an infected crustacean, the metacercaria excysts in the small intestine and partially penetrates the intestinal wall. Young adults remain at this site for several days before entering the coelom. Then, traversing the diaphragm and pleura, they enter the peribronchiolar tissues of the lungs, where they become encapsulated in pairs by host connective tissue and develop to sexual maturity within 8–12 weeks. During migration, young adult worms often become lodged in other organs, producing ectopic lesions before succumbing to host reactions.

Epidemiology

While *P. westermani* is worldwide in distribution, human infections are confined mainly to Oriental countries such as Japan, South Korea, Thailand, Taiwan, China, and the Philippines. A number of animals, including dogs, cats, some rodents, and pigs, can serve as reservoirs. In humans as well as reservoir hosts, infection results from the consumption of raw, improperly pickled, or undercooked infected freshwater crustaceans. Although the pickling process coagulates muscle protein, giving the meat the appearance of being cooked and therefore harmless, it actually has no effect upon the encysted metacercariae. Metacercariae dislodged from the crustacean during the cleaning process may adhere to utensils, which then become a source of infection to food handlers. Humans may also become infected by consuming the juices obtained from crushed crabs, a medicinal practice common in parts of the Orient.

Two other members of the genus *Paragonimus*, *P. ohirai* and *P. iloktsuenensis*, infect the lungs of humans and other mammals in the Orient. Their life cycles are similar to that of *P. westermani*, except that the second intermediate hosts are estuarine crabs that inhabit the brackish waters at the mouths of rivers, primarily in Japan.

Symptomatology and Diagnosis

Paragonimus westermani adults and eggs stimulate the formation of connective tissue capsules in the host, both in the lungs and at ectopic sites. In addition to adult worms, the capsules contain eggs and infiltrated host cells in a hemorrhagic, semifluid mass. The capsules often ulcerate, giving the lungs a peppered appearance. Early symptoms include a cough producing blood-tinged sputum, pulmonary pain, and even pleurisy. A low-grade fever usually accompanies these symptoms. At present, paragonimiasis is difficult to distinguish from other pulmonary disorders such as pneumonia and tuberculosis.

Encysted worms may be found at such ectopic sites as the abdominal wall, lymph nodes, heart, and portions of the nervous system. Infection of the abdominal wall may produce abdominal pain, diarrhea, and bleeding. In the brain, infection may produce a variety of neurological symptoms including epilepsy and paralysis. Fatalities have been recorded from cardiac involvement as well as from heavy pulmonary infections.

Identification of eggs in sputum, pleural aspirate, or feces is the most reliable diagnostic procedure. Patients from endemic areas who show symptoms such as pulmonary distress, blood-tinged sputum, and eosinophilia should be examined carefully. For ectopic infections, immunological tests with *Paragonimus* as a source of antigens have proven useful.

Treatment

A 24-hour course of treatment with praziquantel is recommended.

SELECTED READINGS

Boray, J. C. 1969. Experimental fascioliasis in Australia. *Advances in Parasitology* 7, 96–210.

Koniya, Y. 1966. *Clonorchis* and clonorchiasis. *Advances in Parasitology* **4,** 53–106.

Lloyd, S., and Soulsby, E. J. L. 1998. Other trematode infections. In *Zoonoses* (Palmer, S. R., Soulsby, E. J. L., and Simpson, D. I. H., Eds.), pp. 731–746. Oxford University Press, Oxford, England.

Murrell, K. D., Cross, J. H., and Chongsuphajaisiddhi, T. 1996. The importance of food-borne parasitic zoonoses. *Parasitology Today* **12,** 171–173.

Rim, H.-J., Farag, H. F., Sommani, S., and Cross, J. H. 1994. Food-borne trematodes: Ignored or emerging? *Parasitology Today* **10,** 207–209.

Tielens, A. G. M. 1994. Energy generation in parasitic helminths. *Parasitology Today* **10,** 346–352.

Yokagawa, M. 1969. *Paragonimus* and paragonimiasis. *Advances in Parasitology* 7, 375–387.

Chapter Eleven

BLOOD FLUKES

FIGURE 11-1
(Left) Global distribution of schistosomiasis due to *Schistosoma mansoni* and *S. intercalatum*. (Right) Global distribution of schistosomiasis due to *Schistosoma haematobium, S. japonicum,* and *S. mekongi*.

The human disease complex known as **schistosomiasis** is also referred to as **bilharziasis** or **snail fever**. It is caused primarily by three members of the genus *Schistosoma* (family Schistosmatidae): *S. haematobium*, *S. mansoni*, and *S. japonicum*. There are several other species that infect humans, but they are much less common or even rare. Human infections by these flukes number in excess of 250 million worldwide, and in spite of efforts to control this disease, the level of incidence has shown no significant decrease. In the People's Republic of China alone, a recent estimate indicated at least 15 million cases of schistosomiasis japonica, representing the single most serious disease in that country. As a result of concerted control measures, the incidence in China has been somewhat reduced. Egypt has one of the most heavily infected populations in the world, since not only is *S. haematobium* endemic to that country, but *S. mansoni* also occurs with

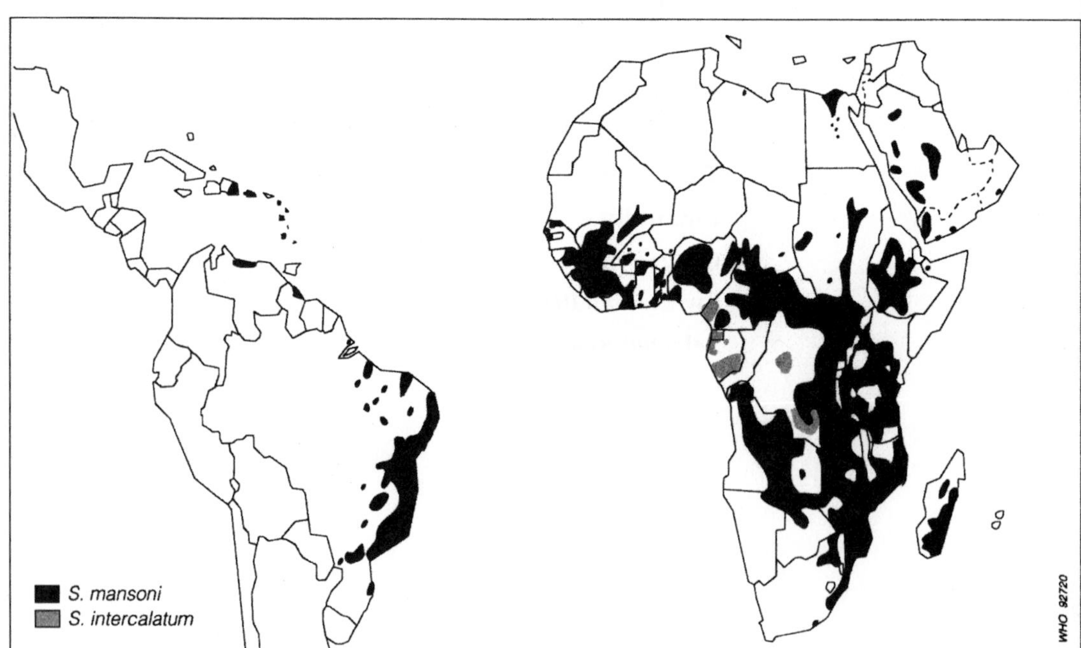

great frequency. Among the inhabitants of some endemic areas of the Nile Valley, the infection rate exceeds 80%. Other areas of high incidence include tropical and subtropical Africa, parts of South America, and several of the Caribbean islands (Fig. 11-1).

It was not until 1852 that the young German parasitologist Theodor Bilharz, working in Egypt, discovered one of the parasites (*S. haematobium*) responsible for urinary schistosomiasis. However, there are recorded accounts of the disease dating from pharaonic times. In the Ebers papyrus from 1500 B.C.E., there is a reference to treatment of hematuria (bloody urine), and calcified eggs of *S. haematobium* have been found in the viscera of Egyptian mummies dating from 1200 B.C.E.

Fossilized bulinid snails that may have served as intermediate hosts for *S. haematobium* have been unearthed in the ancient biblical city of Jericho. An interesting hypothesis based on this discovery is that the city's well was infested with infected snails, producing a high incidence of schistosomiasis among the citizenry. Too debilitated by the disease to defend their city or repair its decaying walls, they were easily defeated by Joshua's army. Without knowing the cause of this heinous disease but wishing to prevent its spread, Joshua destroyed Jericho and proclaimed a curse

FIGURE 11-1 **Continued.**

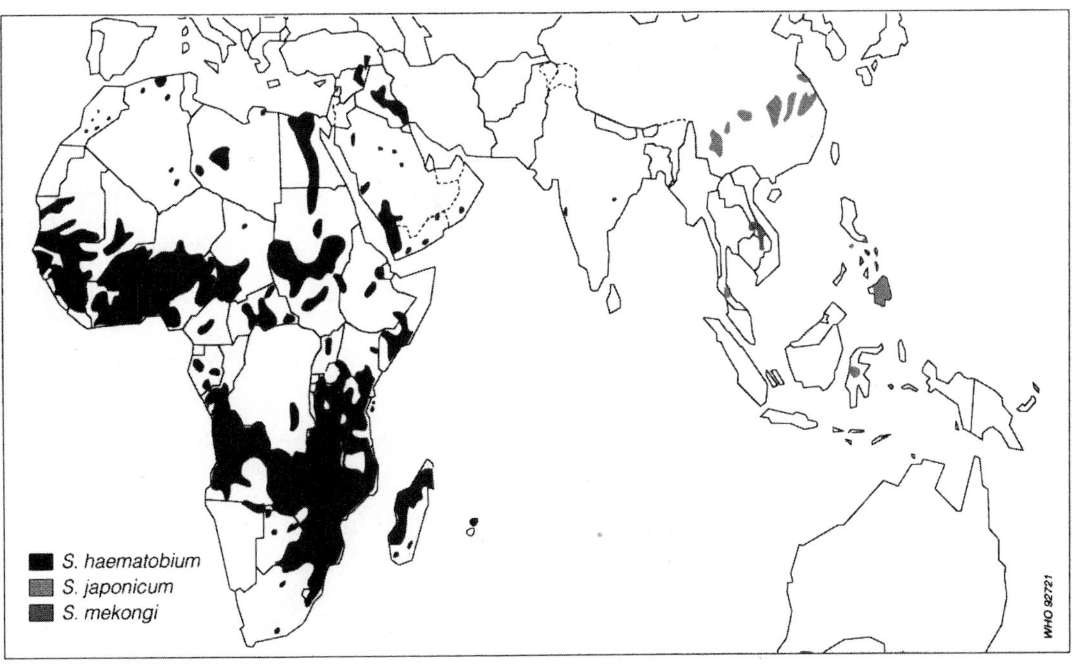

upon any who would rebuild it, thus precluding subsequent repopulation. The city remained deserted for more than 500 years. Centuries of recurring drought apparently destroyed the snails, and the city has remained free of the parasite to this day.

The French invasion of Egypt during the latter part of the eighteenth century was probably one of the first large-scale contacts people of the Western world had with schistosomiasis. Besides amoebic dysentery, the French had to contend with two other diseases previously unknown to them, hematuria and the eye disease known as trachoma. The former, as we now know, is caused by *S. haematobium*, while the latter is caused by a fly-transmitted microorganism (see p. 423). Both diseases remain firmly entrenched in Egypt.

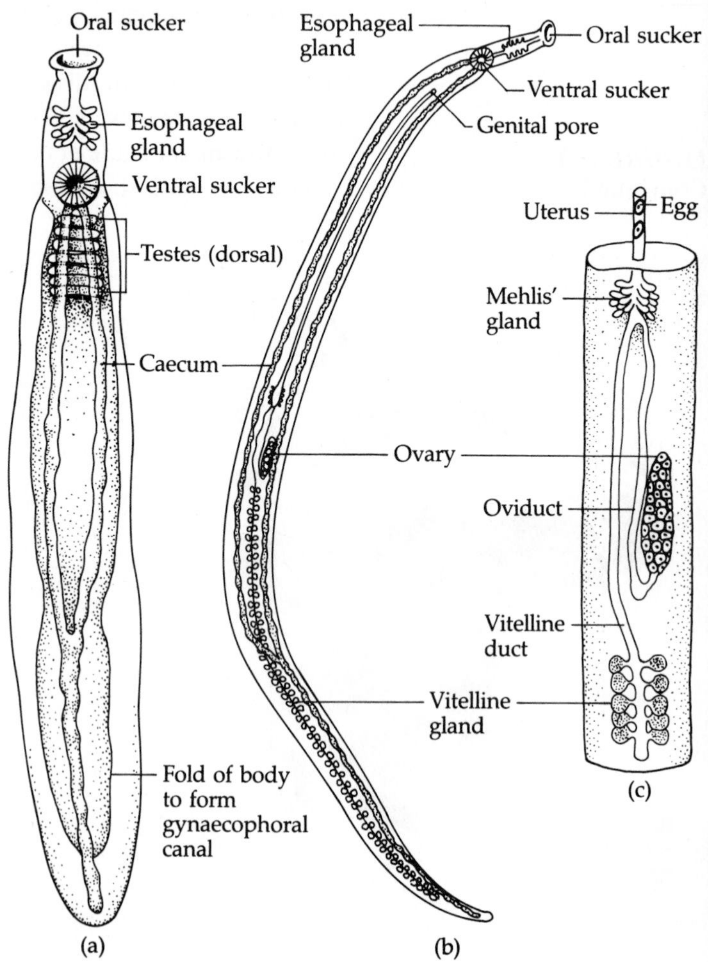

***FIGURE 11-2* Generalized adult schistosomes.** (a) Male. (b) Female. (c) Enlargement of female reproductive system.

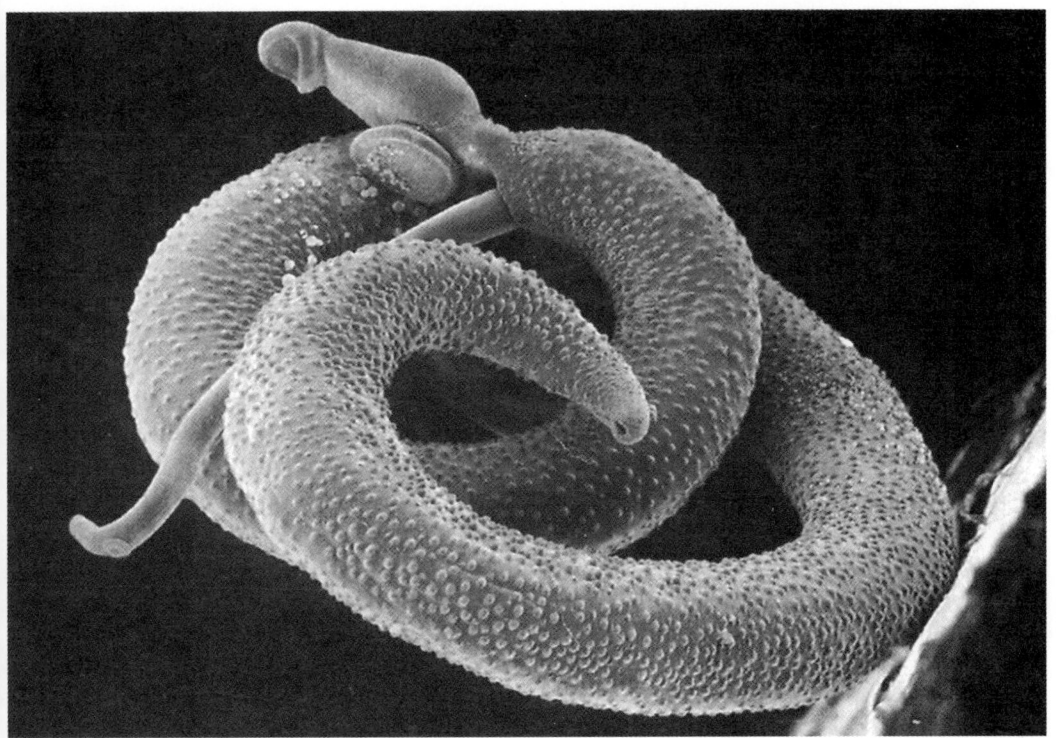

FIGURE 11-3
Scanning electron micrograph of *Schistosoma mansoni* adult worms *in copula*.

MORPHOLOGY

Figure 11-2 depicts adult male and female worms. An oral sucker surrounds the mouth of the adult schistosome, and a ventral sucker is located immediately posterior to the level of bifurcation of the gut. Although no pharynx is present, there is an esophagus with prominent **esophageal glands**. The paired caeca reunite posteriorly, forming a single caecum that extends the remaining length of the body. Schistosomes are unique among digeneans in being dioecious and sexually dimorphic. The adult male is more robust than the female and possesses a ventral fold or groove called the **gynaecophoric canal**. The female, longer and more slender than the male, is held in this canal, permitting almost continuous mating (Fig. 11-3).

The male possesses from five to nine testes, and the male genital pore opens ventrally, immediately posterior to the ventral sucker. There is no cirrus. In the female, the position of the single ovary varies according to species, and the uterus may be long or short, depending on the position of the ovary relative to the female genital pore.

LIFE CYCLE

The life cycles of the three species of *Schistosoma* (Fig. 11-4) are virtually identical and will be so treated. Individual differences will be noted in the section following description of the life cycle.

Adult schistosomes reside in mesenteric veins that drain the intestine (*S. mansoni* and *S. japonicum*) or in vesicular veins serving the urinary bladder (*S. haematobium*). In single-sex infections, the sexual organs of female worms are underdeveloped, leading to the hypothesis that one or more male factors are essential for complete maturation of the female.

The female usually migrates to smaller venules before depositing eggs. The morphology of the egg is distinctive in each species and serves as a diagnostic criterion (see Fig. 9-16). The enclosed miracidium is poorly developed at the time of oviposition but is well formed before it reaches the lumen of the infected organ. To escape to the outside, the egg must penetrate the venule endothelium and then traverse the intervening tissues and mucosal lining before entering the lumen of the gut or the bladder. The method by which the egg passes through these tissues remains speculative but probably involves hydrolytic enzymes emitted through the porous shell. The process is obviously inefficient because only about one-third of the eggs produced reach the exterior; the remaining eggs are either trapped in the urinary bladder or intestinal walls or are carried by the blood to ectopic sites such as the liver (Fig. 11-5) and, occasionally, the spleen and other tissues. After reaching the lumen, the egg passes to the exterior in either feces or urine.

Upon reaching fresh water, the egg escapes the inhibitory osmolarity of the host's body fluids, thereby activating the miracidium to hatch. Because schistosome eggs have no operculum, hatching occurs through a rupture of the eggshell along a line known as the **suture**.

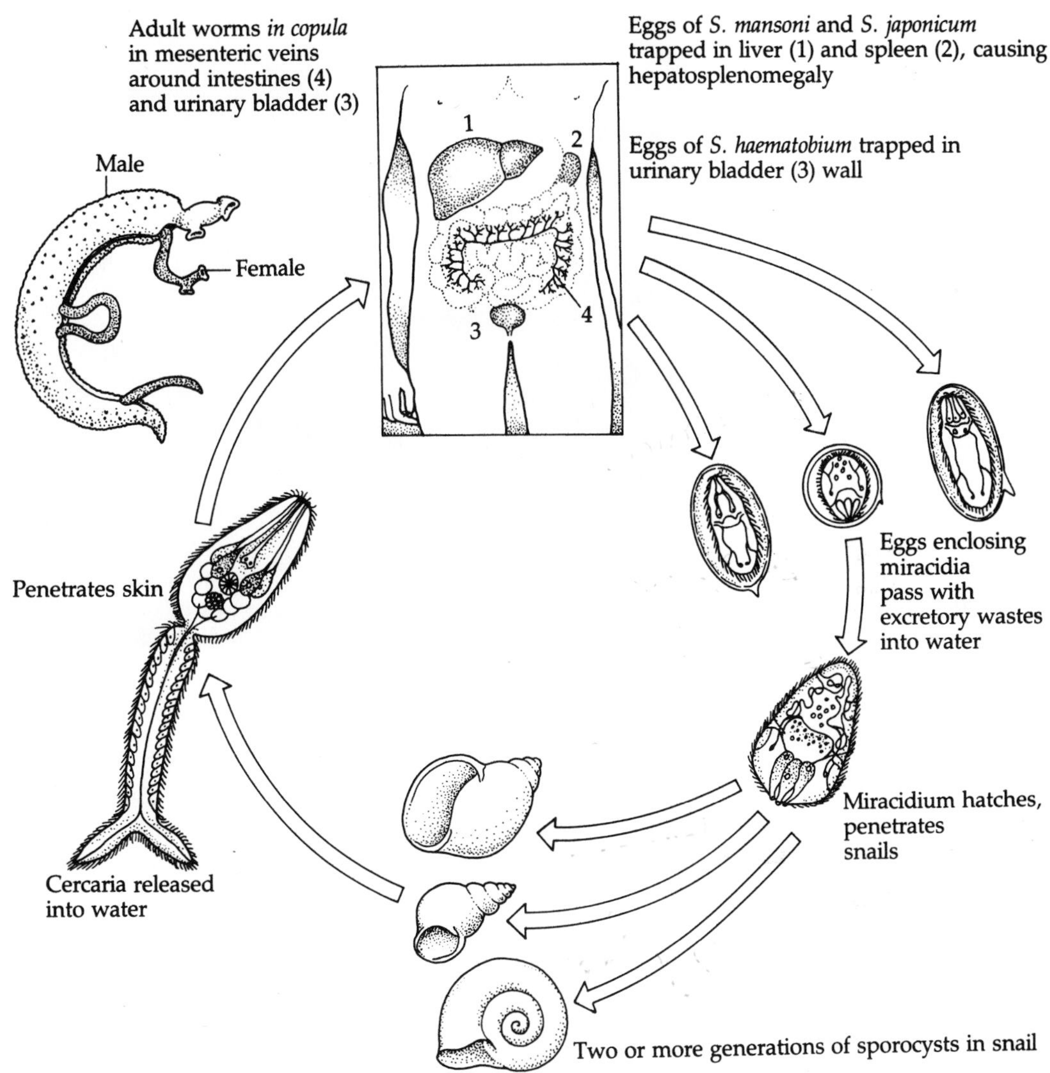
Adult worms *in copula* in mesenteric veins around intestines (4) and urinary bladder (3)
Eggs of *S. mansoni* and *S. japonicum* trapped in liver (1) and spleen (2), causing hepatosplenomegaly
Eggs of *S. haematobium* trapped in urinary bladder (3) wall
1
2
3
4
Male
Female
Penetrates skin
Eggs enclosing miracidia pass with excretory wastes into water
Miracidium hatches, penetrates snails
Cercaria released into water
Two or more generations of sporocysts in snail

FIGURE 11-4
Life cycles of *Schistosoma* spp.

To survive, the free-swimming miracidium (Fig. 11-6) must penetrate a suitable snail intermediate host within a few hours after hatching. After penetration, the miracidium transforms into a sporocyst in the head-foot of the snail (Fig. 11-7). A second generation of migratory sporocysts is produced that move to the digestive gland or gonads, where they either reproduce additional generations of sporocysts or give rise to the cercarial generation.

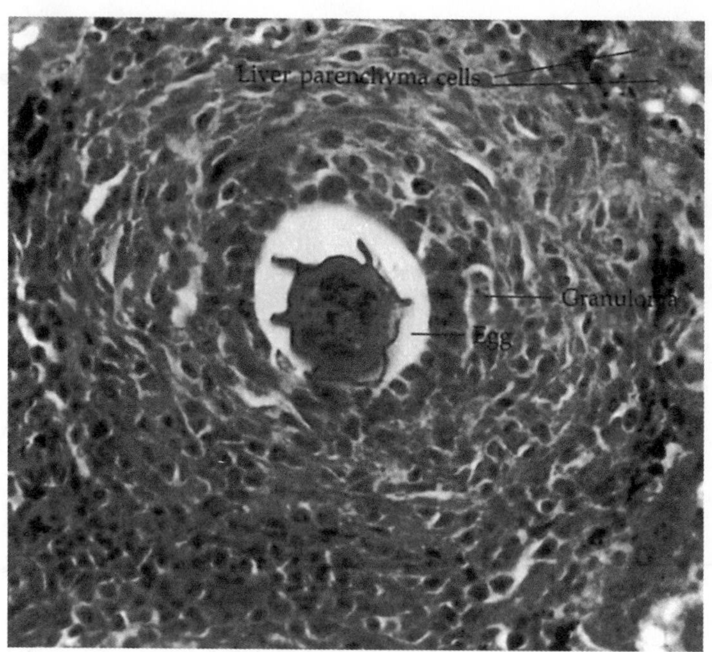

FIGURE 11-5
Schistosoma mansoni **egg in liver granuloma.**

The cercariae leave the sporocyst in which they have developed via a birth pore and pass through the tissues of the snail to the exterior. This passage is facilitated by secretions from a pair of **escape glands** located in the cephalic region of the cercaria (Fig. 11-8a).

Actively swimming cercariae possess distinctive forked tails and move in a figure-eight pattern characteristic of schistosomes. They may swim upward to the surface of the water and then sink slowly toward the bottom, or they may adhere to the surface film and come to rest while they await contact with their next host. The cercariae are stimulated to attach to and penetrate their host by the secretions of the mammalian skin. In fresh water, a mucoid surface coat protects the free-swimming cercariae from the hypoosmolarity of the environment. Cercariae have five pairs of unicellular glands. Two of these, the **preacetabular glands**, are anterior to the ventral sucker, while the other three, the **postacetabular glands**, lie behind the ventral sucker. Each gland cell is equipped with a duct that empties separately at the anterior margin of the oral sucker (Fig. 11-8b).

The cercaria adheres to the skin of the definitive host by means

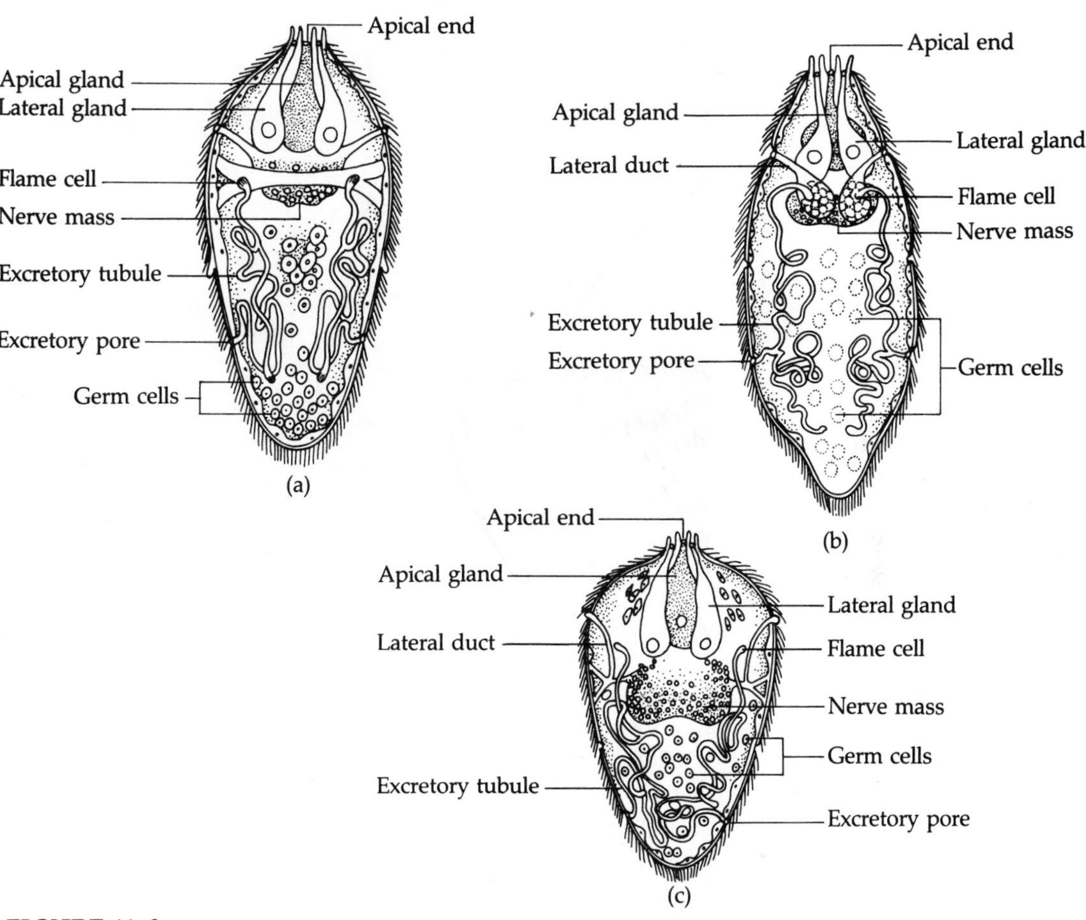

FIGURE 11-6
Miracidia of three major schistosomes that infect humans.
(a) *Schistosoma haematobium.* (b) *S. mansoni.* (c) *S. japonicum.*

of both its muscular suckers and the mucoid secretions of the postacetabular glands. Secretions from the preacetabular glands are more highly enzymatic, facilitating lysis of host skin during the penetration process.

Once the cercaria enters the skin, it burrows to the peripheral capillary bed or enters the lymphatic system; in either case, the worm migrates to the right side of the heart and then enters the lungs. During the penetration process, three significant morphological changes occur in the cercaria: the tail is lost, the surface coat is lost, and the contents of the penetration glands are spent.

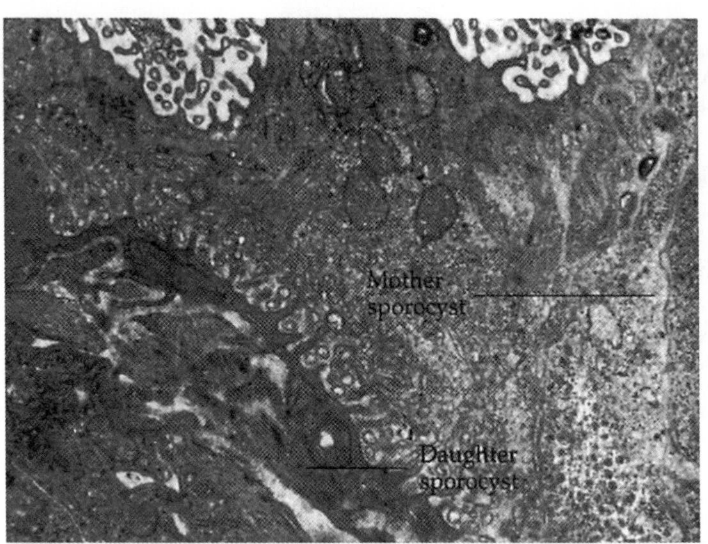

FIGURE 11-7
Transmission electron micrograph of the tegument of a mother sporocyst with enclosed daughter sporocyst of *Schistosoma mansoni*.

Following these changes, the transformed cercaria is called a **schistosomule** (Fig. 11-9).

Schistosomules appear in pulmonary capillaries by the third day after penetration. On day 4, these juveniles begin feeding on host erythrocytes, initiating a period of rapid growth and development. The period spent in the host's lungs varies even within the same schistosome species. After a week to 10 days, the schistosomules move through the pulmonary vein to the left side of the heart and then into the systemic circulation. Approximately 3 weeks after penetration, the worms reach the hepatic portal veins, where they reach sexual maturity and mate after 40 days. Males with females enclosed in their gynaecophoric canals then migrate against the portal flow to venules at the definitive sites. The sex of the worms is genetically determined at the time of fertilization.

VARIATIONS

Although the morphology and life cycles of the three major schistosomes are basically similar, there are certain clinical differences that are useful in diagnosis.

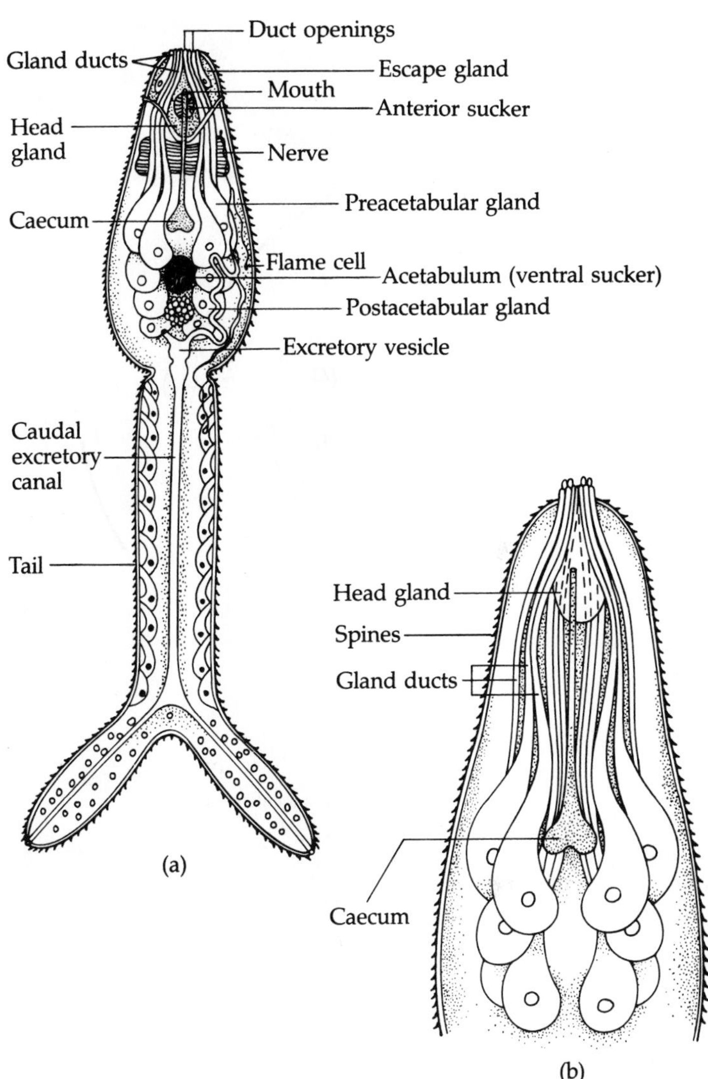

FIGURE 11-8
Cercaria of a schistosome.
(a) Entire cercaria. (b) Anterior end showing head gland.

SCHISTOSOMA HAEMATOBIUM

In India and Portugal, intermediate hosts for *S. haematobium* belong to the snail genera *Ferrissia* and *Planorbarius*, respectively; in all other major endemic areas, from North to South Africa (particularly the Nile Valley), Central and West Africa, and a number of countries in the Middle East, several species of the snail genus *Bulinus* serve as intermediate hosts. The male worm

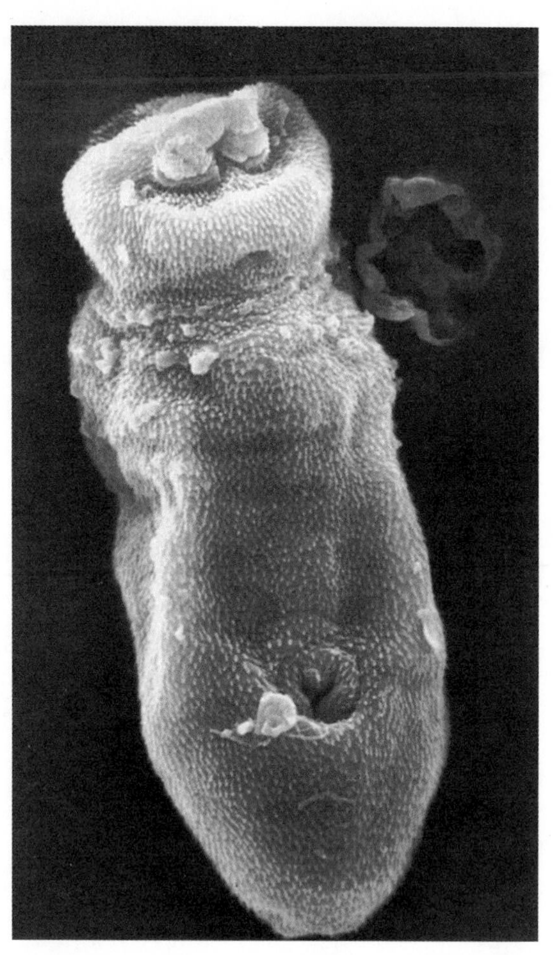

FIGURE 11-9
Scanning electron micrograph of *Schistosoma mansoni* schistosomule.

may attain a length of 15 mm, while females may reach 20 mm (Fig. 11-10a). There are four or five testes in the male; in the female, the single ovary is situated at about the midpoint of the body. The tegument of the male has many knoblike tubercles on the dorsal surface, while the tegument of the female is smooth. In both sexes, the caeca reunite posteriorly at a point about two-thirds of the way down the length of the body.

Females deposit about 30 eggs daily, each egg measuring 112–170 μm by 40–70 μm. The *S. haematobium* egg is readily identifiable by its small, distinct terminal spine (see Fig. 9-16). Intramolluscan development requires approximately 4–6 weeks after penetration by the miracidium. The prepatent period for *S. haematobium* in the human host is 10–12 weeks.

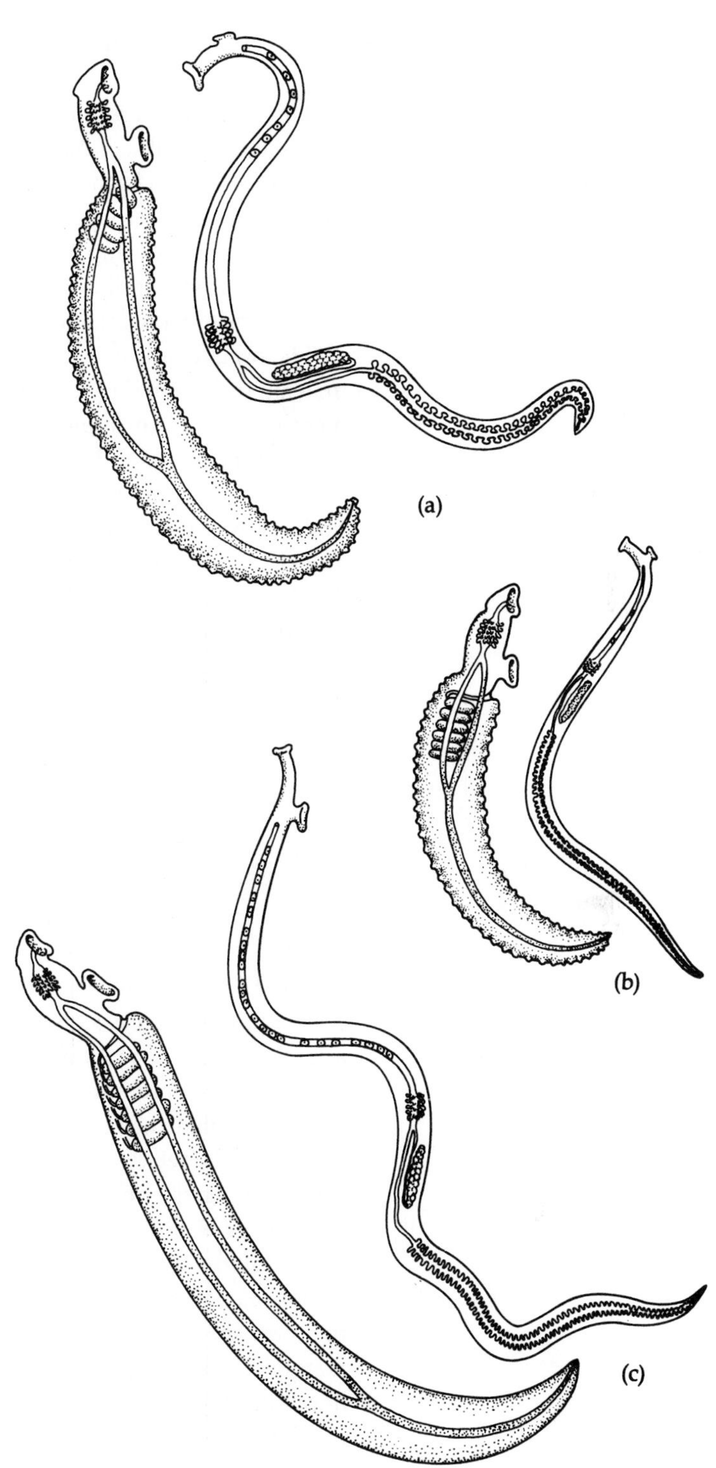

FIGURE 11-10
Adults of three major schistosomes that infect humans.
In each pair, the male is on the left, the female on the right. (a) *Schistosoma haematobium*. (b) *S. mansoni*. (c) *S. japonicum*.

SCHISTOSOMA MANSONI

This species occurs widely throughout Africa and South America, especially in Brazil, Venezuela, Surinam, and Guyana, and on several Caribbean islands, including Puerto Rico, St. Lucia, Martinique, and Guadeloupe. It may have been brought to the Western Hemisphere during the time of the African slave trade when a number of susceptible snail hosts were introduced, possibly in casks of drinking water accompanying the infected slaves.

The male worm measures up to 10 mm in length and the female up to 14 mm (Fig. 11-10b). As in *S. haematobium*, the tegument of the male has tubercles on the dorsal surface, while that of the female is smooth. The male has six to nine testes, while in the female a single ovary is situated in the anterior half of the body. Female worms deposit 190–300 eggs daily, each measuring 114–175 μm by 45–68 μm and bearing a prominent, lateral spine (see Fig. 9-16). Many species of the genus *Biomphalaria* are suitable snail hosts in endemic areas throughout the world except in Brazil, where members of the snail genus *Tropicorbis* serve as intermediate hosts. Intramolluscan development requires 3–4 weeks, and the prepatent period in humans is 7–8 weeks.

SCHISTOSOMA JAPONICUM

This schistosome is found in the Far Eastern countries of China, the Philippines, Taiwan, Indonesia, and to a lesser extent, Japan. The snail host belongs to the genus *Oncomelania*. Adult worms are the largest schistosomes infecting humans, with males attaining a length of 20 mm and females 26 mm. The tegumental surface of both sexes is smooth. The male has seven testes, while the female has a single ovary lying in the posterior half of the body. The relatively long uterus may contain as many as 300 eggs at any given time. The female is a prodigious egg-producer, capable of depositing 3500 eggs per day; unlike those of *S. haematobium* and *S. mansoni*, the eggs are deposited in clusters rather than singly. The eggs of *S. japonicum* are the smallest of the three species, measuring 70–100 μm by 50–65 μm, and they may bear a minute, lateral spine (see Fig. 9-16). Intramolluscan development requires 4–9 weeks, while the prepatent period in humans is 5–6 weeks.

SYMPTOMATOLOGY AND DIAGNOSIS

The first symptom of schistosomiasis is localized dermatitis, often appearing after cercariae penetrate the skin. The characteristic itching and local edema usually disappear after 4 days. Following skin penetration, the symptoms of human schistosomiasis appear in three phases. The first is the migration phase, characterized by toxic reactions and pulmonary congestion accompanied by fever. This phase may last 4–10 weeks, during which the worms migrate from the lungs to the liver, where they reach sexual maturity and mate. Mated pairs of *S. mansoni* and *S. japonicum* then migrate to the mesenteric veins via the hepatic portal system. The second phase is considerably longer, lasting 2 months to several years. Characteristic symptoms, such as bloody stools (schistosomiasis mansoni and japonica) and hematuria (schistosomiasis haematobium), are caused by the passage of eggs through the intestinal and urinary bladder walls. Pathological alteration of these organs accompanies these incursions. The last phase, the most serious, is characterized by severe intestinal, renal, and hepatic pathology, caused primarily by the reaction of the host to the schistosome eggs.

Hepatosplenomegaly (enlargement of the liver and spleen) is a common symptom of advanced schistosomiasis. Eggs trapped in the walls of the intestine and urinary bladder as well as in ectopic regions, notably the liver and spleen, trigger leukocytic and fibroblastic infiltration, which elicits inflammatory reactions, cirrhosis, and anemia. Eventually, a **granuloma** (pseudotubercle) forms around each egg or cluster of eggs (Fig. 11-5). Small abscesses accompanied by occlusion of small blood vessels lead to necrosis and ulceration.

In endemic areas, where reinfection is common, repeated penetration of the intestinal and urinary bladder walls by migrating eggs results in excessive scar tissue formation, which impedes the normal functioning of these organs. For example, *S. haematobium* infections alter absorptive properties of the urinary bladder wall, predisposing it to malignancy; as a result, *S. haematobium* infection is commonly associated with bladder cancer among male agricultural workers in Egypt. Because formation of scar tissue also blocks the migration of eggs through infected organs, more eggs are swept back to other sites, producing organ enlargement, including hepatosplenomegaly.

The surest means of diagnosis is finding and identifying characteristic eggs in excreta or in tissue biopsies, particularly rectal biopsies. In chronic cases in which very few if any eggs are passed, biopsies can be used advantageously, but they are expensive and require the services of trained specialists. Current research efforts emphasize the development of inexpensive, reliable diagnostic procedures adaptable to primitive conditions. Currently, the most promising procedures utilize immunodiagnostic techniques; however, positive results from these tests should be confirmed by identification of eggs, because false positives sometimes result from concomitant infections with other parasites or exposure to various animal schistosome cercariae. The latter sometimes produces a severe dermatitis called **swimmer's itch** (see p. 246).

TREATMENT

No reliable prophylactic regimen is presently available other than the observance of proper hygiene and sanitation procedures, avoidance of cercaria-infested waters, and prevention of water contamination by human excreta. The chemotherapeutic agent recommended for all species of human schistosomes is praziquantel (see p. 203). By disrupting the integrity of the schistosome tegument, this drug apparently exposes otherwise inaccessible antigens as targets for host antibodies.

According to the World Health Organization, the key to eventual schistosomiasis control lies in a four-pronged attack: population-based chemotherapy, with repeated drug administration to infected individuals; use of molluscicides; introduction of biological controls, such as carnivorous snails and fish; and education of the population. Evidence has surfaced of differences in the parasites' degree of susceptibility to drugs and of the development of drug resistance. Therefore, research efforts to improve existing drugs and to synthesize new, more effective ones must continue, at least until a vaccine becomes available.

IMMUNITY

Immunity to human schistosomiasis is not totally understood. It is known that animals experimentally infected with schistosomes normally infective to humans develop immunity to these parasites. The life span of adult schistosomes in the human host can be more than 30 years. As noted earlier, during much of their life time the worms are prolific egg producers, and this output over such a long period elicits a wide range of immune responses, both humoral and cell-mediated. In fact, such responses can be correlated with various parasitic stages in the human host. The first, or skin-penetration stage, is characterized by a reaction to the penetrating cercaria's surface coat and penetration gland secretions, both released into the host's tissues. During the second, or early development stage, there is a response caused by the tegumental changes in the migrating schistosmule. The third, or adult worm and egg stages, precipitates a response to immunogens released from the adult worm's intestine, tegument, and excretory system. The reaction to eggs is in response to immunogens released from either migrating or trapped eggs. The immunogens are macromolecules that diffuse through micropores in the eggshell. While some of these macromolecules facilitate migration of the eggs through the tissues, they also elicit a granulomatous response to eggs trapped in the tissues, causing pronounced pathological changes.

If worms produce immunogens to which the host responds, how do the worms evade this response? Although there is not yet a complete answer to this question, several significant factors provide clues. Perhaps the most remarkable of these is the ability of the worm to acquire host antigens on its surface. These antigens afford protection by disguising the worm's surface so that it escapes detection by the host immune mediators. Antigen acquisition apparently begins during the early schistosomule stage and may be associated with the initiation of feeding on host blood. Logically, therefore, an effective vaccine must target the larval stage before such protection is attained.

OTHER SCHISTOSOMES

Since the mid-twentieth century, new discoveries of metazoan parasites pathogenic to humans have been rare. For many years, pockets of what were thought to be *S. japonicum* infections existed in Southeast Asia, especially in parts of Laos and Cambodia. However, American involvement in Southeast Asia during the

Vietnam War prompted a reevaluation of the causative organism for schistosomiasis in that region; as a result, that parasite is now considered to be a separate species, *Schistosoma mekongi*. While it closely resembles *S. japonicum* in pathology and morphology, there are significant differences: the molluscan intermediate host is a minute snail, *Tricula aperta*, the eggs are smaller, and the prepatent period is a week longer than for *S. japonicum*.

Another schistosome species, *Schistosoma intercalatum*, is known to cause human schistosomiasis in Cameroon and the Democratic Republic of the Congo in Africa. In Cameroon, *Bulinus foskalii* serves as the molluscan intermediate host; in Zaire, *B. globosus* does so. *Schistosoma intercalatum*, normally a blood fluke of cattle, is generally considered more closely related to *S. haematobium* because of the terminal spine on its eggs; like the eggs of *S. mansoni*, however, the eggs of *S. intercalatum* are voided in feces rather than urine. *Schistosoma intercalatum* is also less pathogenic to humans than is *S. haematobium*.

SWIMMER'S ITCH

An interesting phenomenon of schistosome biology is cercarial dermatitis, or swimmer's itch. Although the condition is not life-threatening, it can have a negative impact on the economy of regions where outbreaks occur, especially those popular with tourists. A number of lake and seashore resorts in Michigan, Wisconsin, Minnesota, New Jersey, New England, North Carolina, and Canada have suffered economic losses when outbreaks have driven vacationers away. The condition is caused when cercariae of blood flukes that normally parasitize aquatic birds and mammals penetrate human skin, sensitizing points of entry and causing pustules and an itchy rash. Because humans are not suitable definitive hosts for these flukes, the cercariae do not normally enter the bloodstream and mature. Instead, after penetrating the skin, they are destroyed by the victim's immune responses. Allergenic substances released from dead and dying cercariae produce a localized inflammatory reaction (Fig. 11-11). In freshwater lakes of North America, cercariae of the genera *Trichobilharzia*, *Gigantobilharzia*, and *Bilharziella*, which normally infect birds, are the common dermatitis-producing schistosomes, while the

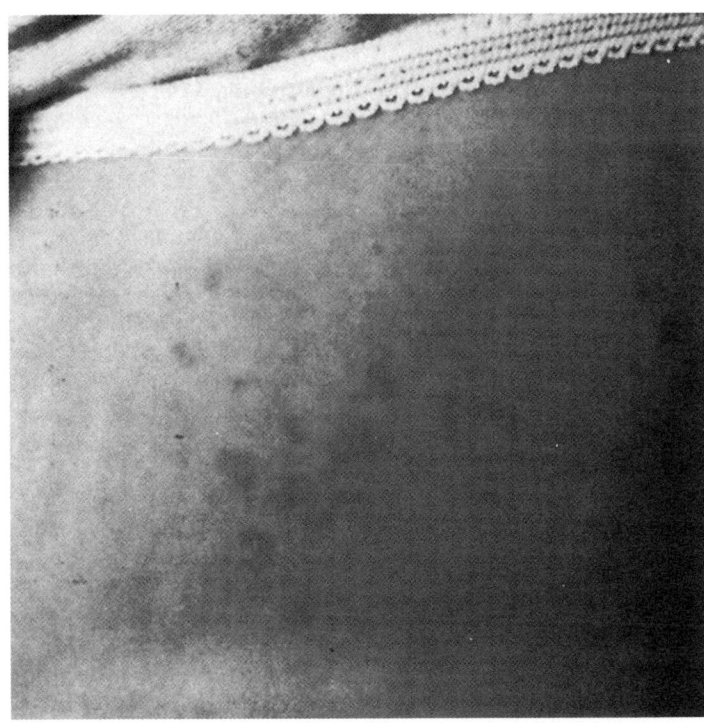

FIGURE 11-11
Swimmer's itch.
Note the localized inflammatory reaction on the thigh.

mammal parasite, *Heterobilharzia*, is the culprit in Gulf Coast states. One of the most common causative agents of marine swimmer's itch on both the east and west coasts of North America is *Microbilharzia variglandis*, a blood fluke of sea gulls; the cercariae of this parasite develop in the mudflat snail, *Ilyanassa obsoleta*. Other marine genera implicated in swimmer's itch are *Austrobilharzia* and *Ornithobilharzia*, which use members of the snail genera *Littorina* and *Batillaria*, respectively, as intermediate hosts. Swimmer's itch is by no means confined to North America; outbreaks have also been reported in Asia, Africa, Europe, and the Middle East.

SELECTED READINGS

Basch, P. F., and Samuelson, J. 1990. Cell biology of schistosomes. I. Ultrastructure and transformations. In *Modern Parasite Biology. Cel-*

lular, Immunological, and Molecular Aspects. (Wyler, D. J., Ed.), pp. 91–106. W. H. Freeman, New York.

Butterworth, A. E. 1990. Immunology of schistosomiasis. In *Modern Parasite Biology. Cellular, Immunological, and Molecular Aspects* (Wyler, D. J., Ed.), pp. 262–288. W. H. Freeman, New York.

Jordan, P., Webbe, G., and Sturrock, R. F. (Eds.). 1993. *Human Schistosomiasis*. (GAB International Publication). Oxford University Press, Oxford, England.

Loker, E. S. 1983. A comparative study of the life-histories of mammalian schistosomes. *Parasitology* **87**, 343–369.

Malone, J. B., Abdel-Rahman, M. S., El Bahy, M. M., Hüh, O. K., Shafik, M., and Bavia, M. 1997. Geographic information systems and the distribution of *Schistosoma mansoni* in the Nile delta. *Parasitology Today* **13**, 112–119.

Popiel, I. 1986. The reproductive biology of schistosomes. *Parasitology Today* **2**, 10–15.

Redman, C. A., Robertson, A., Fallon, P. G., Modha, J., Kusel, J. R., Doenhof, M. J., and Martin, R. J. 1996. Praziquantel: An urgent and exciting challenge. *Parasitology Today* **12**, 14–20.

Rollinson, D., and Simpson, A. J. G. 1987. *The Biology of Schistosomes: From Genes to Latrines*. Academic, New York.

Stirewalt, M. A. 1974. *Schistosoma mansoni*: Cercaria to schistosomule. *Advances in Parasitology* **12**, 115–182.

Taylor, M. G. 1998. Schistosomosis. In *Zoonoses* (Palmer, S. R., Soulsby, E. J. L., and Simpson, D. I. H., Eds.), pp. 717–729. Oxford University Press, Oxford, England.

PART THREE

THE CESTOIDEA

Chapter Twelve

GENERAL CHARACTERISTICS OF THE CESTOIDEA

The Cestoidea, or tapeworms, are a class of parasitic flatworms that possess all of the characteristics of the phylum Platyhelminthes presented in Chapter 9. The most striking difference between members of this class and those of the class Trematoda is that tapeworms lack a mouth and digestive tract. All tapeworms belong to one of two subclasses: the Eucestoda, or true tapeworms (cestodes), to which those infecting humans belong, and the Cestodaria, a smaller, less well-known group.

The Eucestoda are the most highly specialized flatworm parasites known. Adults of this subclass are endoparasitic in the alimentary tract and associated ducts of various vertebrates, including humans; the larvae, on the other hand, infect both vertebrates and invertebrates. The life cycle usually requires one or two intermediate hosts, in each of which the tapeworm undergoes a specific developmental phase.

There is much speculation about the origin and phylogeny of tapeworms. One evolutionary scheme proposes that they arose from a stock of aquatic, free-living, bottom-dwelling protomonogeneans that, in turn, evolved from a rhabdocoel-like ancestor similar to the ancestral form suggested for digenetic trematodes. The immediate ancestors of modern tapeworms evolved adhesive organs that enabled them to become attached to, and subsequently ectoparasitic upon, bottom-dwelling vertebrates. Some of these ectoparasitic forms migrated internally to the gut of these vertebrates and became endoparasitic. They evolved protective modifications, such as a glycocalyx on the body surface and quinone-tanned eggshells, that enabled them to resist the actions of the hosts' digestive enzymes. They also underwent physiological adaptations that allowed them to survive in an environment with reduced oxygen tension. At least one branch of these essentially monozoic animals evolved additional modifications, such as the loss of the gut, development of anterior attachment organs, and duplication of reproductive systems; the last feature leads eventually to segmentation of the body. As the group became increasingly diverse, they acquired other modifications, including adoption of intermediate hosts and the appearance of **apolysis**, the release of gravid (egg-filled) body segments to the exterior. A causal relationship appears certain between the development of apolysis and the loss of capacity to form tanned eggshells resistant to host digestive enzymes, although there is a "chicken or egg" kind of question as to which occurred first.

MORPHOLOGY

The body of the typical adult eucestode consists of three distinct regions: **scolex, neck,** and **strobila** (Fig. 12-1). The scolex, located at the anterior end, is the attachment terminal, the morphology and dimensions of which are key features in identification of these worms. The neck, an unsegmented, poorly differentiated region immediately posterior to the scolex, is generally the narrowest part of the worm. It is from the neck region that new segments, or **proglottids**, differentiate. As new proglottids are formed in the neck region, they push the older ones progressively posteriad, creating a chain of proglottids, the strobila. The asexual process of forming segments is termed **strobilization** (Fig. 12-2). As each proglottid is shifted posteriad, its sexual reproductive system matures progressively; hence, the anteriormost proglottids have the least-developed reproductive systems, while the more posteriorly the proglottids are located, the higher their level of development. This progressive maturity of the reproductive system permits a loose subdivision of the strobila into regions of **immature, mature,** and **gravid** proglottids (Fig. 12-2). The reproductive organs in immature proglottids are visible but nonfunctional, while those in mature proglottids are fully functional. At the posterior end of the strobila are the gravid (egg-filled) proglottids. Often, the reproductive organs in gravid proglottids have atrophied. In apolytic species, gravid proglottids detach from the strobila and exit the body of the host with feces. In **anapolytic** species, eggs are released through a uterine (or genital) pore directly into the host's intestine and, subsequently, also are discharged to the exterior in feces. Most anapolytic tapeworms produce protective, tanned eggshells.

TEGUMENT

The tegument of tapeworms (Fig. 12-3) is essentially similar to that of digeneans, with a few notable differences. The surface of

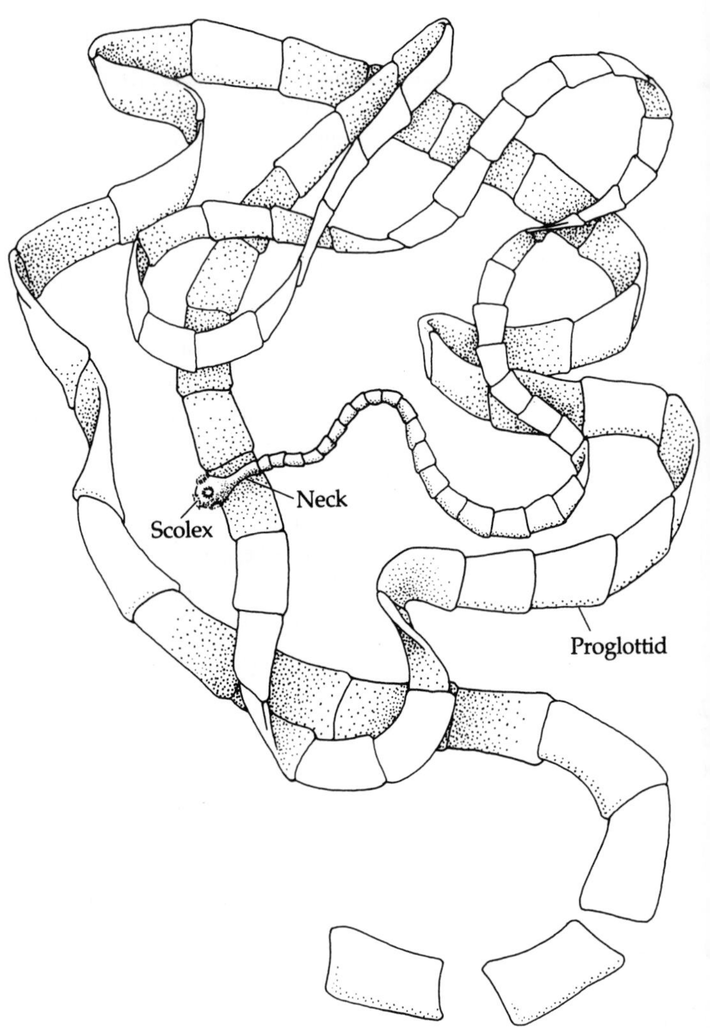

FIGURE 12-1
The three major regions of a generalized eucestode.
Note the scolex and neck regions. The remaining region, made up of many proglottids, is the strobila.

the tapeworm tegument bears specialized microvilli, known as **microthrices** (singular, **microthrix**), that project from the outer limiting membrane of the tegument. The dimensions of these projections vary according to species and location on the strobila. Unlike typical microvilli, each microthrix includes an electron dense, apical tip separated from the more basal region by a multilaminar plate. When applied to the host's intestinal epithelium, these tips provide resistance to the peristaltic movement of the intestine. With each movement of the worm, they also agitate

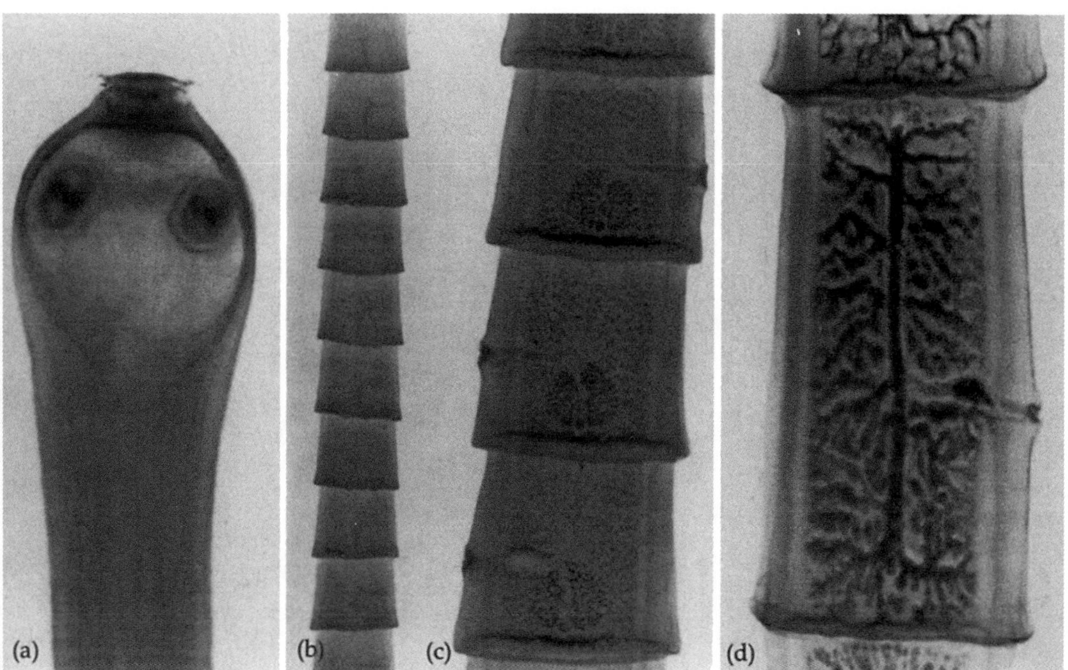

FIGURE 12-2
Regions along the length of a cestode, *Taenia solium*.
(a) Scolex and neck region. (b) Immature proglottids. (c) Mature proglottids. (d) Gravid proglottid.

intestinal fluids in the immediate microhabitat, thus increasing accessibility of nutrients and flushing away waste products. Covering the entire surface of the tegument is a layer of carbohydrate-containing macromolecules, the **glycocalyx,** that serves several important functions, among which are protecting the parasite from host digestive enzymes, enhancing nutrient absorption, and maintaining the parasite's surface membrane.

As in digeneans, the tegumental syncytium of tapeworms consists of two cytoplasmic regions, **distal** and **proximal.** The distal cytoplasm is replete with mitochondria (usually aligned in a broad, basal band), as well as several types of vesicles and scattered membranes. Glycogen granules are also present in this region in some species. The vesicles arise in the nucleated, proximal cytoplasm, or **cyton,** sunk deep in the parenchyma. The cyton contains Golgi complexes, mitochondria, rough endoplasmic reticulum, and other organelles involved in protein synthesis and packaging. Proteins synthesized in the cyton are translocated via

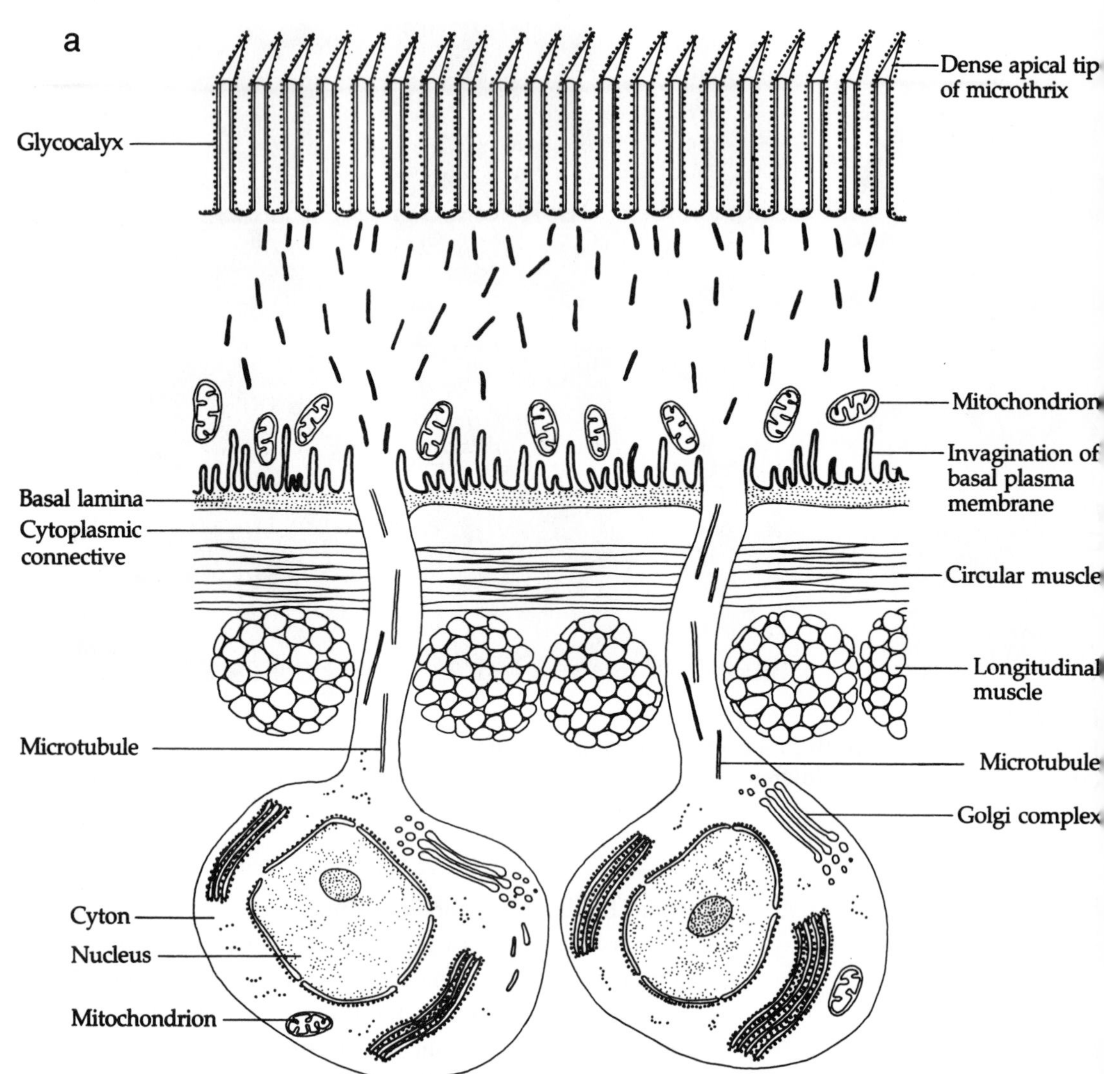

FIGURE 12-3
Tegument of a cestode.
(a) The surface is covered with microthrices, each ending in a thickened, spinelike cap. As is usual among parasitic flatworms, the cell bodies are secretory and produce surface coat constituents among other material. (b) Transmission electron micrograph of the tegumental surface showing microthrices.

cytoplasmic connectives abetted by microtubules to the distal cytoplasm, where they maintain the glycocalyx, membranes, microthrices, and other structures.

Underlying the distal cytoplasm are two layers of muscles, col-

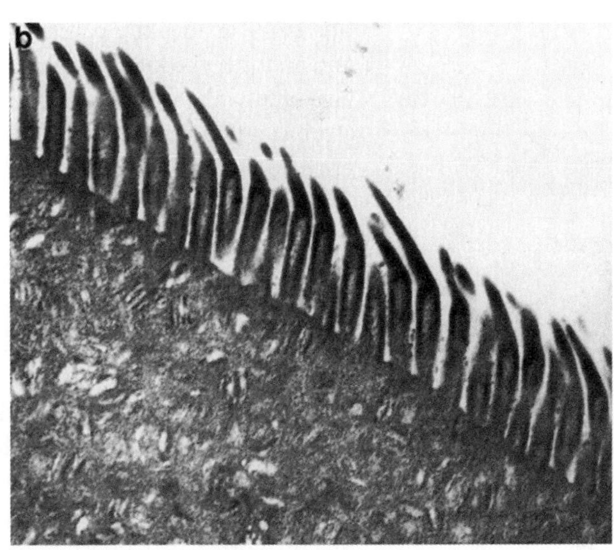

FIGURE 12-3 **Continued.**

lectively known as the **tegumental musculature**, consisting of an outer layer with its contractile fibrils oriented in a circular pattern and an inner layer with contractile fibrils oriented longitudinally.

PARENCHYMA

The space enclosed by the tegument—except for the portion occupied by reproductive organs, osmoregulatory structures, muscle fibers, and nervous tissue—is filled with a spongy tissue known as the **parenchyma.** In live tapeworms, fluid fills the spaces between parenchymal cells. Parenchymal cells are the primary sites for synthesis and storage of glycogen. There is speculation that myoblasts give rise to both the parenchyma and the musculature of most tapeworms.

PARENCHYMAL MUSCLES

Unlike tegumental musculature, **parenchymal musculature** is unique to eucestodes. Bipolar muscle cells and fibers embedded in the parenchyma form a broad band that encircles each proglottid about midway between the outer surface and the central axis;

this band divides the parenchyma into an outer **cortical** region and an inner **medullary** region. In addition to the dominant, longitudinally aligned, contractile myofibers that help stabilize the strobila against peristalsis in the host intestine, circular myofibers are also present.

SCOLEX

To facilitate attachment to the host's intestinal wall, tapeworms utilize several types of structures on their scolices, the most common of which are suckers. Muscles in the scolex make possible the holdfast action of this organ. The musculature of the scolex consists of sets of crisscrossing fibers attached to the inner surfaces of the suckers, enabling the suckers to contract. Scolices of tapeworms that infect humans are categorized as either **acetabulate** or **bothriate**, depending on the type of sucker they possess (Fig. 12-4).

An acetabulate scolex is characterized by the presence of four muscular cups sunk into the equatorial surface of the scolex (Fig. 12-4a). These cups are radially arranged and equidistant from each other. While the rim of each cup is usually round, it may be oval or even slitlike in some species, and it may be flush with the surface or project beyond it. Each cup is covered by a thin layer

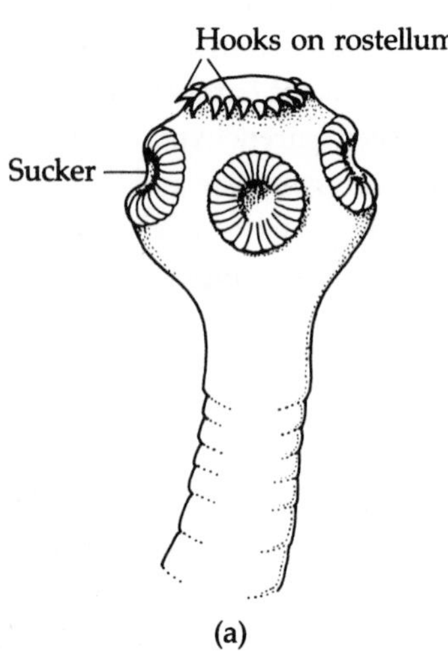

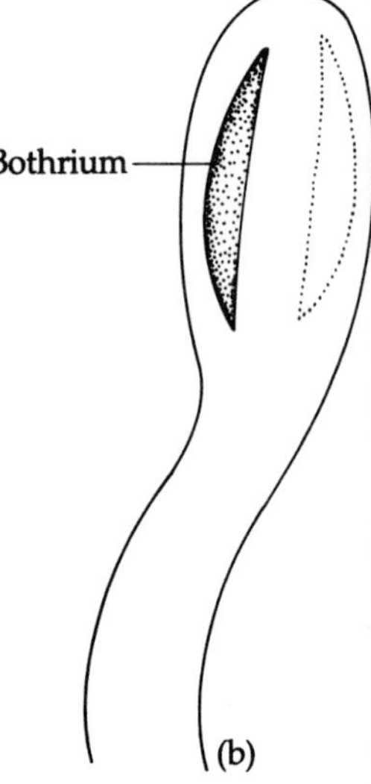

FIGURE 12-4
Types of scolices found on tapeworms that infect humans.
(a) Acetabulate, showing three of the four suckers and an armed rostellum. (b) Bothriate, showing one of the two bothridial grooves.

of tegument continuous with that covering the rest of the body. In addition to the muscular cups, there may be accessory hold-fast structures, such as hooks, that help anchor the scolex to the host's intestinal wall; a scolex with such structures is called an **armed scolex**. The hooks are usually grouped at the apical end of the scolex on a protrusible **rostellum**. The presence, number, size, and shape of the hooks are of taxonomic importance.

A bothriate scolex is characterized by the presence of two, or rarely four or six, longitudinally arranged, shallow depressions called **bothria** (singular, **bothrium**; Fig. 12-4b).

Various types of glandular secretions are associated with the scolices of many tapeworms. The function of these secretions has not been established with certainty, although it has been speculated that they are proteolytic, adhesive, and/or stimulatory, depending upon the species.

CALCAREOUS CORPUSCLES

Large numbers of concretions, known as **calcareous corpuscles**, occur in the parenchyma of numerous cestode species as well as some trematodes. These spherical bodies, most noticeable in larval forms, consist of organic and inorganic components. The organic portion is composed of DNA, RNA, proteins, glycogen, mucopolysaccharides, and alkaline phosphatase; the inorganic portion is made up primarily of calcium, magnesium, phosphorus, and trace metals. Although the functions of these inclusions remain unclear, it has been suggested that they may act as buffers against anaerobically produced acids, serve as reservoirs for inorganic ions required during development, act as enzyme activators, or are excretory products of metabolism.

OSMOREGULATORY SYSTEM

The cestode osmoregulatory–excretory system is essentially the same as the flame-cell, protonephritic type found in digeneans. In most cases, it serves to maintain within the worm an optimal hydrostatic pressure for extensory movements of the strobila and scolex. However, some tapeworms, such as *Hymenolepis diminuta*, are known osmoconformers; that is, they lack the ability to regulate osmotic pressure and therefore adapt or "conform" to the environmental osmotic conditions. In these species, the system appears to be strictly excretory. The morphology of the system varies somewhat among the different taxa, but sufficient similarity exists to justify the following generalized description.

The osmoregulatory–excretory system consists of two components: **collecting canals** and **flame cells.** Four laterally aligned collecting canals, two dorsal and two ventral, extend the entire length of the strobila (Fig. 12-5). All four canals lie just inside the

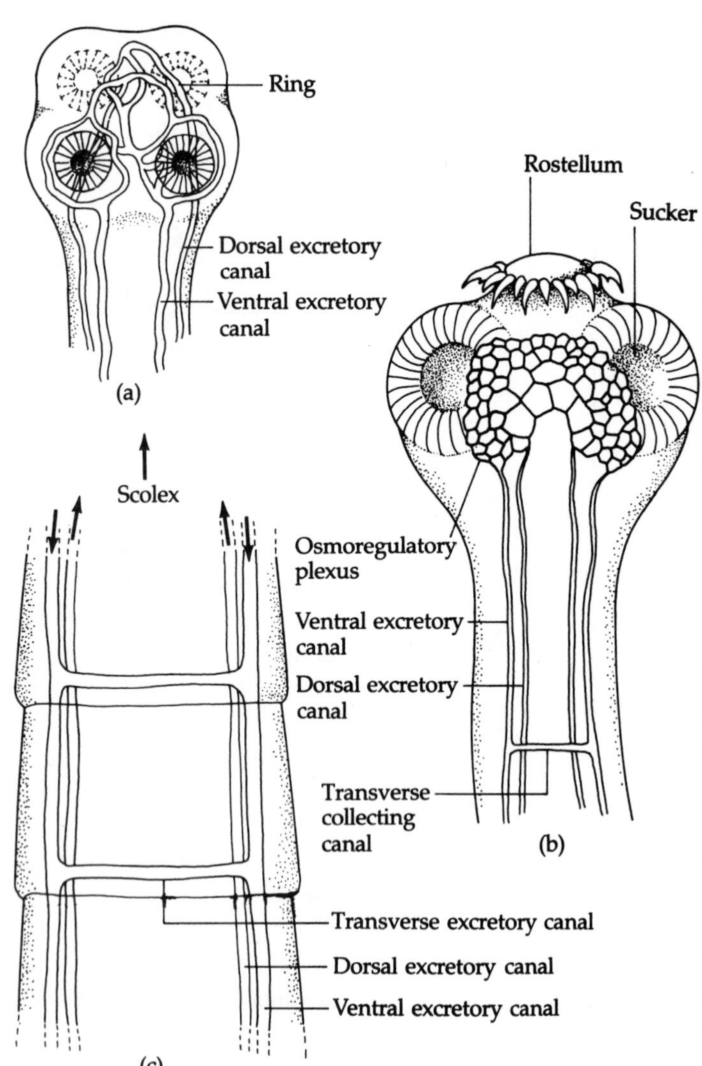

FIGURE 12-5
Morphology of the osmoregulatory–excretory system of cestodes.
(a) Scolex of *Proteocephalus* sp. showing single-ring type of connection of the osmoregulatory canals. (b) Scolex of *Taenia* sp. showing network type of osmoregulatory plexus. (c) Proglottids showing longitudinal collecting canals. Arrows show direction of flow.

medullary margin of the parenchyma, and a single transverse canal connects the ventral canals at the posterior end of each proglottid. The ventral canals carry fluid away from the scolex, while the dorsal canals carry fluid toward it. In some tapeworms, the four longitudinal canals are linked within the scolex by either a network of canals or a single ring vessel; in others, the dorsal and ventral canals on each side are linked by a simple connection in the region of the scolex, with no apparent exchange between the two sides. In the terminal proglottid of young worms, there is an excretory vesicle into which the ventral canals empty. However, in older tapeworms that have sloughed the original posteriormost proglottid, the posterior ends of the ventral canals open independently to the exterior. Flame cells, usually arranged in groups of four, are associated with the ventral canals. Fluid collected by the flame cells passes through secondary tubules into the main canals. Analysis of fluid within the osmoregulatory system of certain species of tapeworm has revealed that it consists primarily of water, glucose, soluble proteins, lactic acid, urea, and ammonia. Reabsorption of essential molecules in this system has not been verified.

NERVOUS SYSTEM

The cestode nervous system is relatively complex. The "brain," located in the scolex, is a rectangular or circular arrangement of nerve tissue varying in complexity from a simple ganglion to a combination of several ganglia and commissures (Fig. 12-6). It gives rise to a system of short anterior and posterior nerves that richly supply various portions of the scolex with motor fibers and receive sensory fibers from the rostellum, suckers, and tegument. Several pairs of longitudinal nerve cords extend posteriorly from the brain along the length of the strobila, lateral to the osmoregulatory canals. The cords are connected in each proglottid by cross-connectives, producing a ladderlike appearance. Small motor nerves emanating from the cords and cross-connectives innervate the reproductive organs and musculature, and small sensory nerves supplying the tegument merge with the cords and connectives. Certain organs of both the scolex and the proglottids, such as parts of the reproductive system and suckers, are more extensively innervated than others.

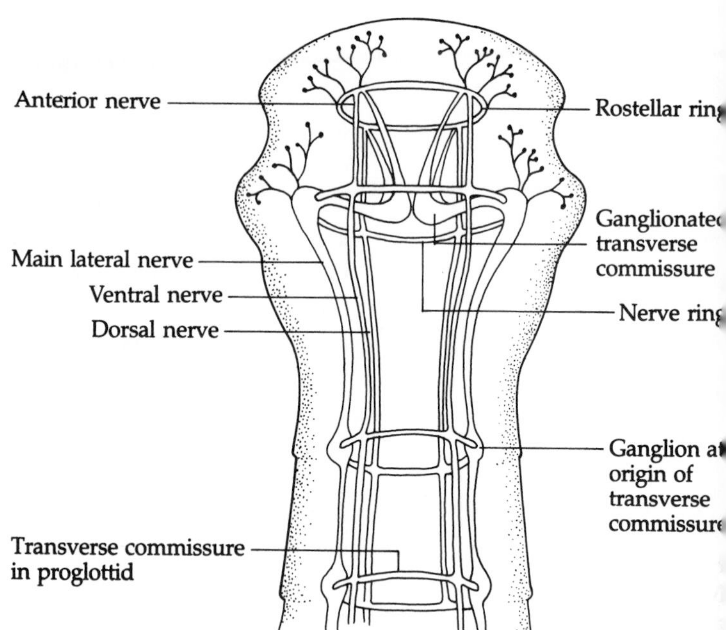

FIGURE 12-6
Cestode brain.

REPRODUCTIVE SYSTEM

The general pattern of the reproductive system of cestodes resembles that of digenetic trematodes, except for the **cul-de-sac uterus** in some forms (cyclophyllideans), the presence of a separate vaginal canal, and often a laterally situated genital pore. A generalized description of the cestode reproductive system follows, with specific variations noted.

Male System

The male reproductive system consists of from one to many testes embedded in the medullary parenchyma of each proglottid (Fig. 12-7). Emanating from each testis is a single vas efferens; in cases of multiple testes, the vasa efferentia unite to form a common vas deferens, which is usually coiled. The distal portion of the vas deferens is modified as a muscular **cirrus**, usually enclosed within a **cirrus sac.** In some species, the cirrus is equipped with spines that hold the organ in place during copulation. The cirrus everts through the male genital pore, which in turn opens into the common **genital atrium.**

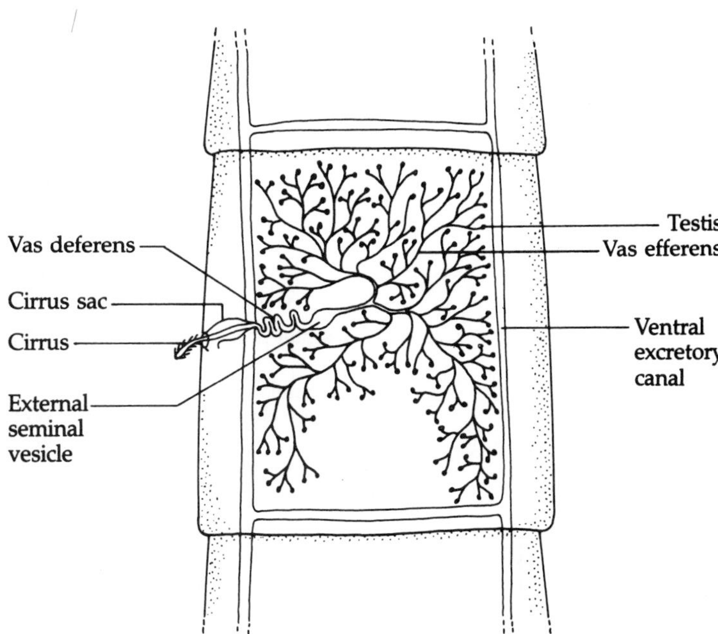

FIGURE 12-7
Male reproductive system of a typical eucestode.

In most species there is an enlarged area of the vas deferens, the **seminal vesicle,** for storage of sperm. When located within the cirrus sac, it is designated an **internal seminal vesicle;** located outside the sac, it is termed an **external seminal vesicle.** Some species possess both.

Female System

Ova are produced in a single, sometimes bilobed ovary (Fig. 12-8). Following fertilization in the proximal portion of the oviduct, the resulting zygote passes into a region of the oviduct, the **ootype,** equipped with structures involved in eggshell formation similar to those found in digeneans. A **Mehlis' gland** surrounds the ootype and secretes into it material essential to formation of the eggshell; a single, common **vitelline duct** enters the oviduct in the vicinity of the ootype. As in digeneans, the common vitelline duct is formed by the union of many **primary vitelline ducts** arising from vitelline glands, which vary in size and location according to species. The vitelline glands (collectively designated as the **vitellaria**) may form a compact body or consist of numerous follicles scattered throughout the medullary region of the parenchyma. With few exceptions, secretions of the vitelline

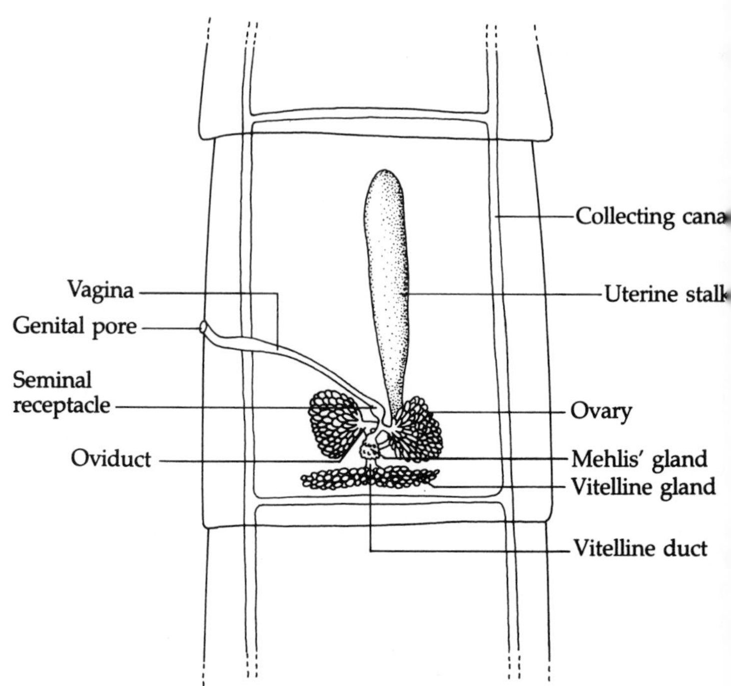

FIGURE 12-8
Female reproductive system of a typical eucestode.

glands contain shell precursors and provide nourishment for the developing larva. The uterine wall may also contribute materially to extraembryonic membranes and capsules.

The **vagina**, a tubular organ that joins the oviduct at the level of Mehlis' gland, provides a passage for sperm between the genital atrium and the oviduct, and fertilization occurs in the region where the vagina and oviduct join. Sperm are stored in an enlargement of the vagina known as the **seminal receptacle.** The oviduct continues as the uterus, which opens to the outside of the proglottid through a **uterine pore** in some tapeworms, such as the anapolytic members of the order Pseudophyllidea. Eggs are produced continuously and are expelled through this opening. In other species, including members of the order Cyclophyllidea, the uterus is a blind sac in which developing eggs accumulate; the uterus becomes distended with eggs, filling the medullary region of the proglottid. The gravid proglottid eventually becomes detached from the strobila and is discharged from the host. In some tapeworms (e.g., *Dipylidium*), there is a modification of uterus–egg interaction in which a much reduced uterus, upon receiving a specific number of eggs, begins pinching off **egg capsules** that eventually fill the medullary region of the gravid proglottid.

During copulation, the cirrus of one proglottid may be inserted in the vagina of another proglottid of the same or another worm. Cross-fertilization between two worms is advantageous, at least periodically, to insure vitality and prevent the development of deleterious features due to excessive self-breeding.

The Egg

The morphology of tapeworm eggs is important for species identification. The following is a brief general description of the basic parts of a typical egg (Fig. 12-9).

The **oncosphere**, containing three pairs of hooks, is encased in an **inner envelope** that, in turn, is surrounded by another membranous structure, the **embryophore**. A cellular zone known as the **outer envelope** lies between the embryophore and the **shell** (or **capsule**), usually the outermost covering of the egg. Tapeworm eggs exhibit certain variations within this basic pattern and are classified into four types: pseudophyllidean, dipylidean, taenioid, and stilesian. Of these, all but the last are represented among tapeworms infecting humans.

The pseudophyllidean egg (Fig. 12-10a), of which the eggs of *Diphyllobothrium latum* are representative, is most similar morphologically and developmentally to those of digenetic trematodes. The fully developed egg has a thick, quinone-tanned shell, usually with a lidlike operculum at one end. Numerous vitelline cells are associated with the zygote, providing stored food for subsequent development. The zygote develops into an oncosphere, which is covered by a ciliated embryophore enabling it to swim upon hatching. This ciliated form of the organism is called a **coracidium** (plural, **coracidia**).

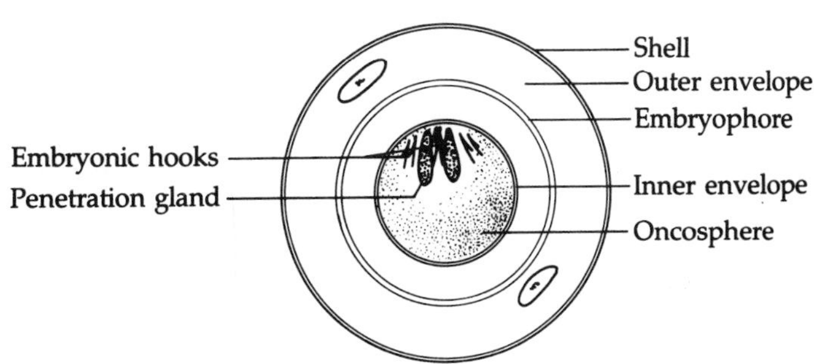

FIGURE 12-9
General structure of a cestode egg and enclosed oncosphere.

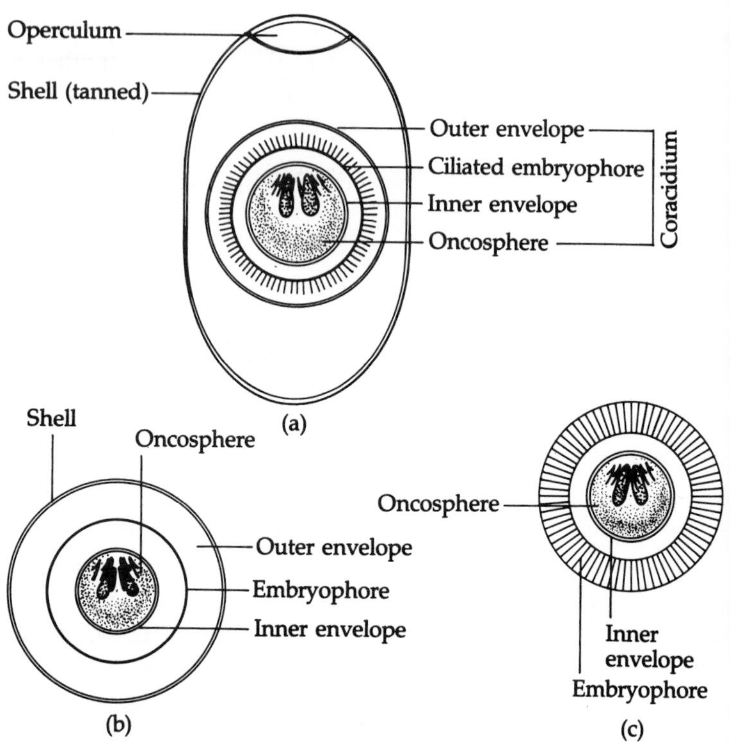

FIGURE 12-10
Variations in cestode egg structure.
(a) Pseudophyllidean. (b) Dipylidean. (c) Taenioid.

The dipylidean egg, seen in the genera *Dipylidium* and *Hymenolepis*, possesses a thin shell, a thin, nonciliated embryophore, and a relatively thick outer envelope (Fig. 12-10b). In the taenioid egg, characteristic of members of the genera *Taenia* and *Echinococcus*, the shell and outer envelope are lacking, and the thick, nonciliated embryophore constitutes the outermost covering (Fig. 12-10c). In *Dipylidium* and taenioid eggs, in contrast to pseudophyllidean eggs, only one or very few vitelline cells are associated with the zygote (Fig. 12-11).

LIFE CYCLE PATTERNS

Tapeworms that infect humans display two basic life cycle patterns, one typical of members of the order Pseudophyllidea, the other typical of members of the order Cyclophyllidea (Fig. 12-12).

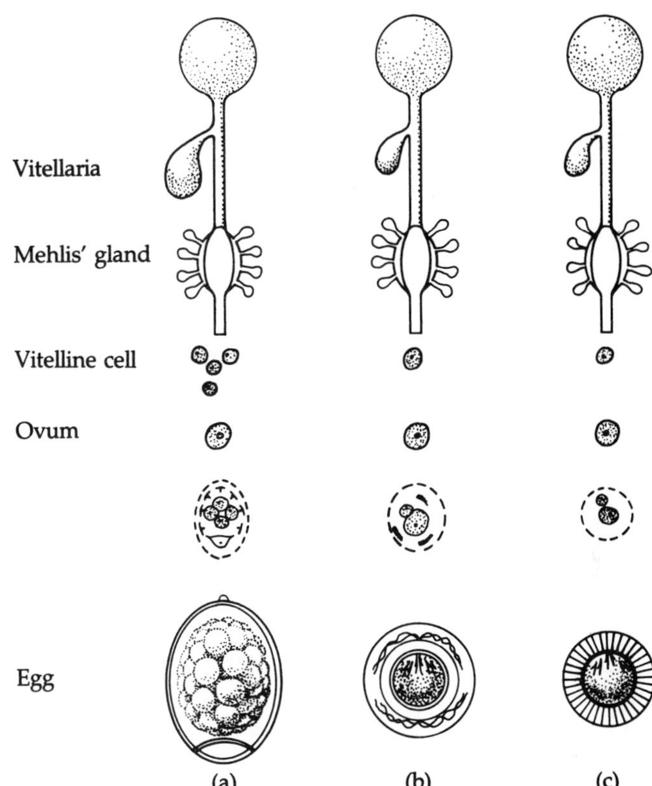

FIGURE 12-11
The three types of egg-forming systems among tapeworms that infect humans.
(a) Pseudophyllidean, e.g., in *Diphyllobothrium latum*. (b) Dipylidean, e.g., in *Hymenolepis nana*. (c) Taenioid, e.g., in *Taenia solium*.

PSEUDOPHYLLIDEAN PATTERN

In members of the order Pseudophyllidea, coracidia-containing eggs leave the host with feces. In water, the coracidium escapes from the eggshell through the operculum and swims for a brief time by means of its ciliated embryophore. Survival of the organism depends upon ingestion of the coracidium by an aquatic arthropod, the first intermediate host, within which the embryo sheds its ciliated embryophore and metamorphoses into a globular **procercoid** in the hemocoel. During this stage of development, the oncosphere hooks are retained, albeit nonfunctionally, in a tail-like structure called the **cercomer**. When the first intermediate host is ingested by a second intermediate host, usually a fish, the procercoid migrates via the peritoneal cavity to any of several parts of the body, principally the musculature, where it grows and develops into a solid, vermiform **plerocercoid** that manifests

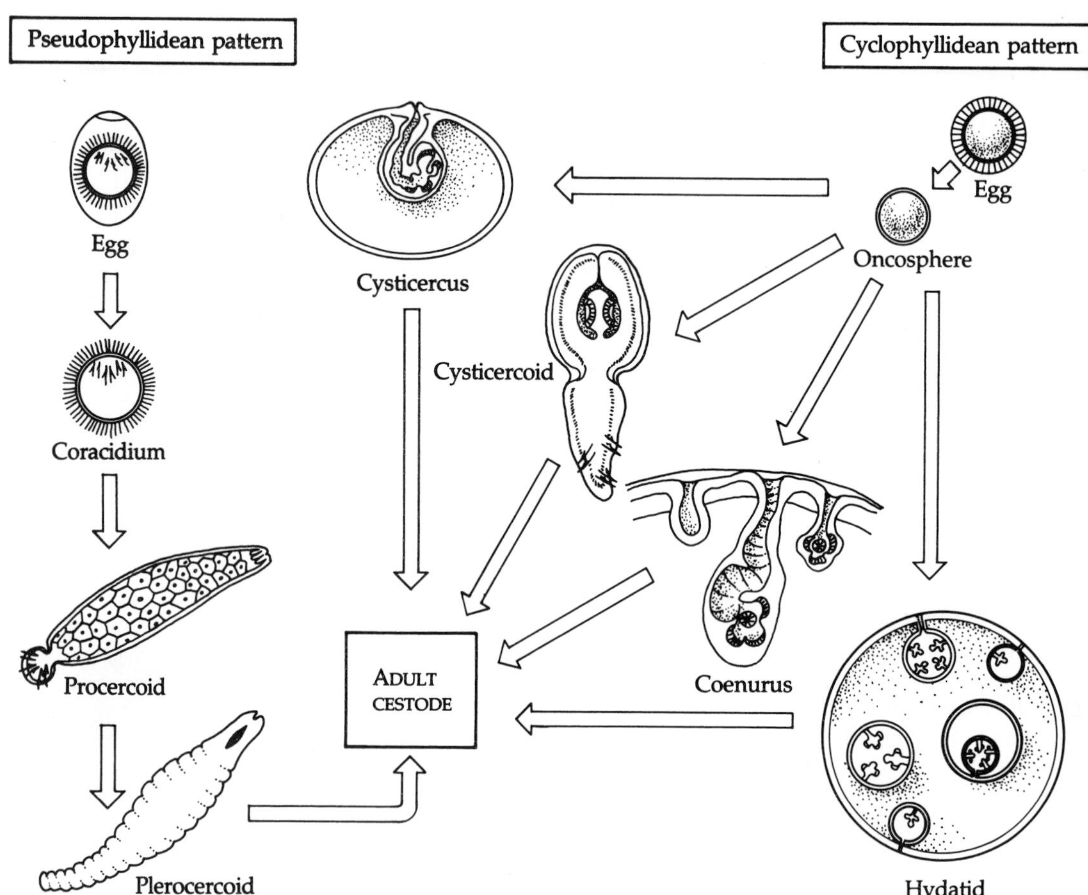

FIGURE 12-12
Life cycle patterns of tapeworms that infect humans.

the beginning of strobilization and a developing adult scolex. The plerocercoid is infective to humans; when ingested, it attaches to the wall of the small intestine, where strobilization occurs. All of the aforementioned stages possess penetration glands that secrete lytic enzymes, which aid in penetration of and migration among the various host tissues and organs.

CYCLOPHYLLIDEAN PATTERN

Adapted as it is to terrestrial hosts, the cyclophyllidean hexacanth embryo, or oncosphere, lacks a ciliated embryophore and must remain passive until the egg is ingested by a vertebrate or invertebrate intermediate host. In species that normally utilize an invertebrate intermediate host (usually an arthropod), the oncosphere, upon hatching in the digestive tract, employs its six hooks and its penetration glands to enter the hemocoel, where it metamorphoses into a **cysticercoid.** This form is solid-bodied and possesses a fully developed acetabulate scolex. It is surrounded by several layers of cystic tissue and has a prominent **cercomer** equipped with hooks. The cystic layers and the cercomer are eaten away in the digestive tract of the definitive host, freeing the scolex and neck to begin strobilization.

In species that utilize vertebrate intermediate hosts, the oncosphere, after ingestion, penetrates the intestinal lining and enters a venule. It is carried by the circulating blood to any of several areas of the body, where it develops into a **cysticercus** with an acetabulate scolex invaginated into a fluid-filled vesicle or bladder; hence, the common name for these parasites is **bladderworm.** Two other forms that follow this developmental pattern are the **coenurus** and the **hydatid** cysts. In the former, the wall of the bladder develops several invaginated scolices; in the latter, secondary cysts are formed as invaginations on the walls. These second-generation cysts are called **brood capsules** because they in turn give rise to scolices, each of which can develop into an adult worm when ingested by a suitable definitive host.

In some tapeworms, certain immature stages—including the cysticercus, coenurus, and hydatid cyst of some cyclophyllideans and the plerocercoid of several pseudophyllideans—are capable of developing in extraintestinal tissues of humans (see Chapter 14).

PHYSIOLOGY

The adaptive morphology of adult tapeworms and the environment in which they dwell are probably the most significant factors influencing their physiology. Lacking a digestive tract, these worms must derive all of their nutrient molecules from the host or from their microhabitat, and such molecules must cross the tegument. The methods by which nutrients cross the tegument include active transport, facilitated diffusion, and simple diffusion. The most important nutrient molecule is glucose, which, after polymerization within the parasite, is stored as glycogen usually in the parenchyma and interstitial fluid. The only other major transported carbohydrate is galactose. The sites on the tegument over which various molecules are transported vary for carbohydrates, amino acids, and purines and pyrimidines, the last two requisite for synthesis of nucleic acids. Most adult tapeworms also absorb lipids, probably by simple diffusion.

The environment in which tapeworms reside, the small intestine, is one of very low oxygen tension, necessitating anaerobic metabolism. Some tapeworms possess a mammalian-style electron transport system, but its role in energy production is minor. Metabolic rates differ in different parts of the strobila. The neck and immature proglottids have a much higher rate of metabolism than mature and gravid proglottids, reflecting the high energy requirements for new proglottid formation and organ development. Most of the energy requirement in mature proglottids is for egg production.

TREATMENT

In most instances, adult tapeworms have little visible effect upon their hosts except in heavy infections, which may result in anemia, weight loss, and various secondary manifestations. The treatment of choice for all tapeworms infecting the small intestine of humans is oral administration of the drug niclosamide, which disrupts proglottids and interferes with the worm's substrate-level phosphorylation, depriving the worm of required ATP. Two other drugs, quinacrine hydrochloride and aminocrine, have also proven effective in treating tapeworm infections. Praziquantel is an excellent broad-spectrum anthelmintic and, like niclosamide, causes disruption of proglottids. As in the case of schistosomes, additional effects of praziquantel upon tapeworms are vacuolization of the tegument and rapid paralysis of the worm's musculature. These drugs should be used cautiously in the treatment of *Taenia solium* infections, because cysticercosis can result from autoinfection by eggs released from disrupted proglottids (see Chapter 14). Five to six weeks after treatment, the patient's feces should be reexamined for the reappearance of eggs (Fig. 12-13), which may indicate that the scolex was retained and developed into a "new" worm.

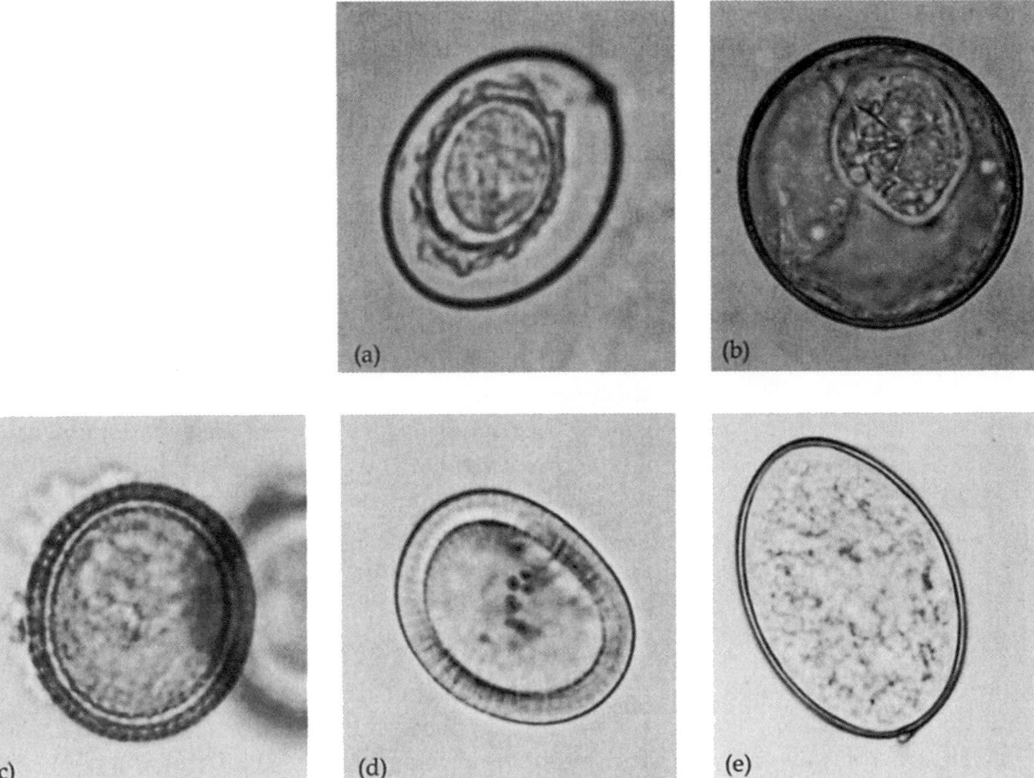

FIGURE 12-13
Some cestode eggs.
(a) *Hymenolepis nana*: the dwarf tapeworm of humans, rats, and mice. (b) *Hymenolepis diminuta*: the rat tapeworm. (c) *Taenia* spp. (d) *Taenia pisiformis*: the dog and cat tapeworm. (d) *Diphyllobothrium latum*: the broadfish tapeworm.

SELECTED READINGS

Coil, W. H. 1991. Platyhelminthes: Cestoidea. In *Microscopic Anatomy of the Invertebrates* (Harrison, F. W., and Bogitsh, B. J., Eds.) Vol. 3, pp. 211–283, Wiley-Liss, New York.

Kuperman, B. I., and Davydov, V. G. 1982. The fine structure of glands in oncospheres, procercoids and plerocercoids of Pseudophyllidea (Cestoda). *International Journal of Parasitology* 12, 135–144.

Lumsden, R. D. 1975. Surface ultrastructure and cytochemistry of parasitic helminths. *Experimental Parasitology* 37, 267–339.

Pappas, P. W., and Read, C. P. 1975. Membrane transport in helminth parasites: A review. *Experimental Parasitology* 37, 469–530

Schmidt, G. D. 1985. *Handbook of Tapeworm Identification.* CRC, Boca Raton, FL.

Smyth, J. D. 1969. *The Physiology of Cestodes.* W. H. Freeman, San Francisco.

CLASSIFICATION OF THE CESTOIDEA*

CLASS CESTOIDEA

All parasitic, being common in all classes of vertebrates except Cyclostomata; intermediate host required for almost all species.

Subclass Eucestoda

Polyzoic flatworms (except orders Caryophyllidea and Spathebothriidea); one or more sets of reproductive organs per proglottid; scolex usually present; shelled embryo with six hooks; parasites of fish, amphibians, reptiles, birds, and mammals.

ORDER CYCLOPHYLLIDEA

Scolex usually with four suckers; rostellum present or absent, armed or not; neck present or absent; strobila usually with distinct segmentation; monoecious (or rarely, dioecious); genital pores lateral (ventral in Mesocestoididae); vitelline gland compact, single (double in Mesocestoididae), posterior to ovary (anterior or beneath ovary in Tetrabothriidae); uterine pore absent; parasitic in amphibians, reptiles, birds, and mammals. (Genera mentioned in text: *Hymenolepis, Echinococcus, Taenia, Dipylidium.*)

ORDER PSEUDOPHYLLIDEA

Scolex with two bothria, with or without hooks; neck present or absent; strobila variable, proglottids anapolytic (senile proglottid detached after it sheds enclosed eggs); genital pores lateral, dorsal, or ventral; testes numerous; ovary posterior; vitellaria follicular as in Trypanorhyncha, occasionally in lateral fields but not interrupted by interproglottidal boundaries; uterine pore present, dorsal or ventral; egg usually operculate, containing coracidium; parasitic in fishes, amphibians, reptiles, birds, and mammals. (Genus mentioned in text: *Diphyllobothrium.*)

* Only those taxa that have genera mentioned in the text are listed.

Chapter Thirteen

INTESTINAL TAPEWORMS

Adult tapeworms belonging to six genera in two orders infect the human intestinal tract. A single representative of the order Pseudophyllidea, *Diphyllobothrium latum*, is included in this group; the remaining genera, representing three families, belong to the order Cyclophyllidea. The family Taeniidae is represented by *Taenia solium* and *T. saginata*; Hymenolepididae is represented by *Hymenolepis nana* and *H. diminuta*; and Dilepididae is represented by *Dipylidium caninum*. At least two other members of the family Taeniidae, *Echinococcus granulosus* and *E. multilocularis*, are of medical importance to humans; however, because only the larvae infect humans, they are discussed in Chapter 14.

DIPHYLLOBOTHRIUM LATUM

Diphylobothrium latum, the broadfish tapeworm, parasitizes several larger mammals, including humans, throughout the world. Its common name is derived from the fact that the proglottids are wider than they are long. It is most prevalent in Scandinavia, the former USSR, and parts of temperate South America. A closely related species, *D. ursi,* may also infect humans in northeastern North America.

On the midventral surface of each *D. latum* proglottid is a common genital atrium into which the male and female genital pores open (Fig. 13-1). The bilobed ovary lies in the posterior portion of the proglottid. The oviduct, arising from the ovary, continues anteriad as a coiled uterus, opening to the exterior through the midventral **uterine pore**. Embryos enclosed in tanned shells are expelled via the uterine pore. The follicular cells that comprise the vitellaria are scattered throughout the cortical fields of the proglottid, and numerous testes are chiefly medullary in their distribution, except for those occupying an area along the midline of each proglottid. Sperm enter the female pore and pass down the vagina to the oviduct, where fertilization occurs.

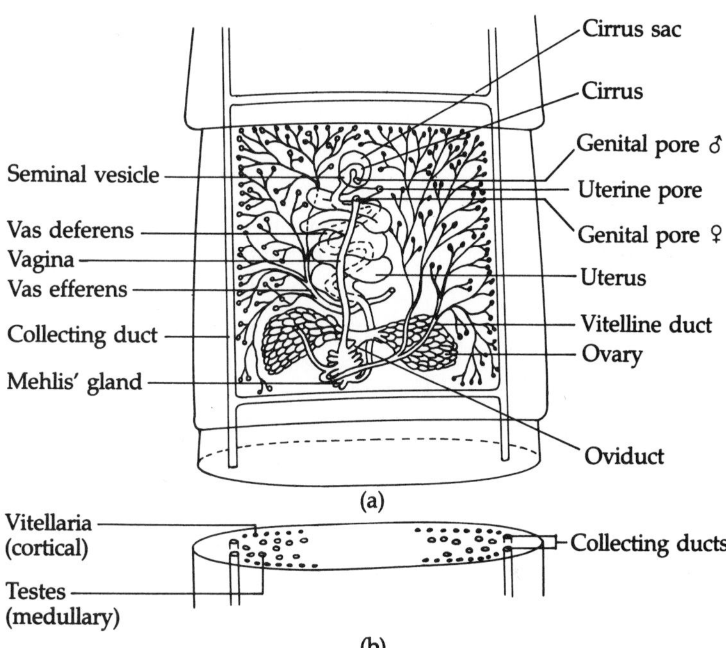

FIGURE 13-1
Mature proglottid of *Diphyllobothrium latum*.
(a) Ventral view. (b) Cross section.

Adult worms may attain a length of 10 meters, may be 10–20 mm wide, and may consist of more than 3000 proglottids, making *D. latum* the largest tapeworm found in humans. The extraordinary size of this tapeworm is partially due to anapolysis, the retention of terminal proglottids; approximately 80% of the proglottids are mature or nearly so. The size of the vertebrate host may also influence the size of the parasite. For example, one of the largest specimens of *D. latum* ever found was 12 meters long; it was recovered at autopsy from a bear from Yellowstone National Park.

Life Cycle

The adult worm attaches to the mucosal lining of the ileum or, sometimes, the jejunum by both bothria (Fig. 13-2). Ovoid, operculated eggs are released from the uterine pore on the ventral surface of the proglottid. At the time of oviposition, the enclosed hexacanth embryo is immature; the eggs must lie dormant in the water for approximately 8–12 days or longer for embryonic development to be completed. Typical of the Pseudophyllidea, the

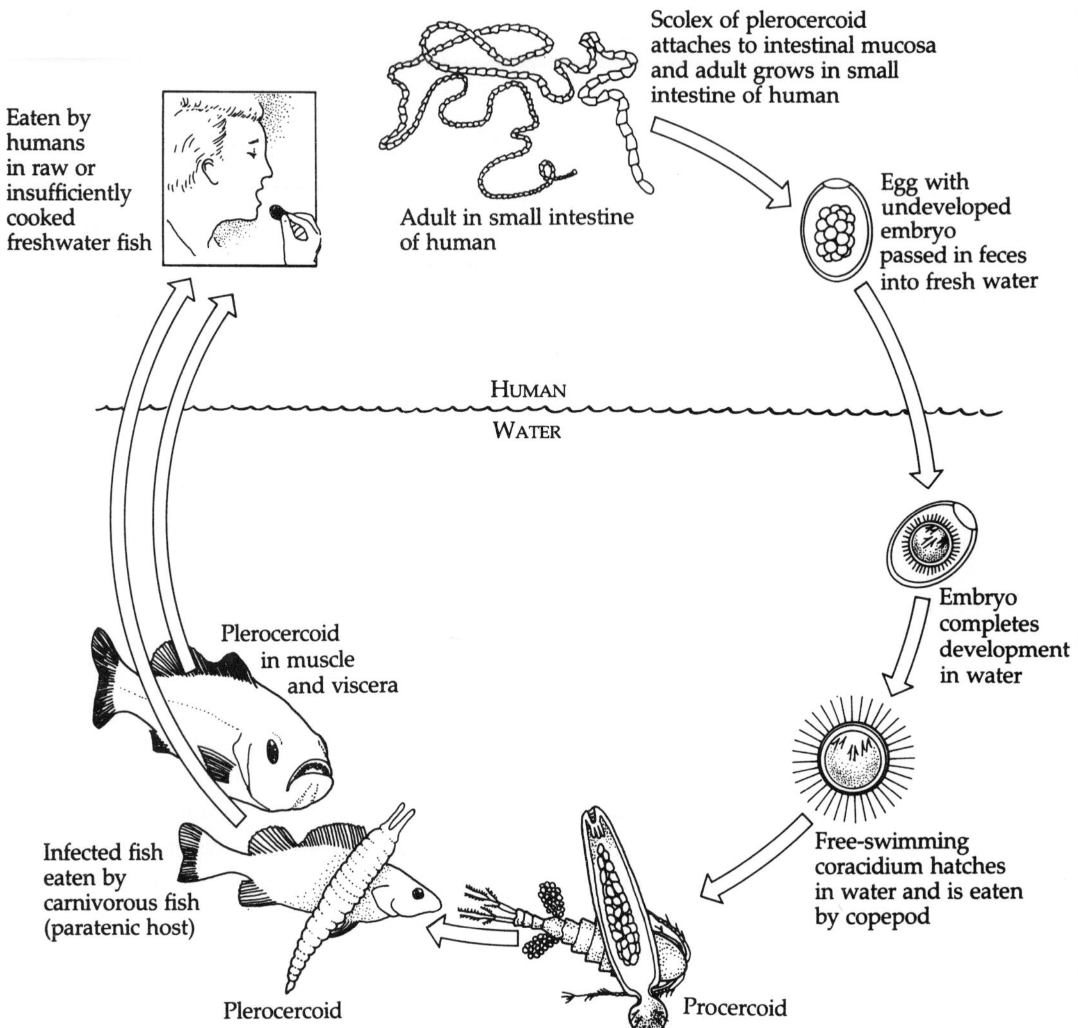

FIGURE 13-2
Life cycle of *Diphyllobothrium latum*.

hexacanth embryo is sheathed in a ciliated embryophore and is called a **coracidium**.

Within 24 hours after hatching, the motile coracidium must be ingested by a freshwater copepod belonging to the genus *Cyclops* or *Diaptomus*, or it will perish. In the digestive tract of the copepod, the ciliated embryophore is shed and the naked hexacanth larva, by means of its hooks and secretions, bores through the intestinal wall into the hemocoel. In 14–18 days, the hexacanth embryos, usually only one or two per infected copepod, metamorphose into elongated, globular **procercoid** larvae, each measuring about 500 μm in length. The prominent cercomer, containing the six hooks, projects posteriorly.

When the infected copepod is ingested by a suitable plankton-feeding freshwater fish, the procercoid larva penetrates the intestinal wall and migrates to the musculature. In 7–30 days, it develops into a long (2–4 cm), solid, pseudosegmented **plerocercoid** larva with a fully developed scolex at one end. Numerous plerocercoids may be present in the musculature of a single fish host.

Unlike most pseudophyllidean plerocercoids, those of *D. latum* are coiled. They may either be encapsulated or, more commonly, lie free in the muscle tissue. Host reaction, such as encapsulation, depends upon the site of plerocercoid invasion. Plerocercoids infiltrating the muscles of the body wall are rarely encapsulated, while those settling in or on the viscera commonly are encapsulated. Definitive hosts, including humans, acquire infection through ingestion of plerocercoids in undercooked, steamed, smoked, pickled, or raw fish. Upon entering the small intestine of the definitive host, the plerocercoid attaches to the mucosa and grows at the rate of about 30 proglottids a day. Although it reaches full sexual maturity in 3–5 weeks, it continues to add proglottids for an extended period.

Epidemiology

Human infection with *D. latum* is primarily, although not exclusively, limited to areas where fresh fishes are a dietary staple or where the cleaning and handling of fish take place. A number of freshwater fishes from cold-water regions, including such prized food fishes as pike, salmon, trout, and whitefish, can serve as second intermediate hosts. In addition to being ingested with raw or improperly cooked fish, plerocercoids that cling to the hands of fish cleaners may be accidentally ingested. Incidence is relatively high, for example, among the residents of Finland and some Baltic communities. In North America, 50–70% of northern and wall-eyed pike found in certain small lakes in the northern United States and Canada harbor plerocercoids of *D. latum*. The parasite is also found in Swiss lakes, the basin of the Danube River, the Middle East, Japan, Chile, Argentina, Peru, and Australia.

Although a number of fish-eating mammals harbor the tapeworm, they are responsible, at worst, for the spread of the parasite in areas devoid of human inhabitants. Coupled with the presence of suitable intermediate hosts, humans are responsible for establishing and maintaining endemicity in the human population through inadequate sanitation and the practice of eating raw or improperly cooked fish. Furthermore, the increased incidence of infected fishes in the United States can be traced directly to the practice of dumping untreated sewage into lakes and streams.

Symptomatology and Diagnosis

Rarely is more than a single worm found in an infected human, and many victims display few, if any, symptoms. Others complain of abdominal pain, weight loss, weakness, and nervous disorders. Many of these vague symptoms are attributable to the patient's reaction to the parasite's metabolic wastes, to degenerating proglottids, or to irritation of the intestinal mucosa; in some cases, they may also be a psychosomatic manifestation after the patient learns of the presence of the worm.

Occasionally, the worm is found in the upper portions of the jejunum, in which case it can compete successfully with the host for ingested vitamin B_{12}. Because this vitamin is important in the synthesis of hemoglobin, patients deprived of it develop an anemia similar to pernicious anemia. In endemic areas such as Finland, 5–10 of every 10,000 individuals infected with *D. latum* suffer from this type of anemia. The anemia subsides if the worm is forced to retreat further down the intestine, by chemotherapy, for instance.

Laboratory diagnosis consists of identifying eggs (see Fig. 12-15) or the characteristic broad proglottids in feces or vomitus.

TAENIA SOLIUM

This parasite, commonly referred to as the "human pork tapeworm," is common among humans in areas where raw or inadequately cooked pork is regularly consumed. The adult worm usually measures 180–400 cm (sometimes up to 800 cm) long and contains 800–900 proglottids. The small scolex (Fig. 13-3a),

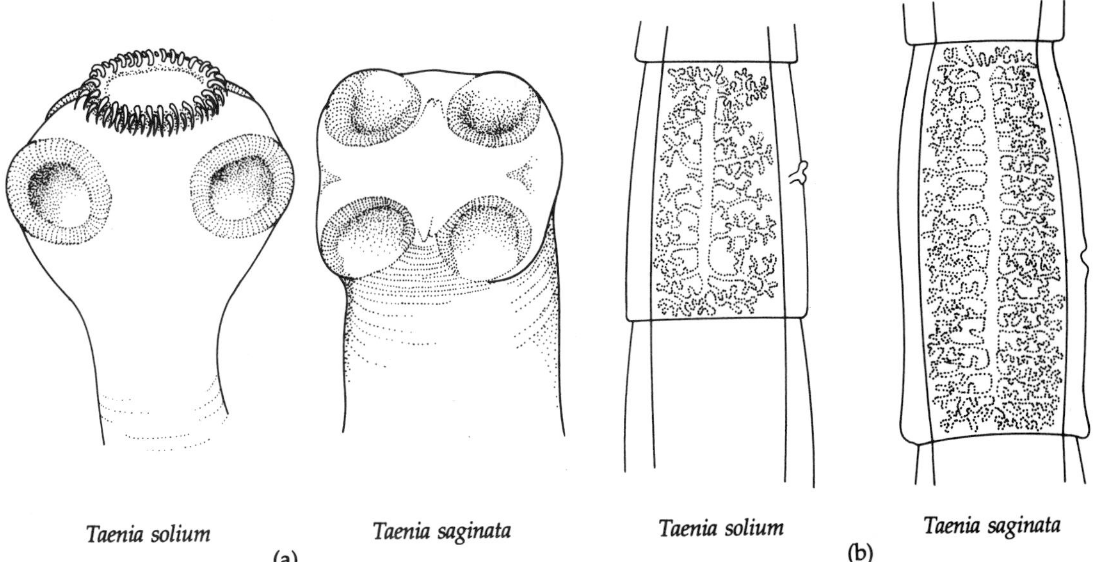

FIGURE 13-3
(a) Armed scolex of *Taenia solium* (left) and unarmed scolex of *T. saginata* (right). (b) Gravid proglottids of *Taenia solium* (left) and *T. saginata* (right).

measuring about 1 mm in diameter, is armed with two circles of 22–32 rostellar hooks. These hooks are of two sizes—long (180 μm) and short (130 μm)—alternating in the two circular rows.

The mature proglottid (Fig. 13-4) is squarish in outline and has a common genital pore situated on the lateral edge, about halfway down. The pores on successive proglottids may be on alternate sides or may be positioned unilaterally. The testes are scattered throughout the medullary region of the proglottid. The ovary consists of two prominent lobes and one small, central lobe. The vitellaria are compact, as is characteristic of cyclophyllideans, and are located in the basal portion of the proglottid just posterior to the ovary. The oviduct arises at the junction of the three ovarial lobes and continues anteriad as the cul-de-sac **uterine stalk**. As eggs are produced, they are pushed up into the stalk, which forms lateral branches as the number of eggs increases. The number of lateral branches serves as a tool for distinguishing *T. solium* from *T. saginata*; *T. solium* has 7–12 lateral branches, while *T. saginata* has more than 12 (Fig. 13-3b).

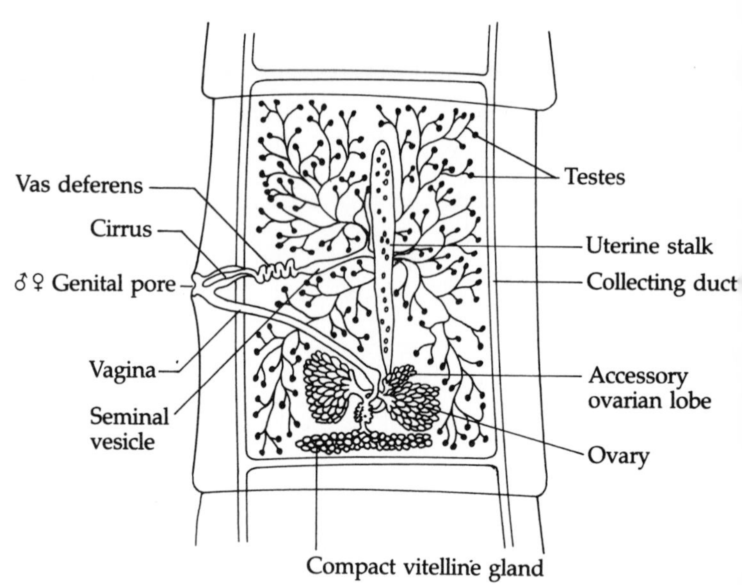

FIGURE 13-4
Mature proglottid of *Taenia solium.*

Life Cycle

Groups of five or six gravid proglottids, each containing thousands of eggs, exit the human host daily (Fig. 13-5). Eggs of *T. solium* are indistinguishable from those of *T. saginata*. The outer egg covering is radially striated and covers the oncosphere. The proglottid may rupture either in the host's intestine or after it leaves the host. When eggs are ingested by pigs, the liberated oncospheres, using their hooks and penetration gland secretions, penetrate the intestinal wall, enter the circulatory system, and are carried by blood or lymph to muscles, viscera, and other organs, where they develop into cysticerci. Each white, ovoid, fluid-filled cycticercus, formerly termed *Cysticercus cellulosae*, measures 6–18 mm in length and contains a single, invaginated scolex. When infected, or measly, pork is consumed by a human, the scolex evaginates and attaches to the jejunal wall; there the parasite develops to sexual maturity in 2–3 months. Humans are the only known natural definitive hosts.

Epidemiology

The prevalence of pork tapeworm infection in humans varies by region. The very low incidence in the United States can be at-

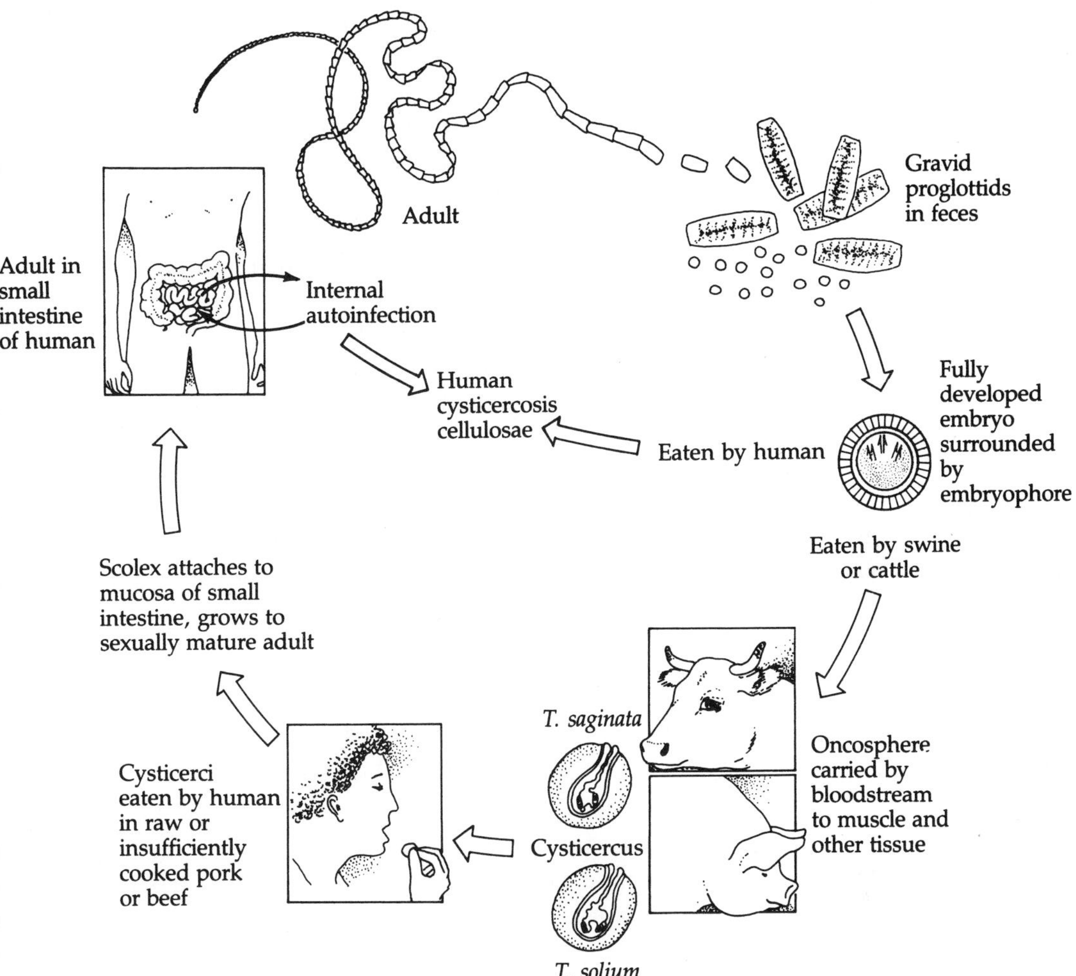

FIGURE 13-5
Life cycles of *Taenia solium* and *T. saginata*.

tributed to the isolation of pigs from human feces. Religious dietary proscriptions forbidding pork consumption by adherents of Islam and Judaism render human infection very rare in Moslem countries and in Israel. However, such infections are common in other parts of Africa, India, China, several countries in South and Central America, and Mexico.

Symptomatology and Diagnosis

Usually only a single adult tapeworm infects a human. The armed scolex may cause irritation of the mucosal lining, and there have been cases in which the scolex perforated the intestine, leading to peritonitis. However, the greatest hazard to human health associated with this parasite is infection with the cysticercus, causing the potentially serious disease, **human cysticercosis** (see Chapter 14).

Identification of proglottids in feces is the most reliable method of diagnosis. Because most taenioid eggs are morphologically indistinguishable (see Fig. 12-15), positive diagnosis is established by counting the number of main lateral uterine branches in gravid proglottids (7–12 in *T. solium*; Fig. 13-3b). The morphology of the scolex, particularly the rostellum, is also useful in diagnosis: *T. saginata* has no rostellum and its scolex bears no hooks, making it easily distinguishable from *T. solium*, which has an armed rostellum.

TAENIA SAGINATA

Taenia saginata is the most common of the large tapeworms of humans. Morphologically, the adult worm resembles *T. solium*. It is usually 35–60 cm long, but specimens as long as 225 cm have been reported. The strobila contains approximately 1000 proglottids. As mentioned earlier, the scolex is unarmed, having neither hooks nor rostellum (Fig. 13-3a). The morphology of mature proglottids in the two species differs primarily in that *T. saginata* has a bilobed ovary and about twice as many testes as *T. solium*. In addition, as previously noted, the gravid uterus of *T. saginata* has in excess of 12 main lateral branches.

Life Cycle

The life cycle of *T. saginata* strongly resembles that of *T. solium* (Fig. 13-5). Adults of both species reside in the jejunum of humans, and gravid proglottids of *T. saginata* detach singly from the strobila and pass to the outside with feces. The eggs of *T. saginata*, indistinguishable from those of *T. solium*, are ingested by a suitable intermediate host, such as a cow or other ugulate. The liberated oncosphere penetrates the intestinal wall and is carried by the lymphatic or blood circulatory system to intramuscular connective tissue, where it develops into a cysticercus known as *Cysticercus bovis*. Humans become infected by ingesting cysticerci in beef, particularly in muscles of the head and heart. Following evagination of the scolex and subsequent attachment to the jejunal wall, the worm develops to sexual maturity in 8–10 weeks.

Epidemiology

Taenia saginata is distributed thoughout the world. Humans acquire infection by eating raw or insufficiently cooked beef infected with the cysticerci, as in dishes such as steak tartare. Cattle acquire *Cysticercus bovis* by grazing in fields upon which human excrement has been deposited, either through fertilization with night soil or from poor sanitation. Pastures flooded by rivers and creeks contaminated with human excrement provide another source of infection for cattle. Under such conditions, eggs may remain viable for 2 months or longer. Thorough cooking of beef at 57°C until the reddish color disappears or freezing at –10°C for 5 days effectively destroys infective cysticerci. The beef tapeworm is comparatively rare in Hindu (Indian) populations, where cows are regarded with reverence and rarely eaten by humans.

Symptomatology and Diagnosis

Saginatus taeniasis (taeniosis) in humans is often characterized by such symptoms as abdominal pain, greatly diminished appetite, and weight loss. These symptoms are especially common in patients already debilitated by malnutrition or other illness. Unlike victims of *T. solium* infection, *T. saginata* victims rarely develop cysticercosis, and the prognosis is generally good. Diagnostic procedures are the same as those for *T. solium*.

HYMENOLEPIS NANA

Known as the dwarf tapeworm of mice and humans, the adult of this species is the smallest of the tapeworms infecting humans.

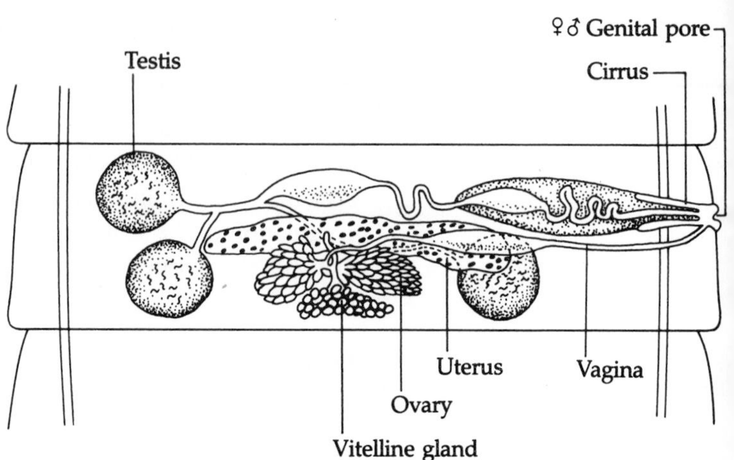

FIGURE 13-6
Mature proglottid of *Hymenolepis nana.*

It measures 7–50 mm in length and may consist of as many as 200 proglottids. The acetabulate scolex has a retractible rostellum armed with a single circle of small hooks. The mature proglottid (Fig. 13-6), approximately four times as broad as it is long, has a single, common genital atrium on the left margin. The male reproductive system consists of three spherical testes, one situated near the genital pore and separated from the other two by the bilobed ovary. The medullary region of the gravid proglottid is entirely occupied by a sacculate uterus containing up to 200 eggs.

Unlike *H. diminuta* (see the following), *H. nana* possesses an armed rostellum. This difference, along with other, less conspicuous differences, leads some to place *H. nana* in a different genus, *Vampirolepis*.

Life Cycle

The life cycle of *H. nana* (Fig. 13-7) is of particular biological significance: it represents a modification of the typical cyclophyllidean life cycle pattern in that the parasite requires only one host to complete its development. Natural definitive hosts, in addition to humans, are rodents, particularly mice and rats. Gravid proglottids from adult worms rupture, releasing oncosphere-containing eggs into the host's intestine, whence they are eliminated with feces. The egg is infective upon release. Its morphology is characteristic of hymenolepid eggs. The oncosphere is enclosed

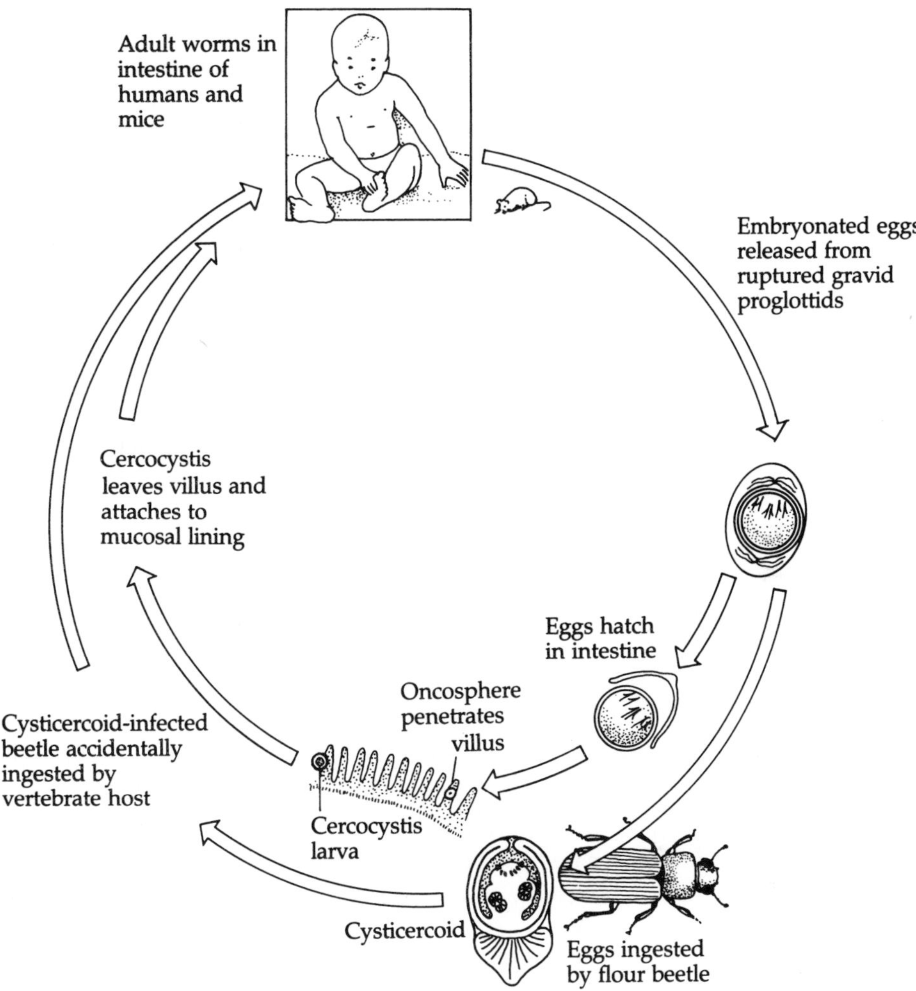
Adult worms in intestine of humans and mice
Embryonated eggs released from ruptured gravid proglottids
Eggs hatch in intestine
Oncosphere penetrates villus
Cercocystis larva
Cercocystis leaves villus and attaches to mucosal lining
Cysticercoid-infected beetle accidentally ingested by vertebrate host
Cysticercoid
Eggs ingested by flour beetle

FIGURE 13-7
Life cycle of *Hymenolepis nana*.

in a thin shell and an embryophore with two polar thickenings, from each of which extend four to eight filaments. Upon being ingested by a new host, the oncosphere, freed in the small intestine from its encapsulating membranes, penetrates a villus and enters the lamina propria. There, about 4 days later, it becomes a modified cysticercoid larva known as a **cercocystis**. The cercocystis erupts from the villus into the lumen of the small intestine, attaches itself to the mucosal lining, and develops into a sexually mature adult in about 30 days. In the case of rodents, an insect, such as the flour beetle, may serve as an intermediate host. In this case, when the insect host is ingested by a rodent, or even accidentally by a human, the cysticercoid attaches to the intestinal wall and develops to sexual maturity. Autoinfection can exacerbate the condition by increasing the number of worms; eggs released from gravid proglottids, instead of passing to the exterior to infect new hosts, hatch in the small intestine and reinfect the same host. The freed oncospheres penetrate villi and repeat the cycle.

Due to certain physiological variations, many authorities recognize two subspecies of *H. nana*: *H. nana nana*, which infects humans, and *H. nana fraterna*, which infects rodents. The life cycle of the rodent subspecies includes fleas and beetles as intermediate hosts in which the infective cysticercoid larva develops. Limited host cross-infectivity does occur.

Epidemiology

Hymenolepis nana is cosmopolitan in distribution and is possibly the more common cestode parasites of humans in the world, especially among children. Worldwide prevalence ranges from less than 1% in the United States to about 9% in Argentina, with an average worldwide prevalence of 4%. The usual mode of transmission in humans is hand-to-mouth; ingestion of contaminated food is also possible, although rare, because infective eggs are very susceptible to heat and desiccation. Infection may also be acquired by accidental ingestion of cysticerci-infected insects. The nature of the life cycle—i.e., no essential intermediate host and a high likelihood of autoinfection—renders prevention difficult. Teaching proper personal hygiene to children is perhaps the most effective preventive measure.

Symptomatology and Diagnosis

Because it is possible for a human victim to harbor massive numbers of these parasites, damage to the intestinal mucosa may be sufficient to produce enteritis. Most infections, however, are light and virtually symptomless, although autoinfection can lead to heavy worm burdens, particularly in children and immunosuppressed patients. In adult patients, the infection is usually self-limiting. In children with a moderate parasite burden, there may be loss of appetite, diarrhea, some abdominal pain, and dizziness. In many patients, a low humoral immune response is detectable. Diagnosis is by identification of eggs in feces (see Fig. 12-15).

HYMENOLEPIS DIMINUTA

Hymenolepis diminuta, a common parasite of rats throughout the world, occasionally parasitizes humans. *H. diminuta* exhibits a typical two-host life cycle, utilizing a grain-ingesting insect, such as a flour beetle, as intermediate host. A single worm may reach a length of 90 cm. The scolex in this species is unarmed, and the width of each proglottid is greater than its length. The morphology of proglottids is markedly similar to that of *H. nana* (Fig. 13-6). Of diagnostic relevance, the eggs are usually yellowish-brown and spherical. Unlike that of *H. nana*, the embryophore in these eggs does not bear conspicuous knobs or filaments at the poles. Insects are infected when they consume rodent feces containing eggs or gravid proglottids that have become detached from the strobila. The oncosphere, utilizing its hooks and secretions from the penetration glands, penetrates the intestinal wall of the insect and enters the hemocoel, where it develops to the cysticercoid stage. The most common intermediate hosts are grain beetles belonging to the genera *Tribolium* and *Tenebrio*, although cockroaches and fleas are also known to harbor infective cysticercoids. Humans acquire infection by eating cereals, dried fruits, and other similar foods contaminated with infected insects. The cysticercoid, once ingested by the definitive host, is freed from the insect's tissues in the small intestine. The scolex escapes from the cysticercoid tissue via a birth pore and attaches to the mucosa of the small intestine. The worm becomes sexually mature within 25 days.

When human infection occurs, children are the most common victims; they may suffer abdominal pain, diarrhea, insomnia, and convulsions.

With a life cycle easily maintainable in the laboratory, *H. diminuta* has been a choice parasite for experimental studies for decades. It is perhaps the most studied of all tapeworms.

DIPYLIDIUM CANINUM

Dipylidium caninum is a common parasite of dogs, cats, and humans, especially children, throughout the world. The parasite can attain a length of 30 cm and possesses on its scolex a conical, retractible rostellum with one to eight (commonly four to six) rows of hooks (Fig. 13-8). This tapeworm is easily recognizable, because each proglottid has two sets of reproductive organs with a genital atrium on each lateral edge. The short, inconspicuous uterus atrophies early, and as eggs are produced, they are enclosed in **egg capsules**, each containing 8–25 eggs. The medullary region of a typical gravid proglottid is packed with hundreds of egg capsules.

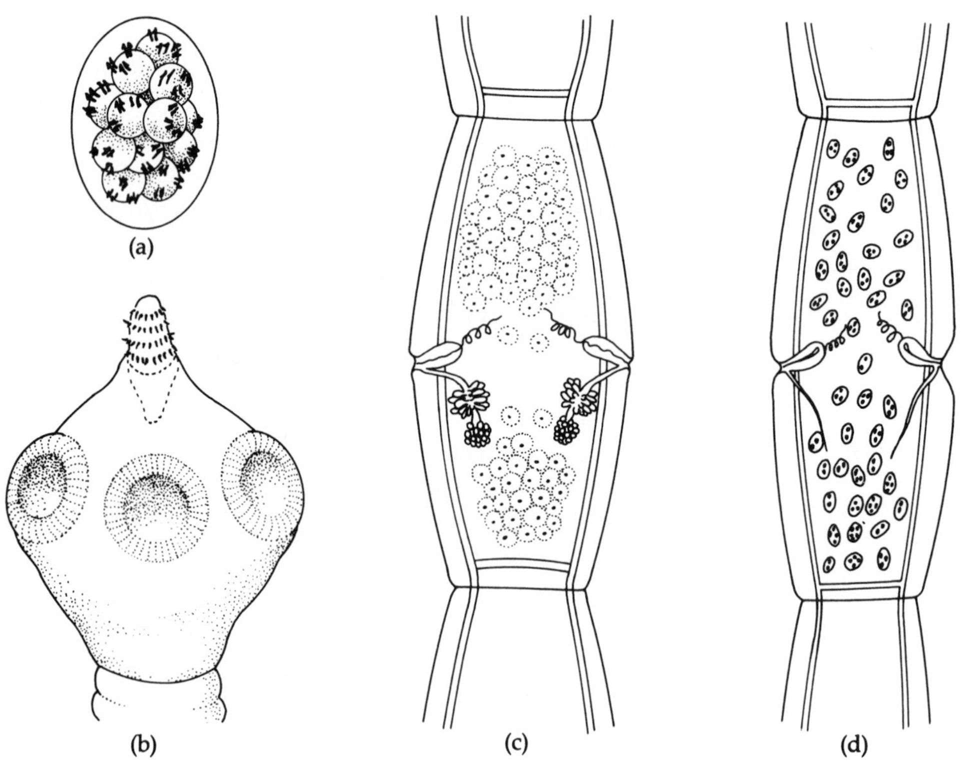

FIGURE 13-8
Dipylidium caninum.
(a) Cluster of eggs in a uterine ball. (b) Scolex with armed rostellum. (c) Mature proglottid with two sets of reproductive organs. (d) Gravid proglottid filled with uterine balls.

Life Cycle

The adult tapeworm lives in the small intestine of the definitive host where large, gravid proglottids (12 mm by 3 mm) separate from the strobila in groups of two or three. The proglottids are capable of moving upon a substrate and can either creep out of the anus or be passed with feces. Eggs and capsules are ingested by larvae of fleas belonging to the genera *Pulex* and *Ctenocephalides* or by the dog louse *Trichodectes canis*. The oncosphere hatches in the gut of the arthropod, burrows through the wall, and develops into a cysticercoid in the hemocoel when the flea or louse metamorphoses to the parasitic adult stage. When the infected arthropod is ingested by a suitable definitive host, the cysticercoid is liberated in the small intestine and the parasite develops to sexual maturity in about 20 days.

Epidemiology

Most human infections are in children younger than 8 years old, with a high percentage falling in the under-6-months age group. This probably is attributable to the fact that a high percentage of dogs are infected, many of which undoubtedly are pets. Transmission to humans usually results from accidental ingestion of infected fleas or lice or from allowing dogs and cats to lick ("kiss") the mouths of children immediately after the pet has bitten an infected arthropod.

Symptomatology and Diagnosis

It is rare for humans to harbor more than a single parasite, and symptoms are seldom apparent. Diagnosis is confirmed by the discovery of characteristic proglottids or eggs in the feces.

SELECTED READINGS

Arai, H. P. 1980. *Biology of the Rat Tapeworm, Hymenolepis diminuta*. Academic, New York.

Arme, C., and Pappas, P. W. 1983. *The Biology of the Eucestoda*. Academic, New York.

Lloyd, S. 1998. Cysticercosis and taeniosis. *Taenia saginata, Taenia solium,* and Asian *Taenia*. In *Zoonoses* (Palmer, S. R., Soulsby, E. J. L., and Simpson, D. I. H., Eds.), pp. 635–649. Oxford University Press, Oxford, England.

Pawlowski, Z., and Schultz, M. G. 1972. Taeniasis and cysticercosis (*Taenia saginata*) *Advances in Parasitology* 10, 269–343.

Tanowitz, H. B., and Wittner, M. 1991. Tapeworm infections. In *Hunter's Tropical Medicine* (Strickland, G. T., Ed.), 7th ed., pp. 834–859. W. B. Saunders, Philadelphia.

von Bonsdorff, B. 1956. *Diphyllobothrium latum* as a cause of pernicious anemia. *Experimental Parasitology* 5, 201–230.

Chapter Fourteen

EXTRAINTESTINAL TAPEWORMS

This chapter deals with tapeworms whose larvae are potentially highly pathogenic to humans. Included in this category are several species of *Diphyllobothrium* and related pseudophyllidean cestodes; *Taenia solium*; and at least two members of the genus *Echinococcus*, namely, *E. granulosus* and *E. multilocularis*. The larvae of two other species, *Hymenolepis nana* and *Taenia multiceps*, sometimes infect humans. However, because human infections by these tapeworms are accidental and relatively rare (*T. multiceps*) or, in the larval stage, produce no serious symptoms (*H. nana*; see p. 286), these species are not considered in this section.

The human disease known as sparganosis is caused by plerocercoid larvae of any of several pseudophyllideans. Human cysticercosis is caused by the cysticercus of *T. solium*. Human hydatidosis results from infection with hydatid cysts of *E. granulosus* or multilocular cysts of *E. multilocularis*.

HUMAN SPARGANOSIS

The plerocercoid larvae of several pseudophyllidean tapeworms are capable of infecting tissues of humans and other vertebrates. One of the more common of these belongs to the genus *Spirometra*, members of which use various carnivores other than humans as definitive hosts. The plerocercoid larva of *Spirometra* was placed originally in the genus *Sparganum* before the association between larva and adult worm was established. The term **sparganosis**, signifying an infection with the plerocercoid larva, stems from the generic name, which is no longer valid.

Life Cycle

Among various pseudophyllidean tapeworms with plerocercoids that can produce sparganosis in humans, *D. latum* has a typical life cycle (see Fig. 13-2). However, it should be emphasized that ingestion of *D. latum* plerocercoids by humans will also eventually produce the adult tapeworms.

Epidemiology

Humans become infected in several ways. A common vehicle is drinking water contaminated with copepods harboring procercoids. Procercoids released in the human gut penetrate the intestinal wall and migrate to various tissues, where they develop into plerocercoids. Backpackers drinking from stagnant pools or lakes are vulnerable to infection in this manner, especially in temperate regions of the world where these parasites are prevalent.

Another way by which humans become infected is through ingestion of insufficiently cooked muscle of fishes, amphibians, reptiles, birds, and mammals such as bears, wild boars, and pigs. Plerocercoids of pseudophyllideans other than *D. latum*, ingested when infected muscle is eaten, are freed in the intestine and migrate to various tissues, most commonly the areas around the eyes, muscles, viscera of the thorax, and subcutaneous regions of the thorax, abdomen, and thighs.

Humans also acquire infection through the use of raw meat poultices, e.g., as a treatment for a black eye. Active plerocercoids from infected meat crawl into the orbit and become established (Fig. 14-1). Similar cases of human ocular sparganosis have been reported from the Orient following treatment of skin ulcers or eye inflammations with poultices made from various infected animals, particularly snakes. In Oriental countries, the most common plerocercoid causing human sparganosis is that of *Diphyllobothrium erinacei*, a tapeworm of carnivores, while in North America, it is that of *Spirometra mansonoides*, a tapeworm of cats. Another species of *Spirometra* that may cause sparganosis in humans displays asexual proliferation of the scolex in the plerocercoid stage; hence its species name *S. proliferatum*.

Because practices such as those described previously are widespread in the Orient, human sparganosis is common there. The disease also occurs, albeit less frequently, in Europe, Australia, Africa, and North and South America.

Symptomatology and Diagnosis

As noted previously, plerocercoids locate in many parts of the body. The movements and secretions of living plerocercoids can

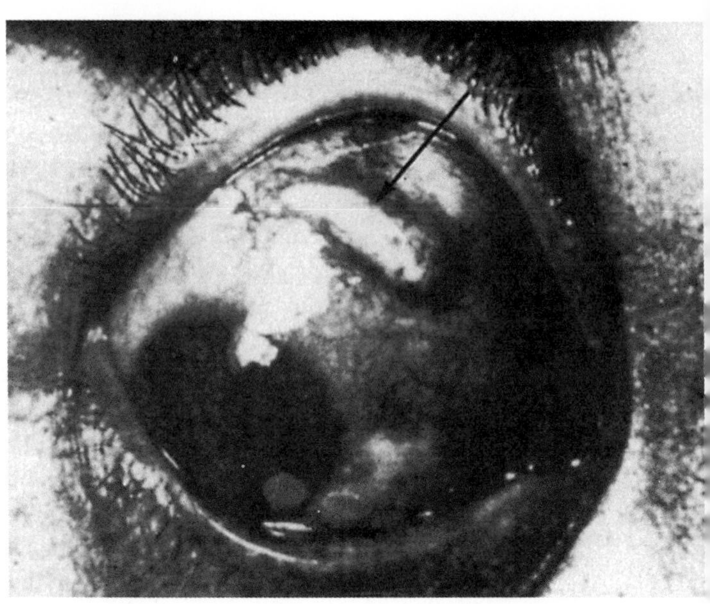

FIGURE 14-1
Human patient with plerocercoid in conjunctiva.

induce localized inflammatory reactions; dead and degenerating larvae sometimes cause edema of the surrounding tissue. Chills and fever may accompany infections. Eye infections, particularly common in the Orient, produce conjunctivitis and swelling. In general, the severity of infection is determined by the location of the larvae and how quickly and completely the patient can be rid of them.

Detection of larvae in the host's tissues constitutes diagnosis.

Treatment

Surgical removal of the larva is the most dependable treatment. Praziquantel, as a supplementary drug, has shown promising results in hastening recovery.

Prevention

A major preventive measure is the thorough cooking of freshwater fishes prior to human consumption. Also, application of animal flesh to human skin should be avoided, and questionable water, especially in endemic areas, should be boiled or filtered before drinking.

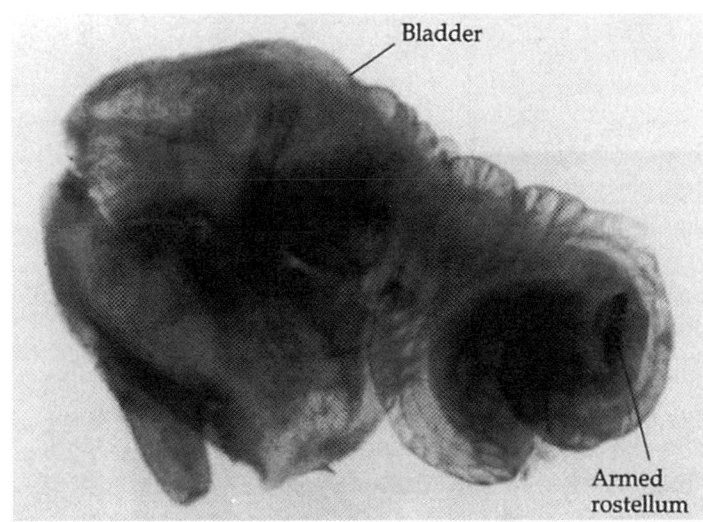

FIGURE 14-2
Cysticercus of *Taenia* sp.

HUMAN CYSTICERCOSIS

The fully developed cysticercus of *Taenia solium* is oval, about 0.5 cm or more in width, and usually enclosed by a capsule of host connective tissue (Fig. 14-2). In areas such as certain parts of the brain, the host capsule may be absent, and the larva may attain a diameter of several centimeters. The ability of the cysticerci of *T. solium* to develop in practically any organ of the body (Fig. 14-3) and the severity of the resulting pathology render it one of the most pathogenic species of tapeworms infecting humans. The life cycle of *T. solium* is diagrammed in Figure 13-5.

Epidemiology

Prevalence of human cysticercosis predictably parallels the incidence of the adult worm. It is quite common in Latin America (particularly in Mexico, where approximately 3 million people are infected), Africa, Indonesia, India, and China. In the United States, its highest prevalence is in southern California, mainly among migrant workers and recent immigrants from Mexico and Central and South America. For some as yet unexplained reason, human males seem more vulnerable to infection than human fe-

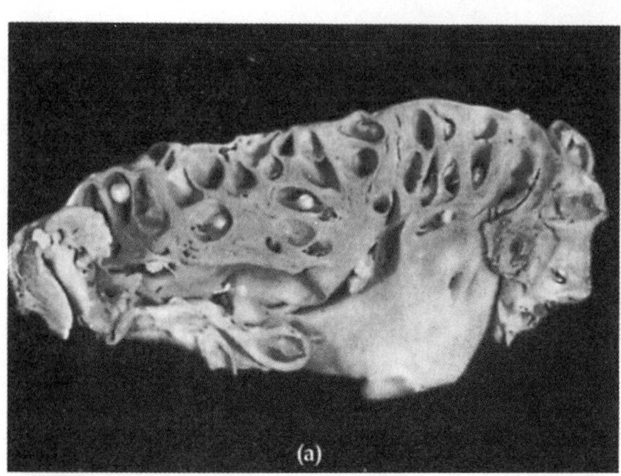

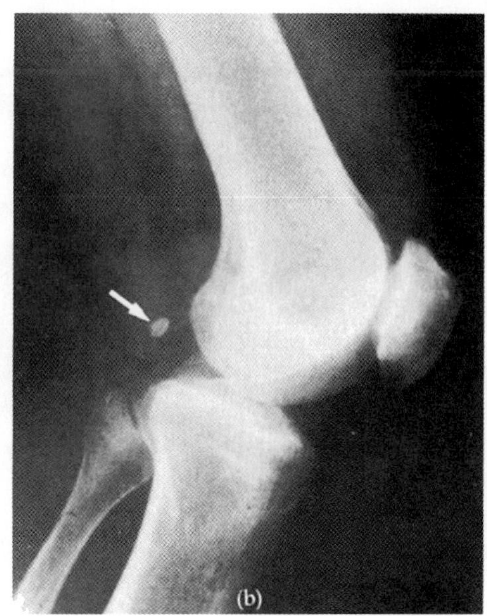

FIGURE 14-3
Human cysticercosis.
(a) Heart containing cysticerci of *Taenia solium*. (b) *Taenia solium* cysticercus close to bone (arrow).

males. Human infection with cysticerci occurs in several ways, perhaps the most common of which is direct ingestion of eggs. This may result from hand-to-mouth self-infection, from eating food contaminated with eggs during unsanitary food-handling practices, or from consuming food or water contaminated with feces containing eggs. Internal autoinfection, whereby eggs are swept back into the stomach by reverse peristalsis, is another method of human infection, although it is of little epidemiological importance because only about 25% of patients with cysticercosis also harbor the adult tapeworm. Eggs, whether ingested or swept back by reverse peristalsis, pass through the stomach and hatch in the small intestine. The escaping oncospheres penetrate the intestinal wall, enter the circulatory system, and are dispersed throughout the body.

Symptomatology and Diagnosis

Although the most common sites for infection are the skeletal muscles and brain, cysticerci may be found in almost any tissue of the body, including the eyes, lungs, and subcutaneous tissues.

Cysts are well tolerated in muscles and subcutaneous tissues, although heavy infections can produce muscle spasms, weakness, and general malaise. Developing cysts elicit a host inflammatory response resulting in fibrous encapsulation although, as noted previously, such a capsule may not be formed when the cyst invades parts of the brain. Calcification of the cyst may occur after 1 year, after which time the disease may become asymptomatic. The most serious symptoms appear 5–10 years after infection as a result of dead and dying cysticerci. The degenerating parasite tissues and associated fluid also elicit a host inflammatory reaction that can be very severe, even fatal.

In addition to eliciting host responses, cysts developing in the central nervous system or sense organs can exert mechanical pressure and cause neurological symptoms. Violent headache, convulsion, local paralysis, vomiting, and optic disturbances are common and, again, are sometimes severe enough to be fatal.

Clinical diagnosis can be made by linking symptoms, such as the late onset of epileptic convulsions, to a history of residence in an endemic area. X-ray examination of infected muscles or central nervous system tissues may confirm diagnosis by revealing calcified cysts. Computerized axial tomography (CAT) scans and magnetic resonance imaging (MRI) have been used to diagnose cysticerci in the brain. Examination of cerebrospinal fluid by ELISA is also useful in diagnosis of patients with cerebral cysticercosis.

Treatment

Surgery is the recommended treatment for cysticerci in the fluid-filled spaces of the body. However, surgery is not generally beneficial in heavy infections of the central nervous system, although removal of some of the cysts has proven helpful. Praziquantel and albendazole with certain steroids (e.g., dexamethasone) are effective in reducing edema and alleviating some of the symptoms of cerebral cysticercosis. Care must be taken during treatment for adult worms to avoid causing severe vomiting, which may induce reverse peristalsis.

Prevention

The most effective preventive measures include strict attention to personal hygiene, sexual habits, and environmental sanitation.

Removal of adult worms from the patient once infection has been ascertained is important in preventing autoinfection. Visitors to endemic areas should observe such preventive measures as the boiling of drinking water and the avoidance of salads and raw fruits and vegetables without rinds.

HUMAN HYDATIDOSIS

The two most important species of *Echinococcus* responsible for human hydatidosis are *E. granulosus*, which causes cystic echinococcosis, and *E. multilocularis*, which causes alveolar echinococcosis. Adults of the genus *Echinococcus* are among the smallest tapeworms, measuring 2–8 mm long with strobilae consisting of three or, rarely, four proglottids (Fig. 14-4). Usually one immature, one mature, and one gravid proglottid make up the strobila. The scolex bears a rostellum with a double row of 28–50 (usually 30–36) hooks, four prominent suckers, and a short neck region. Adult worms inhabit the small intestine of a wide variety of canines and, occasionally, felines. In heavy infections, it is not unusual to find hundreds of worms attached to the mucosa of a dog's small intestine.

Life Cycle

Eggs, measuring 30 μm by 38 μm, reach the exterior by host elimination of gravid proglottids with feces (Fig. 14-5). Released when proglottids disintegrate, the eggs are morphologically indistinguishable from other taeniid ova, and each contains a fully developed oncosphere. The eggs gain entry into the intermediate host when the host ingests water or forage contaminated with egg-containing feces. The usual intermediate host for *E. granulosus* is sheep, but cattle and other herbivores, as well as pigs, can also serve in this capacity. Microtine rodents serve as intermediate hosts for *E. multilocularis*, while cats, dogs, and foxes that prey on rodents harbor the adults. Usually, human infection occurs when eggs are ingested as a result of intimate contact with dogs, notably when dogs are allowed to lick human faces after grooming themselves. Humans can also ingest eggs by putting

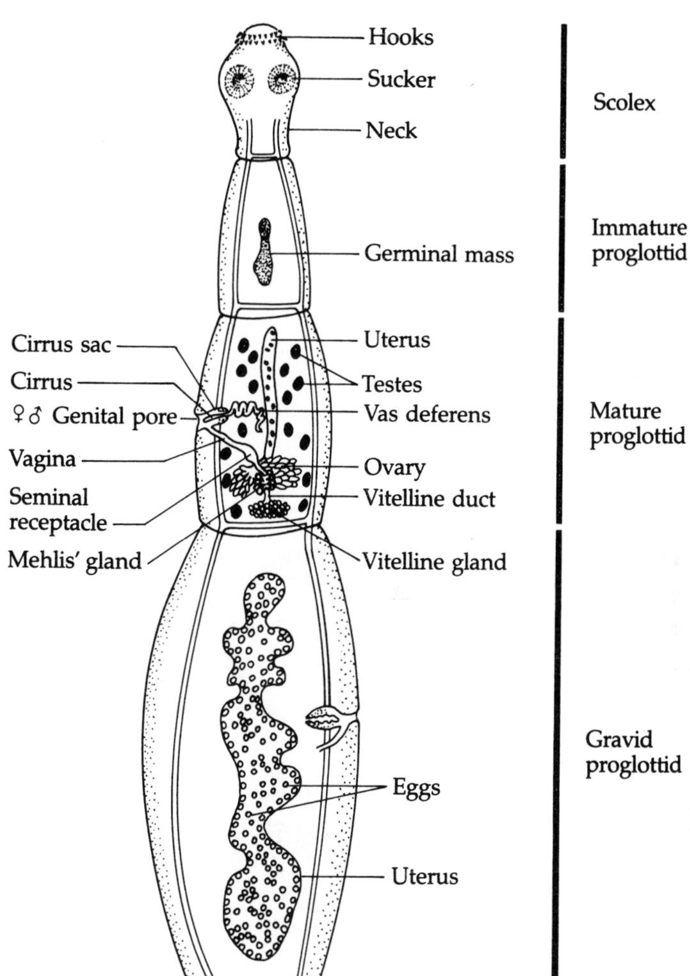

FIGURE 14-4
Morphology of adult *Echinococcus granulosus.*

contaminated fingers into the mouth or by eating raw plants contaminated with feces from foxes, cats, or dogs.

Once swallowed, eggs pass through the stomach and hatch in the small intestine. The freed oncospheres penetrate the intestinal wall, enter the mesenteric venules, and become lodged in capillary beds of various visceral organs. In humans, the developing hydatid cysts favor the liver, but may also invade other tissues, such as the lungs, kidneys, spleen, heart, muscles, brain, and bone marrow. The hydatid cyst grows slowly, reaching a diameter of 10 mm in 5 months. It is not unusual for the cyst ultimately to reach the size of an orange or a small grapefruit and contain a

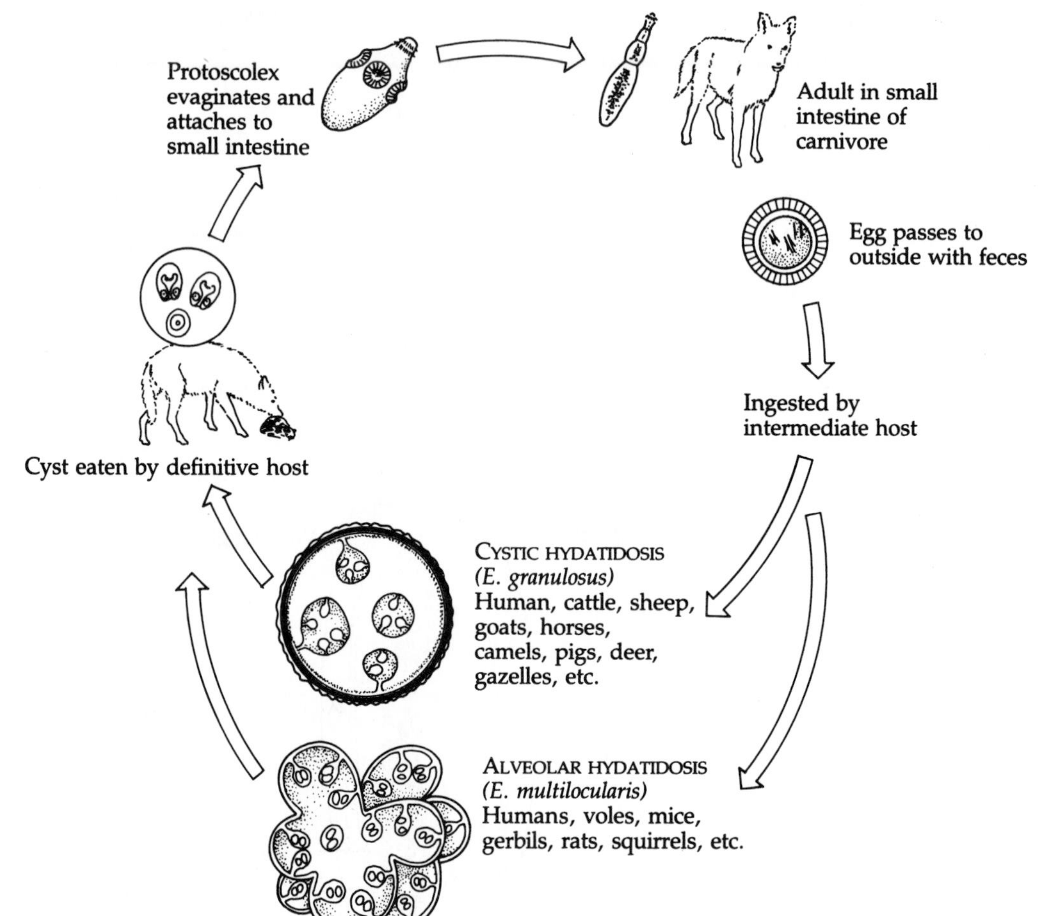

FIGURE 14-5
Life cycle of *Echinococcus granulosus*.

considerable amount of fluid. Within the fully formed cyst, minute larvae with inverted scolices develop. Since these immature, four-suckered scolices lack individual bladders, they are called **protoscolices** (singular, **protoscolex**). The larvae should not be referred to as bladder worms or cysticerci, each of which contains a single scolex within a fluid-filled cyst.

In humans and some domestic animals, formation of hydatid cysts represents a dead end for the parasite. However, many wild animals, such as infected rabbits and squirrels, are potential intermediate hosts as the cysts are ingested when predators feed upon such animals. Upon reaching the small intestine of the definitive sylvatic host (e.g., the predator), each protoscolex has the potential to develop into an adult worm. The average life span of an adult worm is approximately 5 months, although some worms may survive as long as a year.

Hydatid cysts found in humans fall into three categories: (1) unilocular, (2) osseous, and (3) alveolar, the last representing a developmental stage of *E. multilocularis*. Of the three, the unilocular cyst is the most common and least pathogenic, while the alveolar cyst is the most dangerous.

The diameter of the unilocular cyst may reach 20 cm or more in humans, although its usual diameter is 1–7 cm. At maturity, the cyst wall consists of two layers: a thick, laminated, noncellular, outer tegument known as the **ectocyst**; and an inner germinal epithelium that produces the protoscolices and is known as the **endocyst** (Fig. 14-6). Brood capsules attached to the germinal epithelium by a stalk, the **pedicel**, extend into the fluid-filled cavity of the cyst. In large cysts, these capsules may rupture and allow the protoscolices to sink to the bottom of the bladder, where they are commonly known as **hydatid sand**. Each brood capsule contains 10–30 protoscolices. Second-generation daughter cysts often form within the mother cyst. These cysts are replicas of the mother cyst and produce their own generation of protoscolices. Daughter cysts may, in turn, produce still another generation of cysts. It is not surprising, then, that the average fertile primary cyst is estimated to contain more than 2 million protoscolices. If a cyst ruptures within a host, each liberated protoscolex can produce a daughter cyst. Whether the protoscolex itself develops into a cyst or whether small bits of germinal tissue cling to it and generate a new cyst is conjectural.

Osseous cysts are most commonly found in the ribs, vertebrae, and upper portions of long bones. These cysts usually develop in the marrow cavities. They are much smaller than unilocular cysts and contain little or no fluid and no protoscolices.

The outer membrane of the alveolar cyst is very thin, laminated, and difficult to separate from surrounding tissues. Connective tissue septa divide the cyst into numerous irregular compartments, or alveoli, which are filled with a jellylike material. Alveolar cysts are found most commonly in the liver, where they tend to proliferate by evagination of the thin cyst wall. In humans, the cysts usually lack protoscolices.

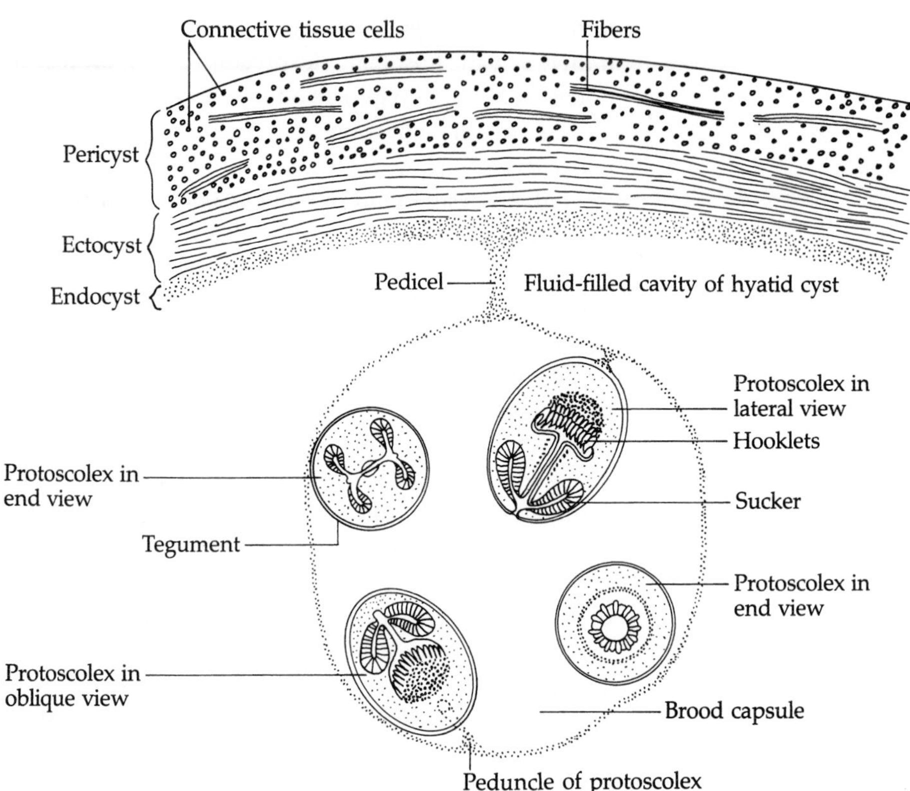

FIGURE 14-6
A section through part of a unilocular hydatid cyst.

Epidemiology

Human hydatidosis is a zoonotic disease that results from intimate contact with dogs. Where dogs are used to herd domestic animals such as sheep, the percentage of infected dogs may run as high as 50%, while the prevalence of hydatid cysts may be as high as 30% in sheep and cattle and 10% in hogs. Incidence among humans in Greece, Romania, Spain, Cyprus, Algeria, Yugoslavia, Argentina, Uruguay, and Chile is relatively high (Fig. 14-7), due to the close association with working dogs such as sheep dogs. Well-organized prevention programs have reduced the incidence in Australia, New Zealand, and Tasmania. Scat-

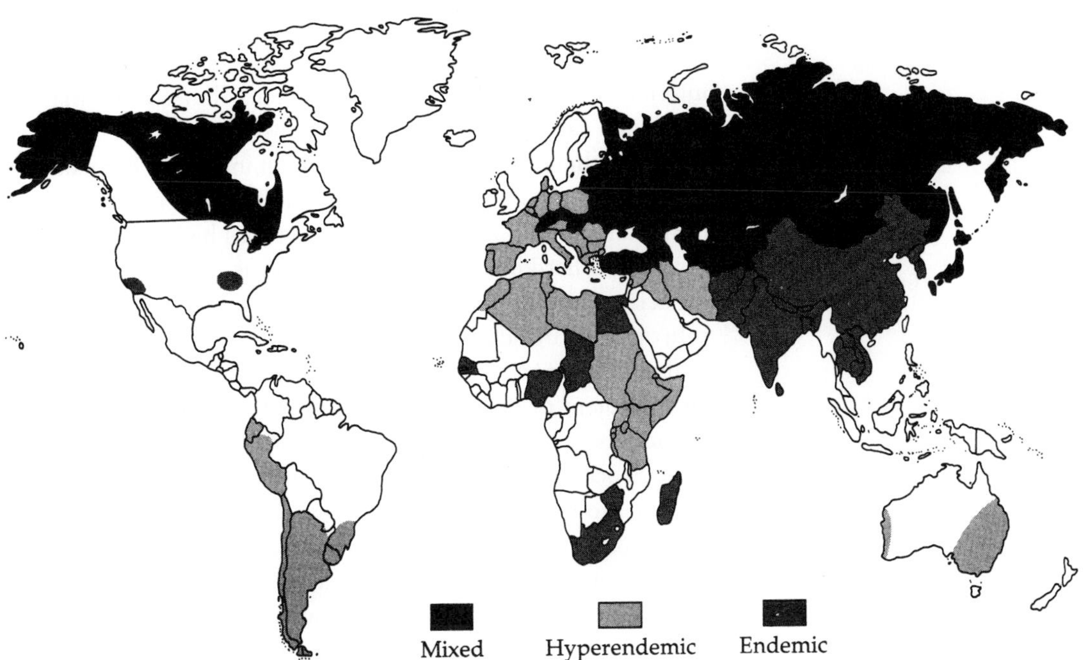

FIGURE 14-7
World distribution of hydatidosis.

tered cases of human hydatidosis have been reported in the United States, especially in the lower Mississippi River Valley, Utah, Arizona, and parts of California. In the Canadian Arctic, moose and caribou, rather than sheep, serve as intermediate hosts and are the main source of echinococcosis in the native Inuit. Isolated areas of heavy incidence have also been reported in the United Kingdom, especially in Wales and in some islands off the Scottish coast. Hydatid disease originating in the Middle East is spreading rapidly in Europe, especially in France and parts of Germany.

In nature, the predator–prey relationship, such as that between wolf and moose, wolf and reindeer, or dingo and wallaby, enables *E. granulosus* to complete its life cycle. This condition is known as **sylvatic echinococcosis.** Humans are seldom involved in this type of cycle. *Echinococcus granulosus* consists of a number of different strains, which are adapted to different intermediate hosts. This fact is important in the epidemiology of the parasite. In Europe, for example, strains in which horses and pigs serve as intermediate hosts do not infect humans, but strains that use sheep and cattle are infective to humans.

Some ethnic customs promote human infection. For example, members of certain primitive tribes in Kenya, where the incidence of human hydatidosis is among the world's highest, utilize dogs not only to herd livestock but also to act as "nurse dogs." In this capacity, the dogs protect babies and clean them after they defecate or vomit by licking their buttocks or faces. The infection rate is also high among leather tanners in Lebanon, since dog feces is an ingredient of the tanning fluid used there. During the preparation process, the tanners' fingers become contaminated, and the tanners accidentally ingest eggs when they put their unwashed fingers into their mouths.

Alveolar echinococcosis is common in regions of the Northern Hemisphere such as Japan, China, the former USSR, western Alaska, and central Europe. Recently, human cases have also been documented in Iran, China, India, and the United States, countries previously free of the disease. In the midwestern United States, a cat–rodent life cycle has been reported for *E. multilocularis*. Foxes are significant reservoir hosts in North America and Europe.

Symptomatology and Diagnosis

The presence of unilocular cysts elicits a host inflammatory reaction that results in encapsulation of the cyst. The primary pathology of the unilocular cyst is impairment of organs from mechanical pressure (Fig. 14-8). Increased pressure resulting from cyst growth may cause surrounding tissues to atrophy. The symptoms, therefore, are not unlike those caused by a slow-growing tumor. Symptoms vary according to the tissues affected and may take many years to appear. For instance, although the liver is the most commonly affected organ, symptoms such as jaundice may take as long as 20 years to emerge. Pulmonary infections, characterized by a cough accompanied by allergic reactions, are also common. The brain, kidneys, spleen, and vertebral column may also be invaded, producing symptoms ranging from seizures to kidney dysfunction over a protracted period.

Freed by the rupture of cysts, protoscolices enter the circula-

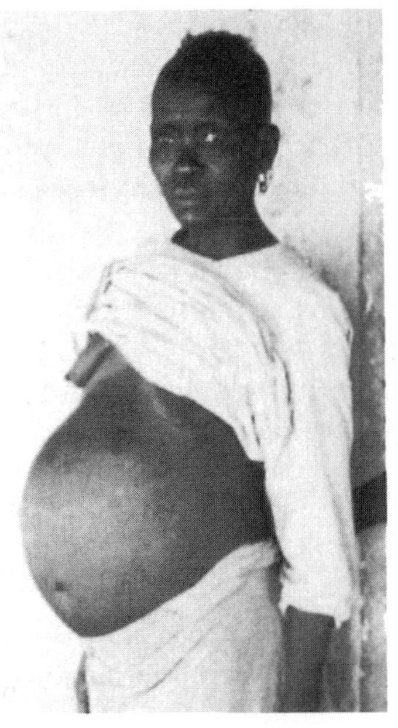

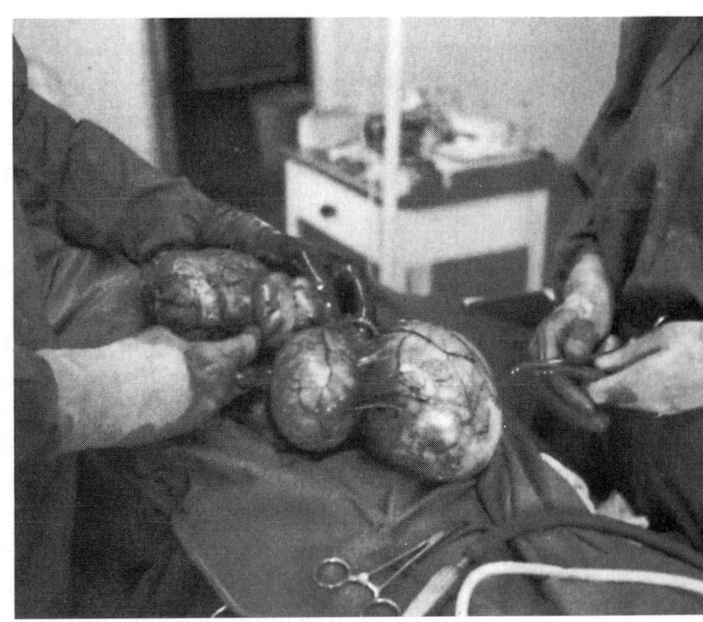

FIGURE 14-8
Human hydatidosis.
(Left) Native Kenyan with disease. (Right) Removal of hydatid cysts by surgical means.

tory system and are transported to tissues throughout the body, where they produce secondary echinococcosis. This condition may not appear for 2–8 years and is far more serious than the primary infection. The rupture of cysts also releases hydatid fluid which sometimes causes severe allergic reactions. If a significant amount of fluid enters the bloodstream, it can precipitate anaphylactic shock.

The alveolar cyst usually is proliferative. Although growth occurs at its periphery, its center may become calcified. Such cysts commonly occur in the liver and are often mistaken for hepatic carcinoma. They are difficult to extirpate, and the condition is usually fatal within 10 years.

Because of its location, the osseous cyst also is difficult to remove. In severe cases, there is often necrosis of the diaphyses of long bones, spontaneous fracture, and distortion of cancellous tissue.

Diagnosis of hydatidosis is based upon a number of criteria, including symptoms (hepatic hypertrophy, etc.), history of residence in an endemic area, and close contact with dogs. X-ray examination is especially useful for revealing calcified cysts, and various ultrasound procedures may locate noncalcified cysts. Laboratory diagnosis, which might be more aptly termed "postsurgical confirmation" of hydatidosis, involves detection of protoscolices. Serological tests are diagnostically useful, the direct hemagglutination test being one of the most commonly used. The intracutaneous test (Casoni's intradermal test) is sufficiently sensitive to be helpful in screening for human hydatidosis; however, negative results are more significant than positive results, as there is about an 18% incidence of false positives.

Treatment

Surgery remains the preferred treatment for unilocular hydatidosis. Following drainage of fluid from the cyst, replacement with 10% formalin for 5 minutes kills the protoscolices and the germinal epithelium. In any surgical procedure for cyst removal, care should be taken to avoid rupturing the cyst. Allergic reactions resulting from stimulation by alveolar fluid respond best to treatment with antihistamines or epinephrine. Most recently, the benzimidazoles (especially albendazole) have been used successfully to reduce the size of both unilocular and alveolar cysts. It is anticipated that, at least in some cases, chemotherapy may eventually replace surgery. A relatively new, nonsurgical approach introduced in Italy involves treatment with albendazole for 12 hours, aspiration of some cyst fluid, injection of the cyst with 95% ethanol, and subsequent aspiration of the alcoholic solution. Developmental and physiological variations among the different strains of *E. granulosus* must be considered when chemotherapy is prescribed, because one regimen may not yield uniform results against all strains.

Prevention

Significant inroads toward prevention of human hydatidosis can be made by reducing contact between dogs and intermediate hosts such as sheep, hogs, and rodents, and by educating the public to the danger of intimate contact with dogs, especially in endemic areas. As added measures, dogs should be treated regularly with anthelmintics and kept away from slaughterhouses, and refuse from slaughterhouses should be disinfected.

SELECTED READINGS

Craig, P. S., Rogan, M. T., and Allan, J. C. 1996. Detection, screening and community epidemiology of taeniid cestode zoonoses: Cystic echinococcosis, alveolar echinococcosis and neurocysticercosis cases. *Advances in Parasitology* **38,** 170–250.

Eckert, J., Pawlowski, Z., Dar, F. K., Vuitton, D. A., Kern, P., and Savioli, L. 1995. Medical aspects of echinococcosis. *Parasitology Today* **11,** 273–276.

Gemmel, M. A. 1977. Experimental epidemiology of hydatidosis and cysticercosis. *Advances in Parasitology* **15,** 311–369.

Gottstein, B. 1992. *Echinococcus multilocularis* infection: Immunology and immunodiagnosis. *Advances in Parasitology* **31,** 321–380.

Lloyd, S. 1998. Other cestode infections. Hymenolepiosis, dyphyllobothriosis, coenurosis, and other adult and larval cestodes. In *Zoonoses* (Palmer, S. R., Soulsby, E. J. L., and Simpson, D. I. H., Eds.), pp. 651–663. Oxford University Press, Oxford, England.

McManus, D. P., and Smyth, J. D. 1986. Hydatidosis: Changing concepts in epidemiology and speciation. *Parasitology Today* **2,** 163–167.

Thompson, R. C. A., and Lymberg, A. J. 1995. *Echinococcus and Hydatid Disease.* CAB International Publication, Oxford University Press, Oxford, England.

PART FOUR

THE NEMATODA

Chapter Fifteen

GENERAL CHARACTERISTICS OF THE NEMATODA

After more than a century of debate, the placement of nematodes, or roundworms, in the phylogenetic scheme remains unresolved. Considered by some to constitute an independent phylum, Nematoda (or Nemata), they are regarded by others as members of the phylum Aschelminthes, with such groups as Rotifera and Nematomorpha. According to still another system of classification, Nematoda and Nematomorpha are designated as separate classes of the phylum Nemathelminthes. In the scheme followed herein, roundworms are assigned to a separate phylum, Nematoda.

Parasitic nematodes are of great importance to biologists because they are abundant and widespread, frequently occur as endoparasites infecting a wide variety of invertebrates and vertebrates, and often have a serious impact upon human health. Nematodes that parasitize humans are assigned to either the class Secernentea (Phasmidia) or the class Adenophorea (Aphasmidia), primarily on the basis of the presence or absence of **phasmids**, minute sensory structures on the body surface. Most nematodes that infect humans belong to the class Secernentea.

Although the origin of nematodes is obscure, there is a marked similarity of structure and of elements of the life cycle among these organisms, whether free living or parasitic. This consistency argues for ancestral uniformity, a descendance from common ancestors. Because most nematodes are not host specific, they are probably largely independent of the evolution of their hosts, using them merely as vehicles for their own evolution. Life-history studies have fostered the view that parasitic nematodes evolved at various times from free-living soil forms, with the free-living ancestor initially utilizing a host for transportation or protection only. Movements of such hosts isolated these nematode populations, preventing interbreeding with their free-living counterparts and thus providing the basis for speciation.

Significant preadaptation of the third-stage larva (see p. 329) to osmoregulation equips certain nematodes to utilize several environments during their life cycle. Such a third-stage larva is characteristic of all secernentean (phasmidian) parasites of animals and serves as a transfer stage from one environment to another. The third-stage larva of aphasmidians, on the other hand, is less diversified and plays no such role.

STRUCTURE OF THE ADULT

Nematodes are generally elongate, cylindrical, and tapered at both ends. The basic body design is a tube within a tube, the outer tube being the body wall and underlying muscles, and the inner tube the digestive tract (Fig. 15-1). Between the tubes is the fluid-filled pseudocoelom, in which the reproductive system and other structures are found. In certain species, the body is almost uniformly cylindrical and is extremely thin. Sexual dimorphism is evident: at the curved, posterior end of the male are a copulatory organ and other specialized organs, such as alae and papillae; males are also usually smaller than females.

Parasitic nematodes vary widely in size according to species. While some are microscopic and others may reach more than a meter in length, most are between 1 mm and 15 cm long. Nematodes are colorless and vary from translucent (smaller nematodes) to opaque (larger nematodes) when examined alive. It is not uncommon for some to absorb colored matter from surrounding host tissues or fluids.

CUTICLE

An elastic **cuticle** covers the body surface of nematodes (Fig. 15-2). The presence of enzymes in the cuticle indicates that it is metabolically active, not an inert covering. Although the cuticle is generally smooth, various structures such as spines, bristles, warts, punctuations, papillae, striations, and ridges may be present on it. Some of these specialized structures are sensory, while others aid in locomotion; their arrangement and position are of taxonomic importance.

The cuticle not only covers the entire external surface, but also lines the buccal cavity, esophagus (pharynx), rectum, cloaca, vagina, and excretory pore. It consists of four basic layers: **epicuticle, exocuticle, mesocuticle**, and **endocuticle** (Fig. 15-3).

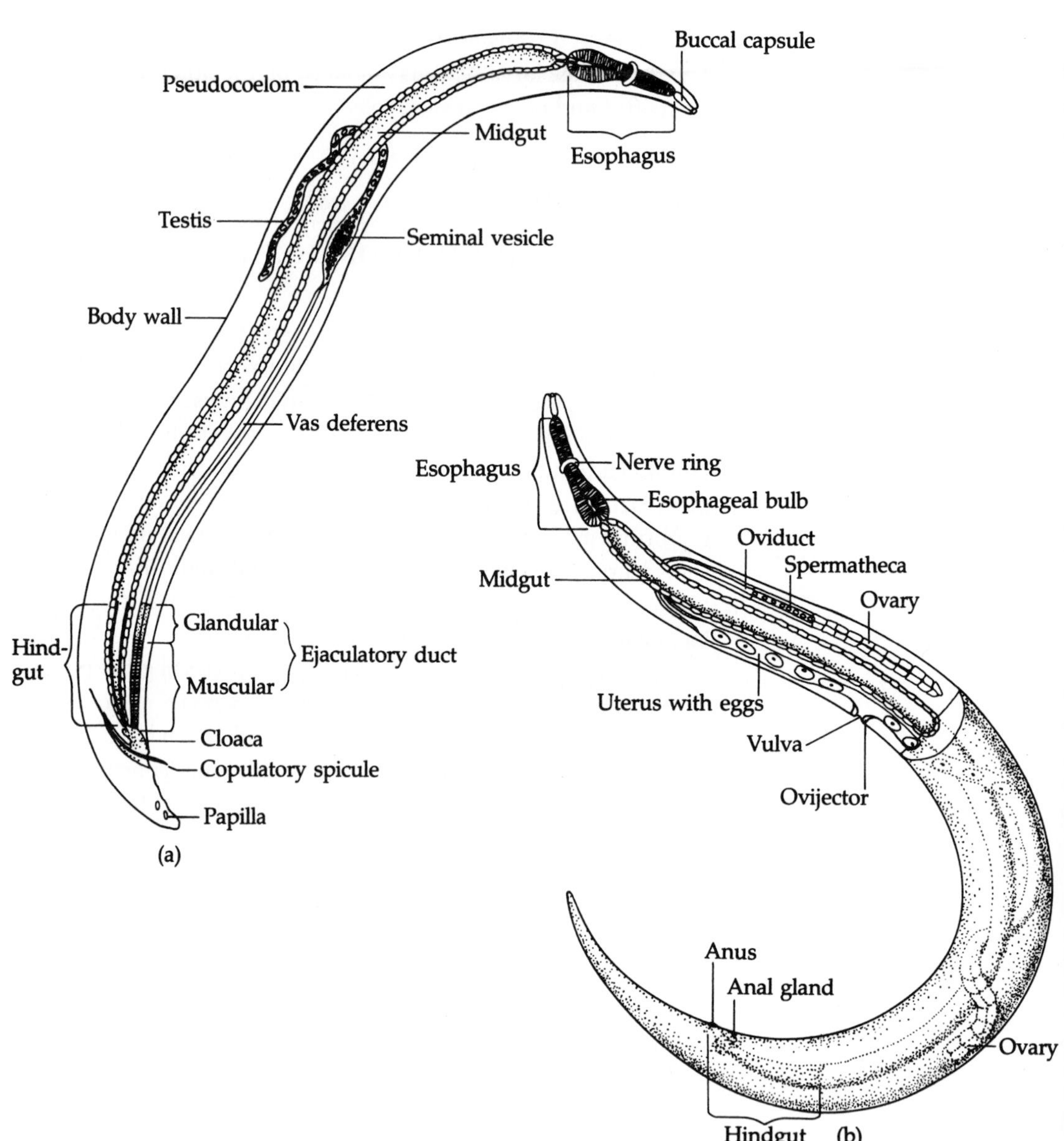

FIGURE 15-1
Morphology of a generalized nematode.
(a) Male. (b) Female.

The epicuticle is a relatively thin layer and is a consistent component of all nematode cuticles. Typically, it is trilaminate with a carbohydrate-containing glycocalyx. Its function is largely un-

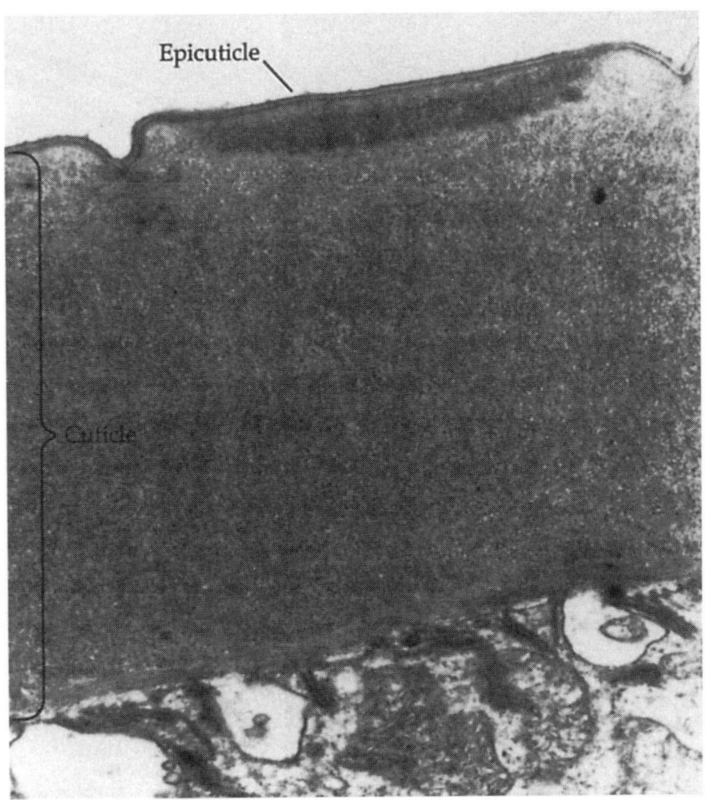

FIGURE 15-2
Transmission electron micrograph of the cuticle of a nematode.

known, although it is believed to act at least in part as a protective barrier.

The exocuticle is usually composed of two distinct sublayers: the relatively homogeneous **external exocuticle**, with no visible substructure; and the radially striated **internal exocuticle.**

The mesocuticle is the most diverse of the cuticular layers. It commonly consists of obliquely oriented, collagenous, fibrous sublayers that vary in number and in angular relationship to each other. The ability of the mesocuticular fiber sublayers to shift their angles of orientation provides flexibility to the cuticle. In some nematodes, the thickness of the mesocuticle is directly proportional to the age of the worm.

The endocuticle is the innermost layer of the cuticle. It is also fibrous, but the orientation of fibers is not as distinct as in the mesocuticle. Often, the pattern is disorganized, with a great deal

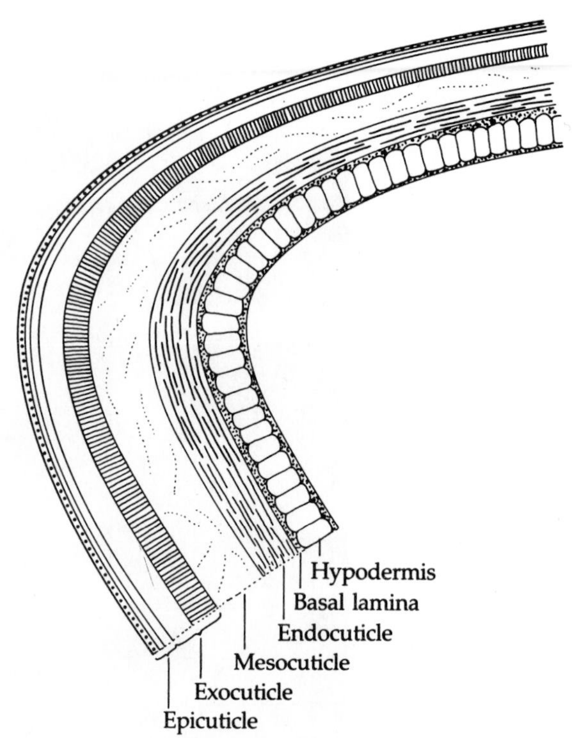

FIGURE 15-3
Layers of the nematode cuticle.

of overlapping between fibers. A basal lamina separates the cuticle from the underlying hypodermis.

HYPODERMIS

Beneath the basal lamina lies the thin, cellular (in adenophoreans) or syncytial (in secernenteans) hypodermis. A major function of the hypodermis is formation of the cuticle. The hypodermis protrudes into the pseudocoelom along the middorsal, midventral, and lateral lines to form the longitudinal **hypodermal cords**. These cords partially divide the pseudocoelom into quadrants. Hypodermal organelles, such as nuclei and mitochondria, are confined to the cords. The lateral cords are the largest and contain the primary excretory canals when these are present, while the dorsal and ventral cords contain longitudinal nerve trunks (Fig. 15-4).

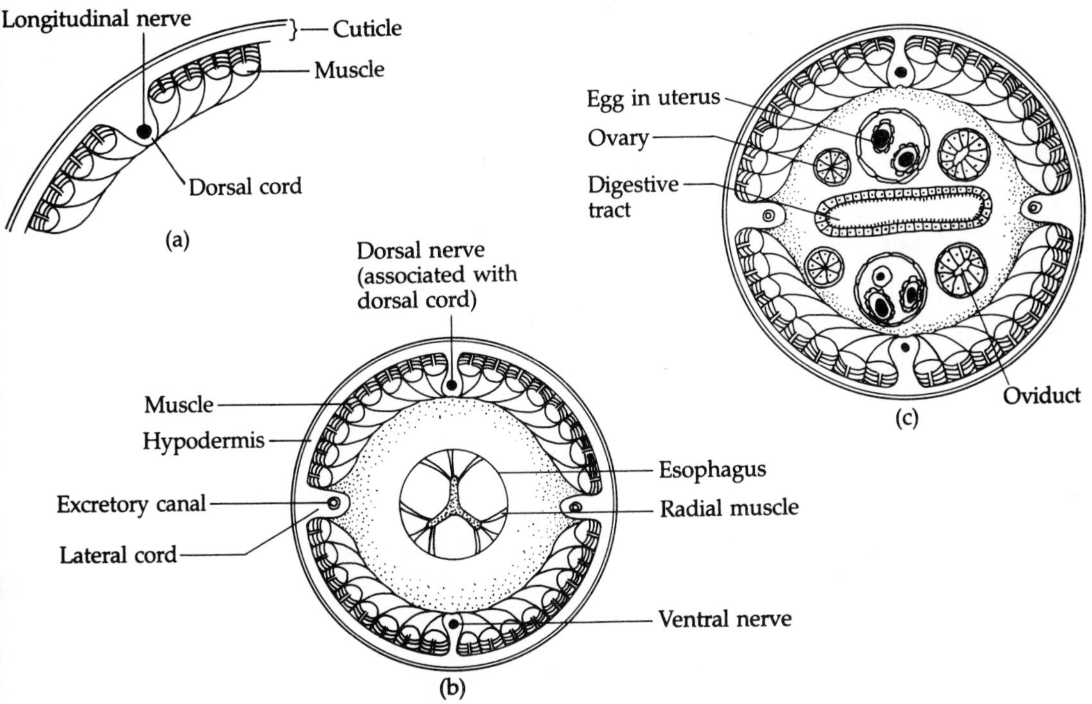

FIGURE 15-4
Nematode morphology.
(a) Portion of the dorsal body wall showing the relationship of the dorsal cord to the cuticle. (b) Cross section through the esophageal region. (c) Cross section through the midgut region.

MUSCULATURE

Within and closely associated with the hypodermis are one or more layers of longitudinally arranged muscle cells, the **somatic musculature.** Collectively, the cuticle, hypodermis, and somatic musculature make up the body wall. A convenient classification system to describe muscle cell arrangement has been devised based upon the number of rows of muscle cells per quadrant (Fig. 15-5). According to this system, an arrangement of multiple, longitudinal rows of muscle cells in each quadrant is termed **polymyarian;** one with no more than two rows of cells is designated **holomyarian;** and one with two to five rows is called **meromyarian.** Each muscle cell is comprised of a contractile portion

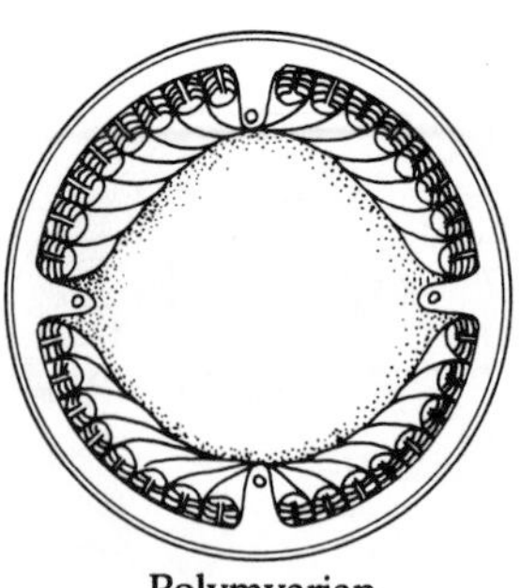

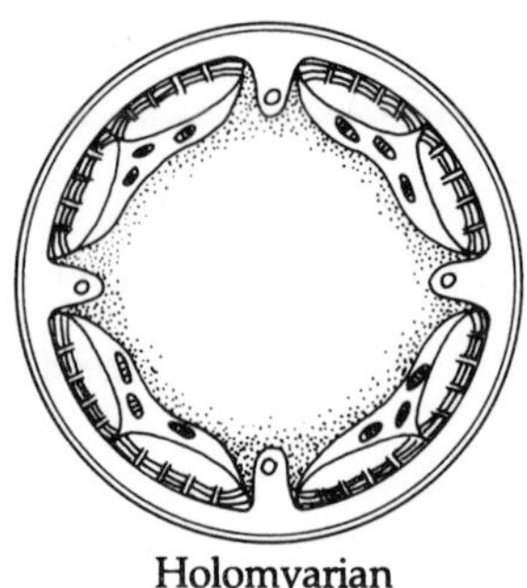

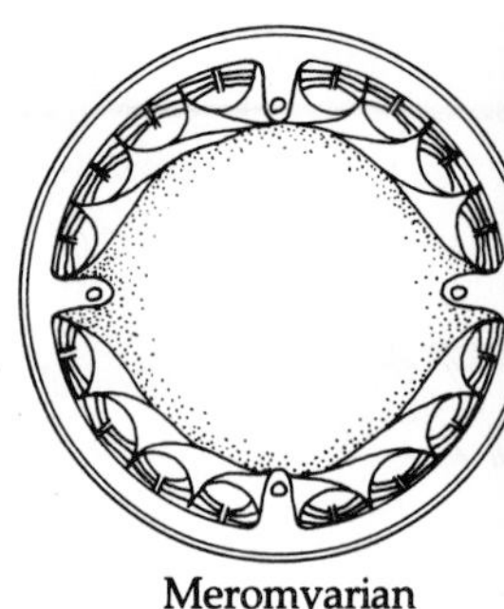

FIGURE 15-5
Muscle arrangements in nematodes.

containing myofibrils and a noncontractile portion, in which are found the various organelles, such as the nucleus, mitochondria, ribosomes, and endoplasmic reticulum, as well as stores of glycogen and lipid (Fig. 15-6). Sensory processes usually extend from the noncontractile portion of each cell to the longitudinal nerve trunks. Fibers originating in the contractile portion pass through the basal lamina and attach to the endocuticle.

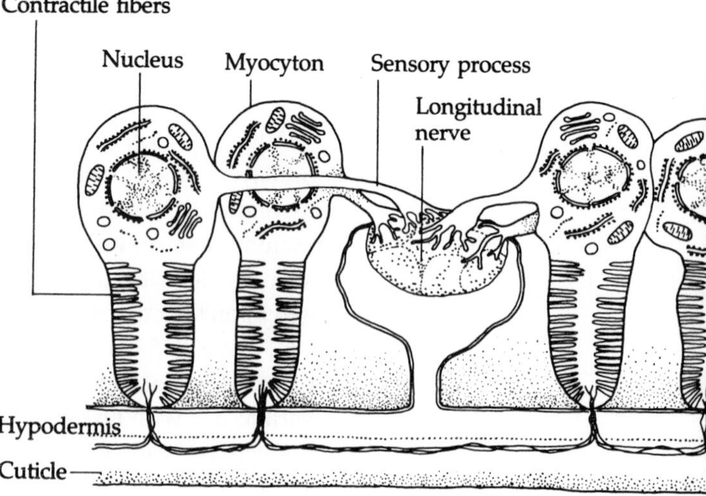

FIGURE 15-6
Arms of four myocytons forming junctions with a nerve.

DIGESTIVE TRACT

The digestive tract of nematodes is complete (Fig. 15-1). It consists of an anterior mouth, a gut, a cloaca, and a subterminal vent. The three major regions of the gut (foregut, midgut, and hindgut) each display a certain degree of specialization.

Foregut

The cuticle-lined foregut begins at the mouth, which opens into a **buccal capsule** in many species and continues as the esophagus. When present, the buccal capsule may contain ridges, rods, and plates that maintain its shape, as well as spears, stylets, or teeth that are used to attach to or penetrate the host or to acquire food.

The buccal capsule, or the mouth if a capsule is absent, leads into the esophagus, an elongate structure of varying length and complexity. The lumen of the esophagus is characteristically triradiate in cross section and is lined with cuticle. The structure of the esophagus varies within the phylum, but its similarity among members of a given taxon makes it an important taxonomic feature (Fig. 15-7). It may be completely muscular or completely glandular, or the anterior half may be glandular and the posterior half muscular. Esophageal action is often enhanced by one or more muscular enlargements called **bulbs**. The glandular portion of the foregut ranges from a few unicellular glands to large, prominent glands lying along the esophagus. The glands secrete several digestive enzymes, including amylase, proteases, and cellulases. In a number of species, these enzymes initiate the digestive process, which is completed in the midgut. Generally, nutrients are ingested and processed in the nematode foregut for eventual digestion and absorption in the midgut.

Midgut

The esophagus empties into the midgut (or intestine) through a junction called the **esophago-intestinal valve**. The midgut is a straight tube lined with a single layer of cells bearing microvilli and a prominent glycocalyx. In smaller nematodes, it is interesting that the number of cells making up the midgut is fixed for each species. This phenomenon makes nematodes useful in certain developmental studies. The cellular layer rests on a basal lamina of connective tissue fibers and myofibers connected to the

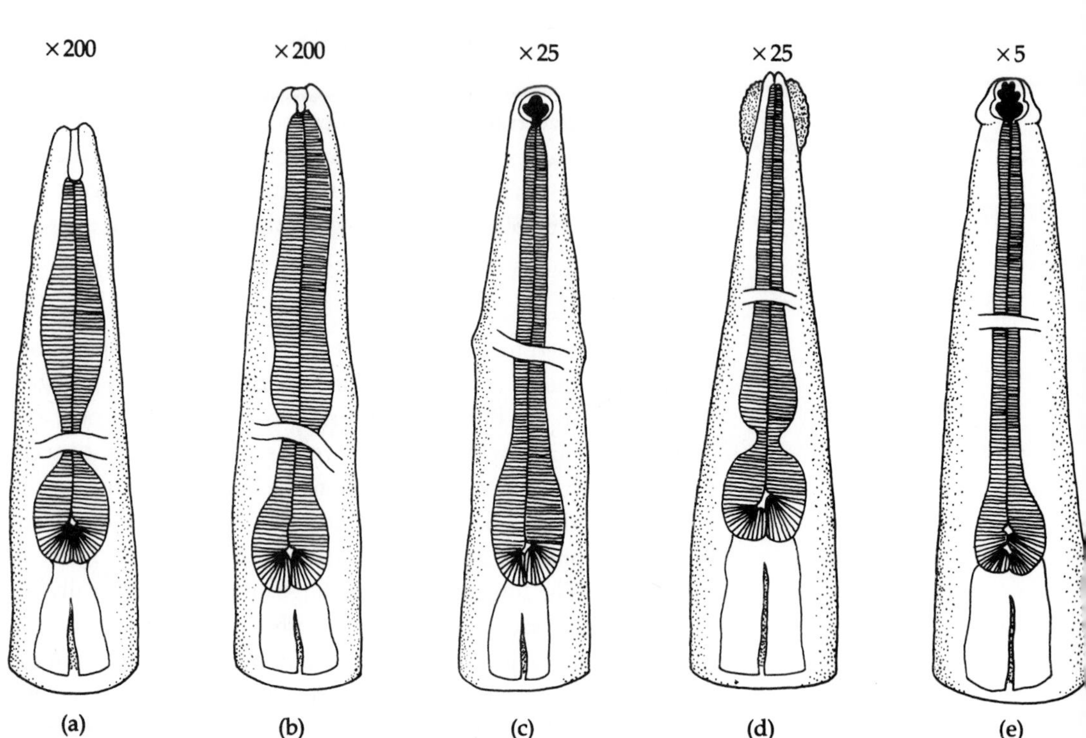

FIGURE 15-7
Variations in foregut of some nematodes.
(a) *Rhabditis hominus.* (b) *Strongyloides stercoralis.* (c) *Ancylostoma duodenale.* (d) *Enterobius vermicularis.* (e) *Ascaris lumbricoides.*

body wall by muscular extensions. The midgut is nonmuscular, the food being moved posteriorly by the muscular activity of the foregut and overall body movements. The form of digestion varies among nematodes. In some, digestion is extracellular; in others, it is both extracellular and intracellular.

Hindgut

In females, the midgut empties into the cuticle-lined hindgut, or rectum, a short, flattened tube joining the midgut and the anus. In males, the posterior-most portion of the hindgut receives the products of the reproductive system via the vas deferens and is therefore called a **cloaca**.

NERVOUS SYSTEM

There are two major nerve centers in nematodes (Fig. 15-8). One, the **circumesophageal commissure,** or **nerve ring,** surrounds the esophagus. In at least one species, the commissure consists of four nerve cells and numerous supporting cells. Associated with the commissure are various ganglia from which longitudinal nerves emanate. The anterior longitudinal nerves innervate the anterior sense organs, such as oral papillae and amphids. The posterior longitudinal nerves, embedded in the dorsal and ventral hypodermal cords, innervate organs in the posterior regions of the body. The ventral longitudinal nerve is the largest nerve in the nematode body; it passes posteriorly as a chain of ganglia, the most posterior of which branches, continues dorsally from the hypodermal cord into the pseudocoelom, and encircles the rectum to form the second nerve center, the **rectal commissure.** Peripheral nerves branch from the main longitudinal trunks and supply sensory organs, such as the phasmids, in the cuticle.

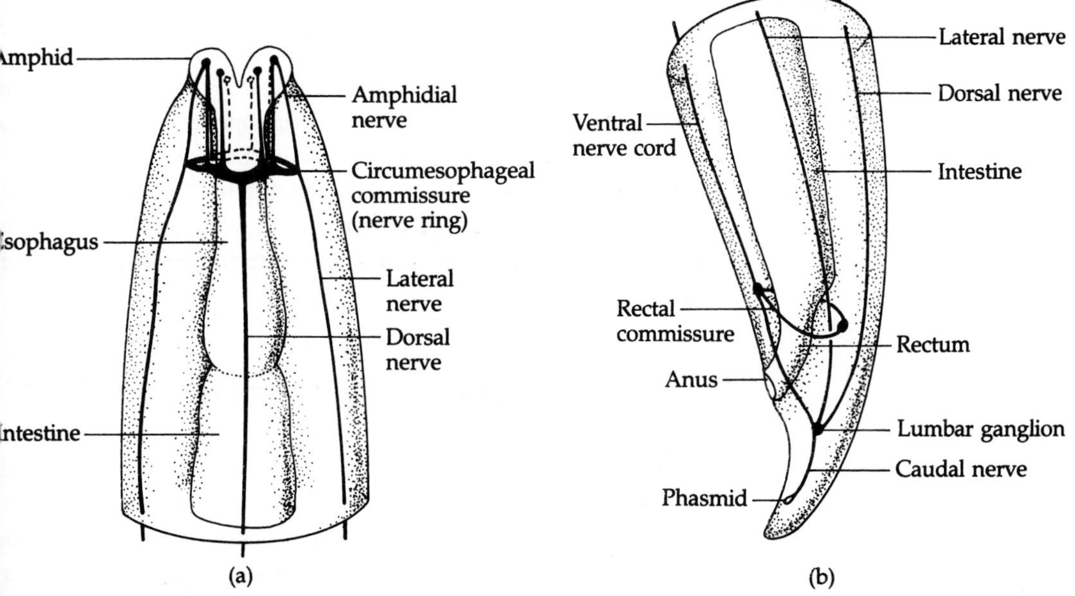

IGURE 15-8
Iematode nervous system.
ı) Anterior end. (b) Posterior end.

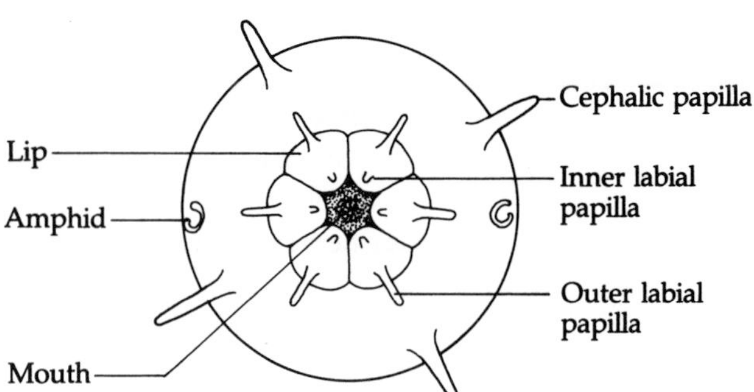

FIGURE 15-9
Labial and cephalic papillae.
En face view of nematode showing relationship of mouth, lips, amphids, and papillae.

Parasitic nematodes possess both mechano- and chemoreceptors. Located near the mouth are papillae of two main types: **labial papillae** on the lips surrounding the mouth and **cephalic papillae** behind the lips (Fig. 15-9). Papillae are mechanoreceptors and are innervated by **papillary nerves** derived from the circumesophageal commissure. Other papillae may be found at different levels of the nematode body. For example, **caudal papillae** observed in many male nematodes, aid in copulation. **Amphids** are chemoreceptors located in shallow, anterior depressions or pits at the same level of the body as the cephalic papillae. The sensory endings in amphids are modified cilia innervated by **amphidial nerves**, which are also associated with the circumesophageal commissure. **Phasmids** comprise another set of chemoreceptors that appear near the posterior end of many parasitic species as a pair of cuticle-lined organs. While morphologically resembling amphids, phasmids have a unicellular gland opening into the depression in addition to the sensory nerve endings.

EXCRETORY SYSTEM

The excretory system of nematodes, when present, is unique the basic component(s) being one or two **renettes**, large unicellular glands that empty through an excretory pore (Fig. 15-10). The renettes and the excretory pore are usually located anteriorly at approximately the level of the circumesophageal commissure Most frequently, renettes are associated with longitudinal excretory canals that course the length of the nematode body in the lat

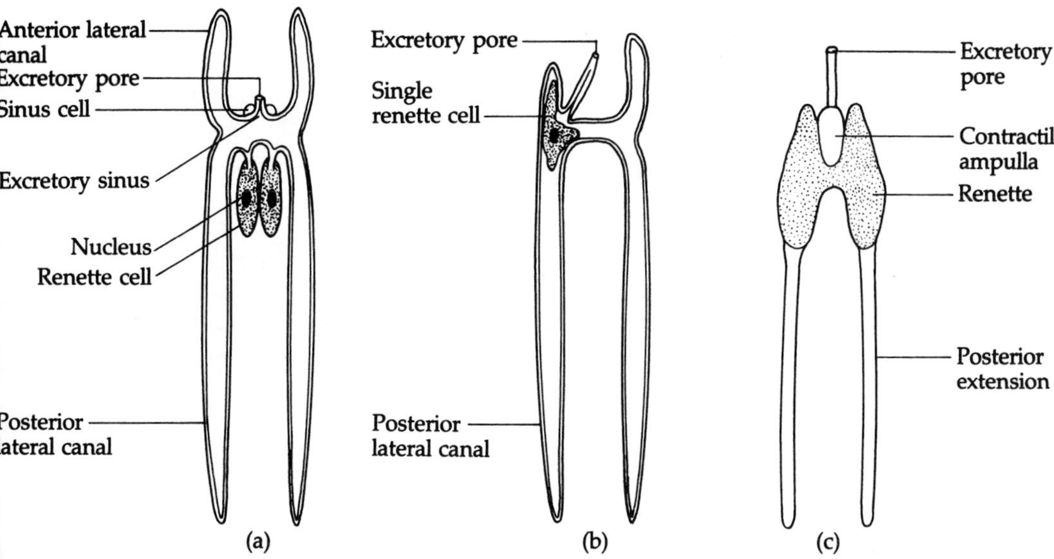

IGURE 15-10
Nematode excretory systems.
a) Rhabditoid type. (b) Ascaroid type. (c) Juvenile *Ancylostoma*.

eral hypodermis. In some genera, however, renettes empty independently to the exterior through an excretory pore, or two renettes join to form an H configuration, with a crossbar that connects with a common contractile ampulla; the pulsation of the ampulla expels the excreta via a duct leading to the excretory pore. In yet another variation, two renettes join anteriorly, and excreta are emptied via a common duct through the excretory pore.

It has not been shown conclusively that this system serves as the primary vehicle for excretion. Indeed, there is strong evidence that the digestive tract is the principal excretory organ and that the system described previously is chiefly osmoregulatory, with merely ancillary excretory and secretory functions.

REPRODUCTIVE SYSTEMS

Although some of the monoecious species of nematodes are self-fertilizing hermaphrodites and others, such as *Strongyloides stercoralis*, are **protandrogonous** (see p. 350), nematodes are usually dioecious.

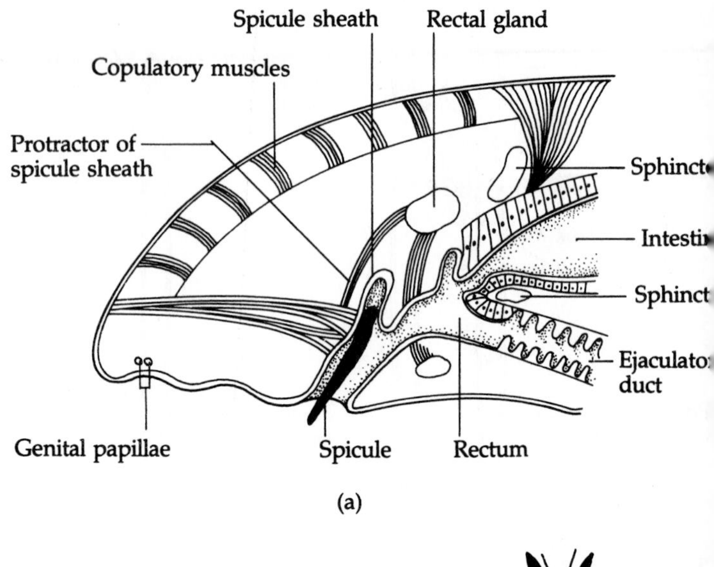

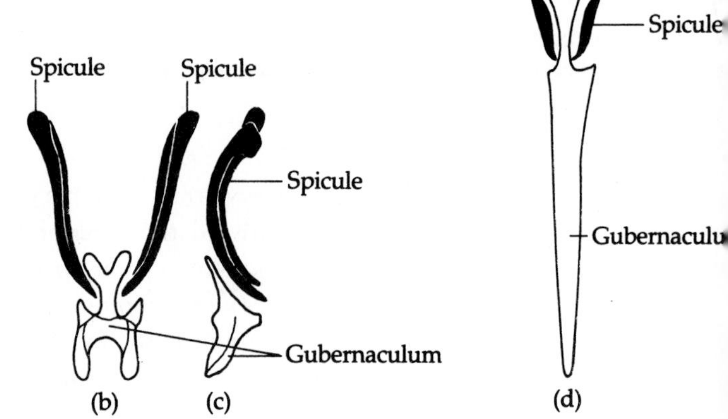

FIGURE 15-11 **Specializations of male reproductive system of nematodes.** (a) Posterior portion showing relationship of spicules to digestive tract. (b–d) Various relationships of spicules to gubernaculums.

Male System

There is most often a single testis, although two are not uncom mon (Figs. 15-1 and 15-11). Tubular and usually convoluted and or recurved, testes can be classified according to the location o their respective **germinal zones**, or regions of sperm formation. I the **telogonic** type, spermatogonial divisions occur at the blin end of the elongate testis, with the remaining portion of the testi making up the **growth zone**; in the **hologonic** type, the germina zone extends the entire length of the testis. The **vas deferen** (sperm duct), a slender tube continuous at its proximal end wit the testis, extends distally to the cloaca. Two specializations of the vas deferens are evident anterior to its junction with the cloaca. These are the **seminal vesicle**, in which sperm are stored, and the **ejaculatory duct**. In certain species, numerous unicellular **prostate glands** are present along the length of the ejaculatory duct.

Male nematodes are equipped with one or, more commonly, two **copulatory spicules** (Fig. 15-11). These cuticular structures, which usually resemble slightly curved, pointed blades, are encased within their respective spicule pouches located laterally in the cloacal wall. Each spicule contains a cytoplasmic core formed by cells lining the pouch. The spicules aid during copulation by keeping the female vulva open, thus facilitating the entry of sperm into the female reproductive tract.

In addition to spicules, other accessory structures may be present, such as a sclerotized **spicule guide** or **gubernaculum**. This structure, located along the dorsal wall of the spicule pouch, typically has inwardly curved margins and serves to guide spicules when they are extended.

Nematode sperm have no flagella, acrosomes, or nuclear envelopes (Fig. 15-12). Sperm can be classified into several morphological types, ranging from small, rounded cells that move by pseudopodia and display distinct anterior and posterior cytoplasmic areas, to cells with distinct heads and cytoplasmic extensions resembling nonmotile tails. In some species, sperm become activated only after being introduced into the female reproductive tract.

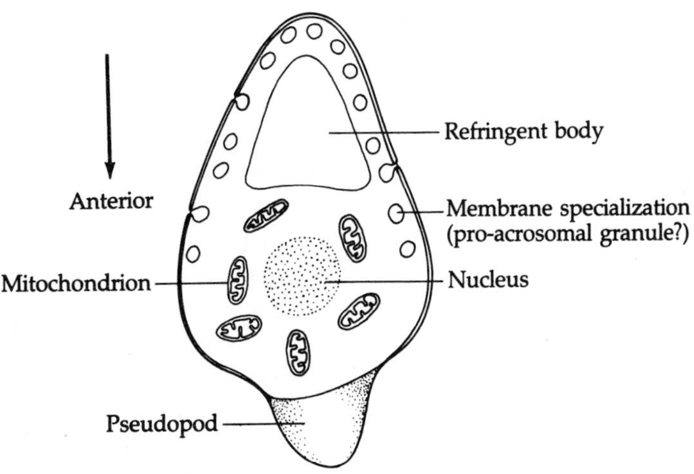

FIGURE 15-12
A generalized nematode sperm.

Female System

Female nematodes are usually **didelphic**, i.e., equipped with two cylindrical ovaries and uteri (Fig. 15-1). **Monodelphic** species, with one ovary and one uterus, occur less frequently, and, rarely, there are **polydelphic** species with multiple ovaries and uteri. The uteri in didelphic and polydelphic species unite to form a common **vagina** that opens through a gonopore, or **vulva,** usually located near midbody. The ovary, a solid cord of cells attached to a central **rachis**, constitutes the first element in the linearly arranged female reproductive system. Oogonia are produced in the germinal zone at the proximal end of the ovary. As the oogonia develop into oocytes, they move distally along the rachis into the growth zone. Approaching the oviduct, oocytes detach from the rachis and pass distally to a portion of the oviduct called the **spermatheca**, where sperm are stored. Initiation of meiosis and shell formation begin almost immediately after penetration by a sperm. The developing "egg" is moved down the tract by a combination of uterine peristalsis and hydrostatic pressure. The usually muscular, distal portion of the uterus, the **ovijector**, acts in conjunction with muscles of the vulva to expel ripe eggs.

Upon oviposition, eggs of parasitic nematodes ordinarily consist of three layers enclosing an embryo that may range from a few blastomeres to a completely formed larva (Fig. 15-13). Immediately following sperm penetration, the oocyte secretes a **fertilization membrane**, which gradually thickens to form the chitinous **shell.** The inner membrane, the **lipid layer**, is formed by the zygote. As eggs pass down the uterus, a **proteinaceous layer** is sometimes secreted by the uterine wall and deposited on the shell surface. This layer may be rough (as in *Ascaris*) or smooth (as in *Trichuris*).

Eggs of parasitic nematodes may hatch either within the host or in the external environment. The eggs of many nematodes hatch only after ingestion by a host, in which case, hatching stimuli generated by the host may be related to carbon dioxide tension, salts, pH, or temperature. These conditions stimulate the enclosed larva to secrete enzymes that partially digest the enveloping membranes. When hatching of eggs occurs in the external environment, a first-stage larva (see section titled Larval Forms) usually emerges. This process is controlled partly by the maturity of the larva and partly by ambient factors such as temperature, moisture, and oxygen tension. An egg will hatch only

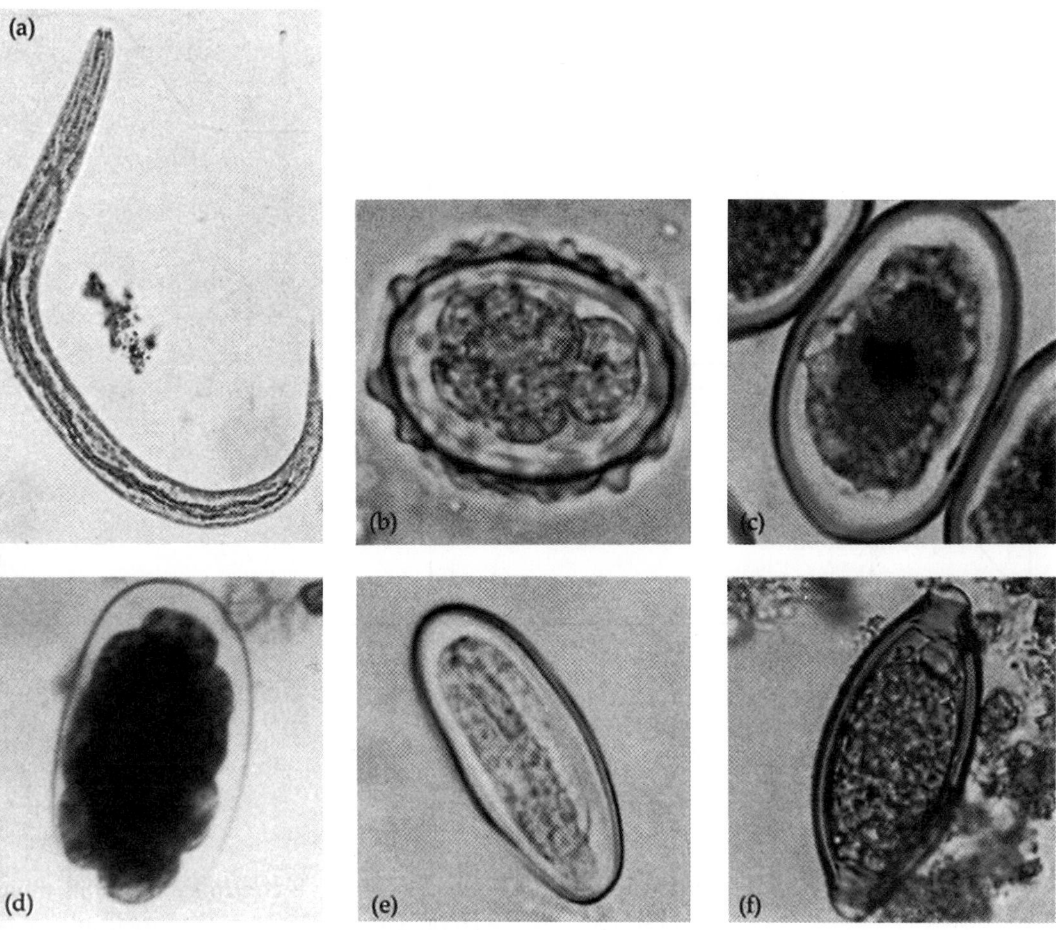

FIGURE 15-13
Some nematode eggs and larvae.
(a) *Strongyloides stercoralis* rhabditiform larva. (b) *Ascaris lumbricoides* normal fertilized egg with developing larva. (c) *Ascaris lumbricoides* unfertilized egg. (d) Hookworm egg. (e) *Enterobius vermicularis* egg. (f) *Trichuris trichiura* egg.

when external conditions are favorable, thus ensuring that the emerging larva does not enter an unduly harsh environment.

Molting

Nematodes undergo four molts (Fig. 15-14), each of which involves four events: (1) formation of a new cuticle, (2) loosening of the old cuticle, (3) rupturing of the old cuticle, and (4) escape

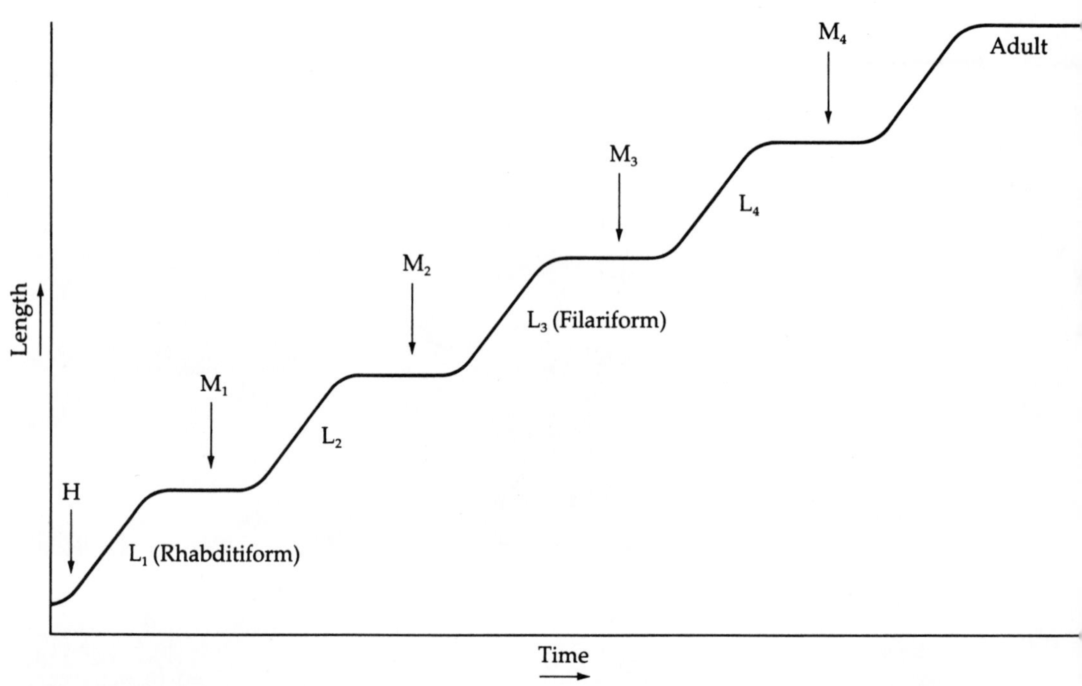

FIGURE 15-14
Nematode growth pattern.
H, hatch; M, molt; L, larva.

of the larva. The sequence of events is controlled by **exsheathing fluid** secreted by the larva. This fluid digests the cuticle at specific sites on the inner surface, causing it to loosen. The larva's ability to form a new cuticle in the hypodermis before shedding the old one allows the nematode to develop continuously between molts; however, growth occurs most rapidly just after molting. This pattern of development strongly resembles that of arthropods.

In some nematodes, there is a lag at some stage of development, during which a phase of the life cycle is temporarily arrested. Known as **hypobiosis**, this phenomenon is thought to be an adaptation that allows the larva to withstand adverse environmental conditions while awaiting access to a new host. Renewal of the life cycle following hypobiosis depends upon stimuli that accompany events such as penetration of host skin or being swallowed by the host. In some species, hypobiosis may occur in the definitive host.

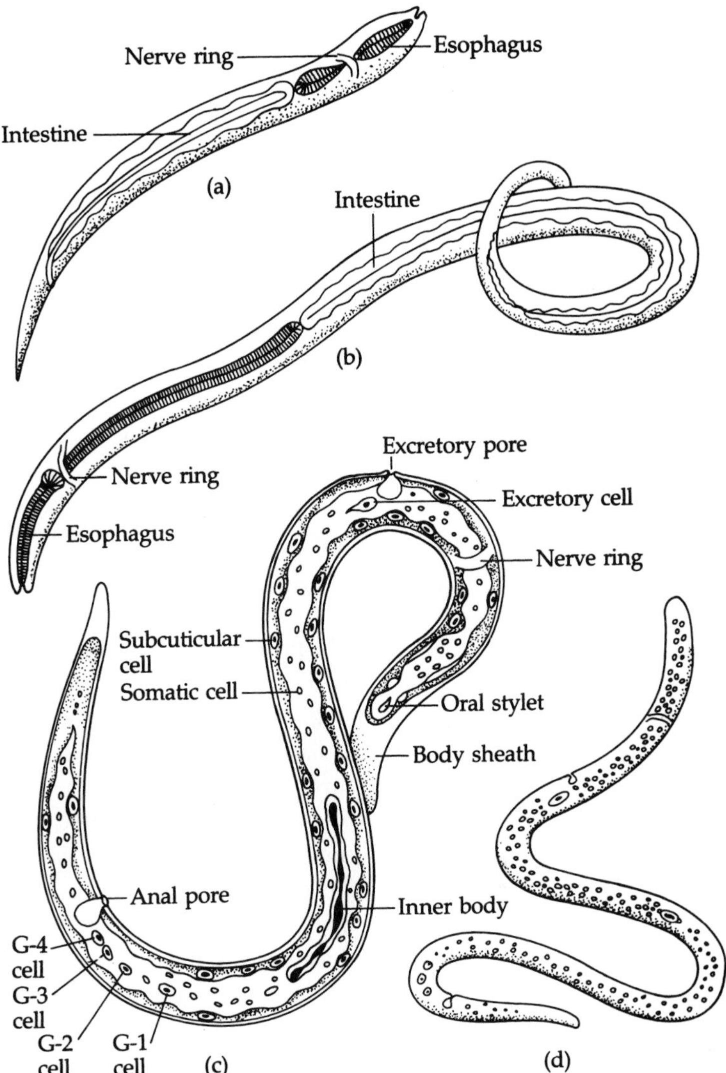

FIGURE 15-15
Nematode larvae.
(a) Rhabditiform larva. (b) Filariform larva. (c) Sheathed filariform larva of *Wuchereria*. (d) Unsheathed filariform larva of *Onchocerca*.

LARVAL FORMS

Larval stages (Fig. 15-15) in the life cycle of parasitic nematodes are generally referred to as first-, second-, third-, and fourth-stage larvae (L_1–L_4), the first-stage larva being prior to the first molt. Various other designations also are used for specific nematode larval forms.

Rhabditiform Larva

The first-stage larvae of parasitic nematodes such as *Strongyloides* and hookworms are called **rhabditiform larvae** (Fig. 15-15a). The esophagus of these small larvae is joined to a terminal esophageal bulb by a narrow isthmus.

Filariform Larva

After molting twice, the rhabditiform larvae of *Strongyloides* and hookworms normally retain the remnants of their last cuticle and become ensheathed, third-stage or **filariform larvae** (Fig. 15-15b). In this stage, the esophagus is typically elongate and cylindrical with no terminal bulb. The filariform larva is usually the stage that is infective to the definitive host.

Microfilaria

The prelarvae or advanced embryos of filarial nematodes such as *Wuchereria bancrofti* and *Loa loa* are known as **microfilariae** (Fig. 15-15c). The larval body surface is covered by a thin layer of flattened epidermal cells. The primordia of various adult structures are visible within the pseudocoelom in the form of a conspicuous cord of nucleated cytoplasm that extends the length of the body and represents the developing digestive tract. This larva, generally found in circulating blood and cutaneous tissues, is microscopic, measuring 0.2–0.4 mm in length. Unlike tissue-dwelling microfilariae (see p. 382), those that inhabit host blood are usually surrounded by a thin, cuticular **sheath**.

PHYSIOLOGY

Parasitic nematodes derive much of their energy from the metabolism of glycogen. This carbohydrate reserve is stored primarily in the hypodermis, the intestine, the noncontractile parts of the muscles, and parts of the reproductive system. It is difficult to establish with certainty whether adult intestinal nematodes are exclusively aerobic or anaerobic in their usage of carbohydrate or whether free-living larvae are invariably aerobic. Experimental data strongly suggest the importance of determining not only whether each species uses oxygen but also the manner in which it is utilized. For instance, intestinal nematodes belonging to the genus *Ascaris* can use oxygen if available; however, it serves only as a terminal electron acceptor in a system independent of an electron transport system or a functional Krebs cycle. On the other hand, both larvae and adults of *Trichinella spiralis* use oxygen in metabolic pathways that include the Krebs cycle. Thus, the former organism generates ATP by means of substrate-level phosphorylation, while the latter organisms do so primarily through oxidative phosphorylation. The eggs and first- and second-stage larvae of *Ascaris* spp. carry out aerobic metabolism with a functional Krebs cycle. Indeed, optimal larval development in most species that have been studied is dependent upon relatively high concentrations of oxygen.

Certain relatively large nematodes possess some sort of oxygen-binding system, including utilization of the respiratory pigments myoglobin and hemoglobin. Such pigments are usually found in the pseudocoelomic fluid and the hypodermis.

SELECTED READINGS

Ashton, F. T., and Schad, G. A. 1996. Amphids in *Strongyloides stercoralis* and other parasitic nematodes. *Parasitology Today* **12**, 187–194.

Bird, A. F. 1971. *The Structure of Nematodes*. Academic, New York.

Gibbs, H. C. 1986. Hypobiosis in parasitic nematodes—An update. *Advances in Parasitology* **25**, 129–174.

Lee, D. L., and Atkinson, H. J. 1977. *Physiology of Nematodes*. Columbia University, New York.

Roberts, M. C., and Modha, J. 1997. Probing the nematode surface. *Parasitology Today* **13**, 52–56.

Rosenbluth, J. 1965. Ultrastructural organization of obliquely striated muscle fibers in *Ascaris lumbricoides*. *Journal of Cell Biology* **25**, 495–515.

Rosenbluth, J. 1965. Ultrastructure of somatic cells in *Ascaris lumbricoides*. II. Intermuscular junctions, neuromuscular junctions, and glycogen stores. *Journal of Cell Biology* **26**, 579–591.

Wright, K. A. 1987. The nematode's cuticle—Its surface and the epidermis: Function, homology, analogy—A current consensus. *The Journal of Parasitology* **73**, 1077–1083.

CLASSIFICATION OF THE NEMATODA*

PHYLUM NEMATODA

Bilaterally symmetrical, unsegmented pseudocoelomates; body generally elongate, cylindrical, covered by cuticle; mouth terminal surrounded by lips; sexes separate; anterior body characteristically with 16 setiform or papilliform sensory organs and two amphids (chemoreceptors); digestive tract complete, with subterminal anus; excretory system, when present, empties through anterior, ventromedian pore; body musculature limited to longitudinally oriented muscles; no respiratory or circulatory system; eggs with determinate cleavage; oviparous or ovoviviparous; stages in life cycle are egg, four juvenile (larval) stages, and adult.

CLASS ADENOPHOREA

Amphids postlabial, variable in shape (porelike, pocketlike, circular, or spiral); cephalic sensory organs setiform to papilloid, postlabial and/or labial; setae and hypodermal glands present; papillae usually present on body; hypodermal cells uninucleate; cuticle usually smooth, but transverse or longitudinal striations sometimes present; excretory organ, if present, single-celled, ventral, without collecting tubules; caudal glands (three) usually present (absent in most members of Dorylaimida, Mermithida, and Trichocephalida); usually two testes in males, with single, ventral series of papilloid or tuboid preanal supplements; male tail rarely with caudal alae; parasitic species associated with invertebrates, vertebrates, and plants; many free living; includes most marine nematodes.

ORDER TRICHOCEPHALIDA

With protrusible axial spear in early larval stages; amphids adjacent to lip region; posterior esophageal glands in one or two rows along esophageal lumen, not enclosed by stichosome; stichosome and individual gland openings posterior to nerve ring; males and females with single gonad; germinal zones of male and female gonads extend entire length and form a serial germinal area on one side or around gonoduct; males with one or no spicule; eggs operculate; life cycle either direct (often requiring canni-

*Only those taxa that include parasitic species mentioned in text are defined.

balism), or indirect (involving arthropod or annelid intermediate host); adults parasitic in vertebrates.

SUPERFAMILY TRICHUROIDEA

Stichosome of adults as single row on each side of esophagus (two rows in early larval development); body divided into elongate, narrow anterior end with esophagus with stichosome, and posterior end with reproductive system beginning at esophagointestinal junction; bacillary band (glandular and nonglandular cells of unknown function) occurs laterally; glandular tissue emptying to exterior through cuticular pores; males and females with single gonad, reflexid; males with single spicule; eggs operculate; females oviparous; males small and degenerate in some species, in uterus of female; parasitic in humans and other mammals; life cycle direct or indirect. (Genus mentioned in text: *Trichuris*)

SUPERFAMILY TRICHINELLOIDEA

Stichosome as single, short row of stichocytes; body not distinctly divided into two regions; no bacillary band present; female genital pore opening far anterior, in region of stichosome; ovary posterior to stichosome; males with single testis but no spicule; females viviparous. (Genus mentioned in text: *Trichinella*)

CLASS SECERNENTEA

Amphids usually opening to exterior through pores located dorsolaterally on lateral lips or anterior extremity (amphidial apertures oval, cleftlike, slitlike, or located postlabially in some species); generally 16 cephalic sensory organs situated on lips, porelike or papilliform, arranged in two circles (a circumoral circle of six and an outer circle of 10), but may be reduced in some species; caudal phasmids present; hypodermis uninucleate or multinucleate; cuticle from two to four layers, almost always transversely striated, laterally modified into a "wing" area marked by longitudinal striae or ridges, generally raised slightly above body contour; lateral alae may extend out a distance equal to body diameter; esophagus of most species with three esophageal glands, one dorsal (opening in anterior half of body) and two subventral (opening in posterior half of body); excretory system emptying ventromedially through cuticularized duct on one or both sides of body; somatic setae or papillae absent on females; caudal papillae may occur on males; male preanal supplements paired, often elaborate; some males with medioventral preanal supplementary papillae; males commonly with caudal alae (known as copulatory bursa).

Subclass Rhabditida

Esophagus of juveniles divided into corpus, isthmus, and valved postcorporal bulb; lumen of esophageal bulb expanded into trilobed reservoir lined with cuticle; buccal cavity (stoma) without movable armature and composed of two parts (cheilostome and esophastome), each possibly subdivided into two or more sections; males generally with well-developed bursae supported by cuticular rays or papillae.

ORDER RHABDITIA

Number of lips six, three, two, or none; buccal cavity generally tubular but may be separated into five or more sections; esophagus divided into corpus, isthmus, and bulb; terminal excretory duct lined with cuticle with paired, lateral collecting tubules running posteriorly; females with one or two ovaries; intestinal cells uni-, bi-, or tetranucleate; caudal alae (copulatory bursa), if present, contain papillae rather than supporting rays; parasites of invertebrates and vertebrates.

Suborder Rhabditina

Buccal cavity usually cylindrical, without distinct separation, generally two or more times as long as wide; lips usually distinct, with cephalic sensory papillae and porelike amphids; esophagus divided into corpus (procorpus and metacorpus) and postcorpus (isthmus and valved bulb); females with one or two ovaries; males generally with paired spicules and gubernaculum; caudal alae (copulatory bursa) common (absent in some families); parasites of invertebrates and vertebrates.

SUPERFAMILY RHABDITOIDEA

Well-developed, cylindrical buccal cavity (stoma); lips vary from two to six; esophagus, at least in larvae, include muscular posterior bulb with rhabditoid valve; caudal alae of males supported by five to nine papilloid supplements; parasites of invertebrates and vertebrates. (Genus mentioned in text: *Strongyloides*)

ORDER STRONGYLIDA

Labial region of three or six lips or replaced by corona radiata; stoma well developed or rudimentary (never collapsed and unobtrusive); esophagus of juveniles typically rhabditiform (corpus, isthmus, bulb); esophageal bulb contains typical trilobed rhabdiform valve; esophagus of adults cylindrical to clavate; excretory system includes paired lateral canals and paired subventral glands; females with one or two ovaries and heavily muscular uterus; males with muscular copulatory bursa, paired genital papillae, and paired, equal spicules; adults parasitic in vertebrates.

SUPERFAMILY ANCYLOSTOMATOIDEA

Stoma thick-walled, globose, armed or unarmed anteriorly with teeth or cutting plates; without lips or corona radiata; copulatory bursae of males with greatly reduced branches; adults parasitic in intestine of mammals; L_1 and L_2, free living; commonly known as hookworms. (Genera mentioned in text: *Ancylostoma, Necator.*)

ORDER ASCARIDIDA

Oral opening usually surrounded by three lips (absent in some species); paired porelike amphids present; esophagus of some species with short, swollen region near stoma, followed by cylindrical to club-shaped region, often ending in terminal bulb with three-lobed valve; appendages (caeca) extending from posterior region of esophagus in a few species; excretory system with lateral collecting tubules, in some species extending posteriorly and anteriorly (H-shaped); males usually with two spicules (none or one in others); with or without gubernaculum; females usually with two ovaries (some with multiple ovaries); adults parasitic in vertebrates.

SUPERFAMILY ASCARIDOIDEA

Bodies 1–40 cm long; cuticle thick in larger species, superficially annulated; terminal oral opening usually surrounded by three well-developed lips; porelike amphids on subventral lips; stoma poorly developed (collapsed); esophagus cylindrical to clavate; appendage (caecum) sometimes extending from posterior portion of esophagus over anterior portion of intestine; second caecum sometimes present, extending forward past base of esophagus; females usually with paired ovaries; males with two spicules; small gubernaculum present in a few species; adults parasitic in vertebrates; life cycle direct or indirect. (Genera mentioned in text: *Ascaris, Toxocara, Anisakis.*)

SUPERFAMILY OXYUROIDEA

Lips greatly reduced or absent; cephalic sensilla in whorl of eight or four; ventrolateral sensilla absent; stoma vestibular; esophagus variable but posterior bulb always valved; intestinal caeca absent; males sometimes with precloacal suckers; copulatory spicules sometimes greatly reduced; adults usually parasites of amphibians, reptiles, and mammals. (Genus mentioned in text: *Enterobius.*)

ORDER SPIRURIDA

Frequently with two lateral lips or pseudolabia (some species with four or more lips, rare species without lips); oral aperture variable in shape, encircled by teeth; amphids laterally situated on anterior extremity; stoma varying from cylindrical and elongate to rudimentary; esophagus generally divided into narrow anterior portion and expanded postcorpus enclosing multinucleate glands; hatched larvae generally provided with cephalic hook and porelike phasmids on tail; parasites of annelids, arthropods, molluscs, and terrestrial and aquatic vertebrates.

SUPERFAMILY FILARIOIDEA

Oral aperture circular or oval, usually surrounded by eight sensilla of external circle (internal circle absent or consisting of two or four papillae); stoma small; esophagus rudimentary with multinucleate glands; corpus and postcorpus not distinct; vulva usually in anterior portion of body; copulatory spicules of males equal or unequal; caudal alae present or absent; no gubernaculum; parasites of amphibians, reptiles, birds, and mammals. (Genera mentioned in text: *Wuchereria, Brugia, Onchocerca, Loa, Dirofilaria.*)

SUPERFAMILY DRACUNCULOIDEA

Stoma commonly reduced to small vestibule; full complement of sensilla surrounding oral opening, with internal circle comprised of six well-developed sensilla and external circle of eight separate and well-developed sensilla; vulva in midbody region, atrophied in mature females; posterior intestine atrophied in females; males without well-developed caudal alae (alae small and postcloacal if present); adults parasitic in tissues of fish, reptiles, and mammals. (Genus mentioned in text: *Dracunculus*.)

Chapter Sixteen

INTESTINAL NEMATODES

THE ADENOPHOREA

Parasitic nematodes belonging to the class Adenophorea possess neither phasmids nor an excretory system. Two parasites of the human intestinal tract, *Trichuris trichiura* and *Trichinella spiralis*, belong to this class.

TRICHURIS TRICHIURA

In adult *Trichuris trichiura* (Fig. 16-1), the anterior portion of the body is long and slender, whereas the posterior portion widens abruptly and thickens, giving the worm the appearance of a bullwhip; hence, its common name is "whipworm." Males are slightly smaller than females, the latter measuring 30–50 mm in length. In both sexes, a capillary-like esophagus extends two-thirds of the body length and is encircled along much of its length by a series of unicellular glands, the **stichocytes.** The posterior extremity of males is characteristically coiled and equipped with a single spicule enclosed in a spinose, retractile, cuticular sheath.

Life Cycle

Adult whipworms occur primarily in the human host's colon but also inhabit the appendix and rectum (Fig. 16-2). The female deposits up to 5000 eggs daily; these are typically barrel-shaped with two polar plugs. The eggs measure 50 μm by 22 μm and contain an uncleaved zygote at oviposition, after which the unembryonated eggs pass to the exterior in feces and develop slowly in warm, damp soil. An unhatched, infective, third-stage larva develops in three to six weeks.

New human hosts become infected when these embryonated eggs are ingested with contaminated food or water or from fingers. The larvae hatch in the upper portions of the small intestine and quickly burrow into the cells of the intestinal villi near the crypts of Lieberkühn, where they mature, undergoing two molts

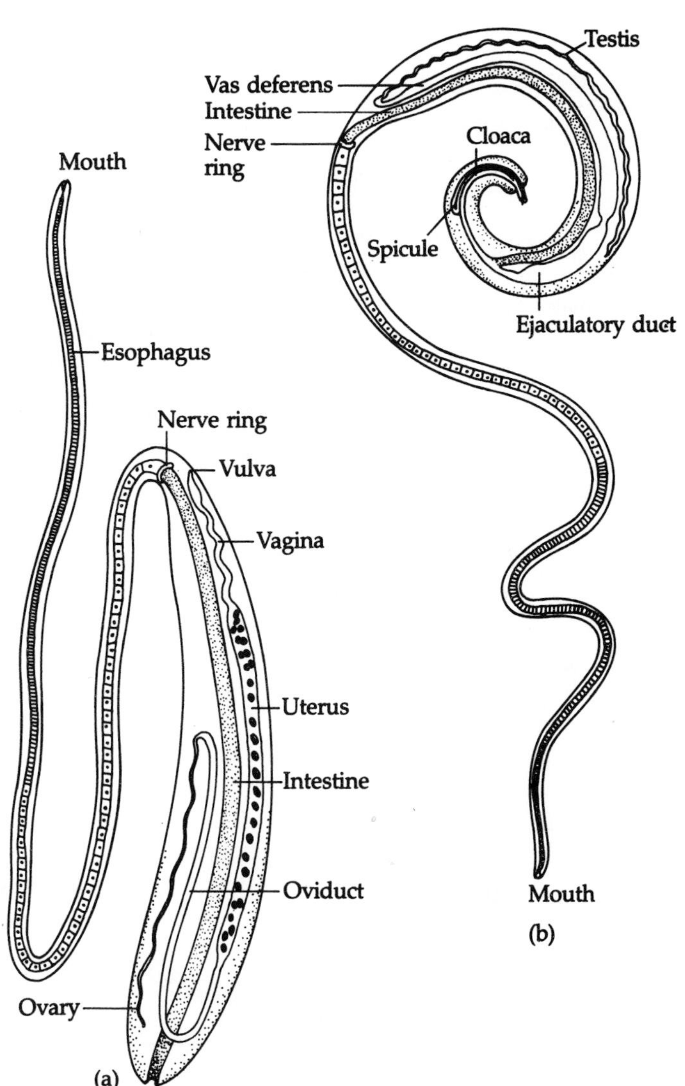

FIGURE 16-1
Adult *Trichuris trichiura*.
(a) Female. (b) Male.

in about 3–10 days. Subsequently, they migrate to the caecal region and develop to sexual maturity in 30–90 days from the time the eggs were ingested. Adult worms embed the long, slender, anterior ends of their bodies deeply into the colon submucosa. Little is known about the parasites' nutritional requirements, but there is no evidence that they feed on host blood. While these worms normally survive approximately 2 years in the human host, there have been reports of infections lasting 8 years or longer.

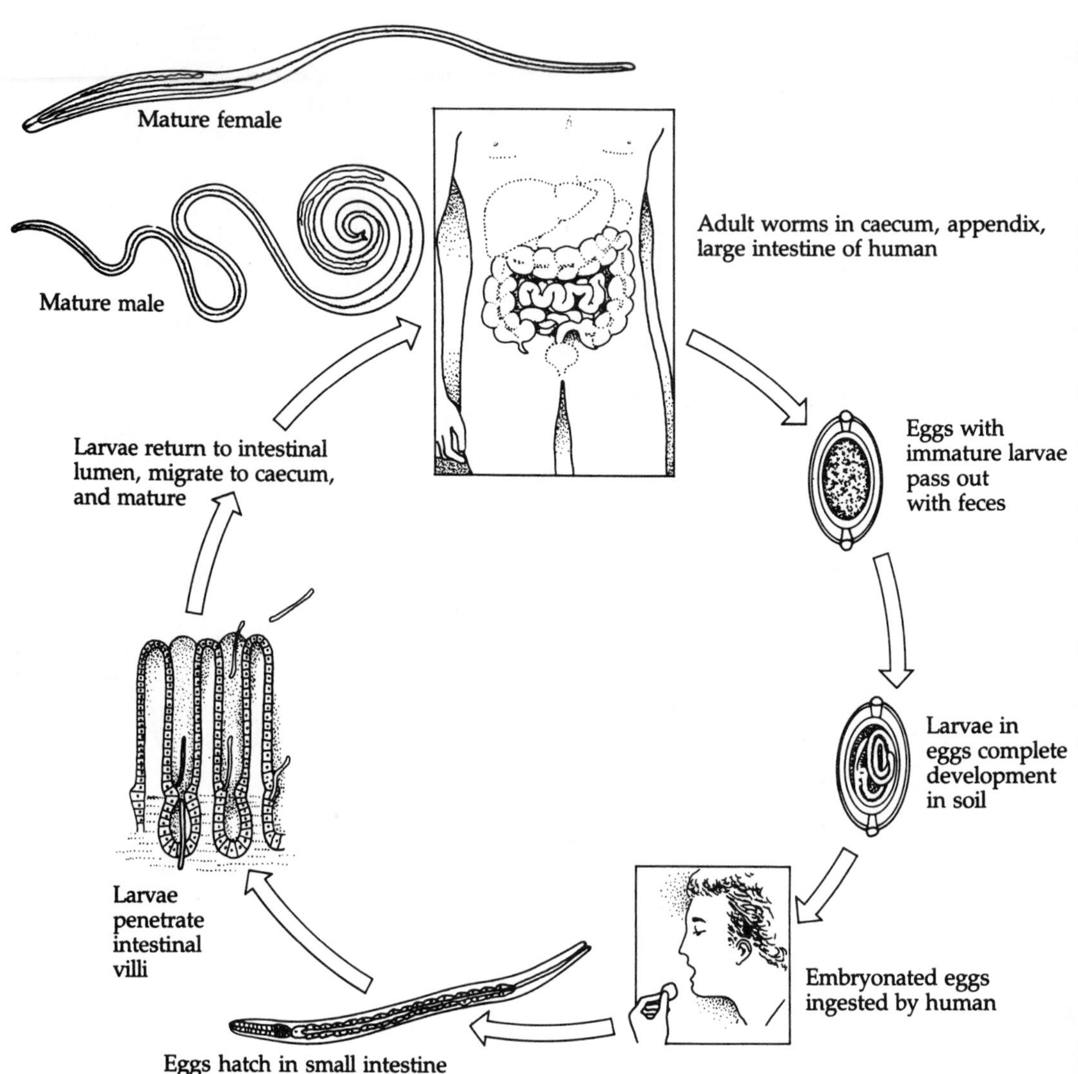

FIGURE 16-2
Life cycle of *Trichuris trichiura*.

Epidemiology

Whipworm infection occurs worldwide, most frequently in tropical countries. It is estimated that whipworms infect several hundred million people, making them the third-most common nematode infecting humans. In the United States, it is the second-most common nematode infecting humans (after *Enterobius*) and is found predominantly in the Southeast, paralleling human *Ascaris* infections. Fortunately, worm burdens are light in the majority of cases. Generally, the worm is found in areas of warm climate, heavy rainfall, dense shade, and sanitary practices conducive to soil pollution. Children are more likely to be infected than adults, because they are more apt to come into close physical contact with contaminated soil.

Symptomatology and Diagnosis

Most infections are light with no clinical symptoms. Heavy infections, however, produce symptoms such as bloody stools, pain in the lower abdomen, weight loss, rectal prolapse, nausea, and anemia. In the case of rectal prolapse, adult worms can be observed externally, embedded in the rectal mucosa. Anemia results primarily from hemorrhage when the worms penetrate the intestinal wall, although some blood loss may be attributable to the worms ingesting host blood. In heavy worm burdens, secondary bacterial infections are common, a result of the worms' penetration of the mucosal lining, which provides entry for pathogenic bacteria. Mixed infections of whipworm and *E. histolytica*, hookworm, or *Ascaris lumbricoides* are not uncommon.

Identification of eggs in fecal material constitutes diagnosis.

Treatment

Mebendazole or albendazole, the drugs of choice, are most effective when administered orally for three consecutive days. These drugs are two of the benzimidazolecarbamate class of compounds that generally cause degenerative changes in the nematode intestine. They are believed to have a depolymerizing effect on cytoskeletal elements, such as microtubules. The drugs are contraindicated during pregnancy or the first year of a child's life.

TRICHINELLA SPIRALIS

Small and slender, adult trichina worms are rarely observed (Fig. 16-3). The male, measuring 1.5 mm by 0.04 mm, has a curved posterior end with two lobed appendages called **alae**. The male reproductive system, with its single testis, is located in the posterior third of the body. The female, measuring 3.5 mm by 0.06 mm, has a bluntly rounded posterior end and is monodelphic, with the vulva in the anterior fifth of the body.

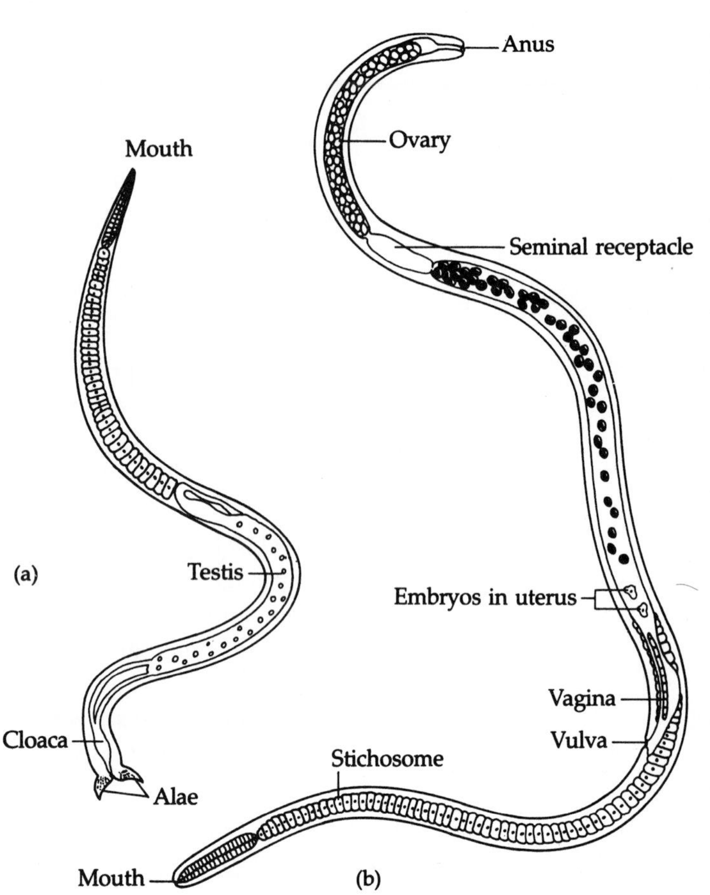

FIGURE 16-3
Adult *Trichinella spiralis.*
(a) Male. (b) Female.

Life Cycle

Trichinella spiralis requires only one host in its life cycle, with larval and adult stages occurring in different organs (Fig. 16-4). Infection results from the consumption of meat, most commonly poorly cooked pork, containing encapsulated first-stage larvae. Once ingested, the larvae are released from their capsules in the duodenum by the action of the host's digestive enzymes. Shortly thereafter, the freed larvae penetrate the absorptive and goblet cells of the mucosa. There they undergo four molts within 24–30 hours and reach sexual maturity.

Soon after copulation, the male passes out of the host, while the female burrows deeper into the mucosa and submucosa, sometimes entering the lymphatic ducts to be carried to the mesenteric lymph nodes. About 5 days after initial ingestion of

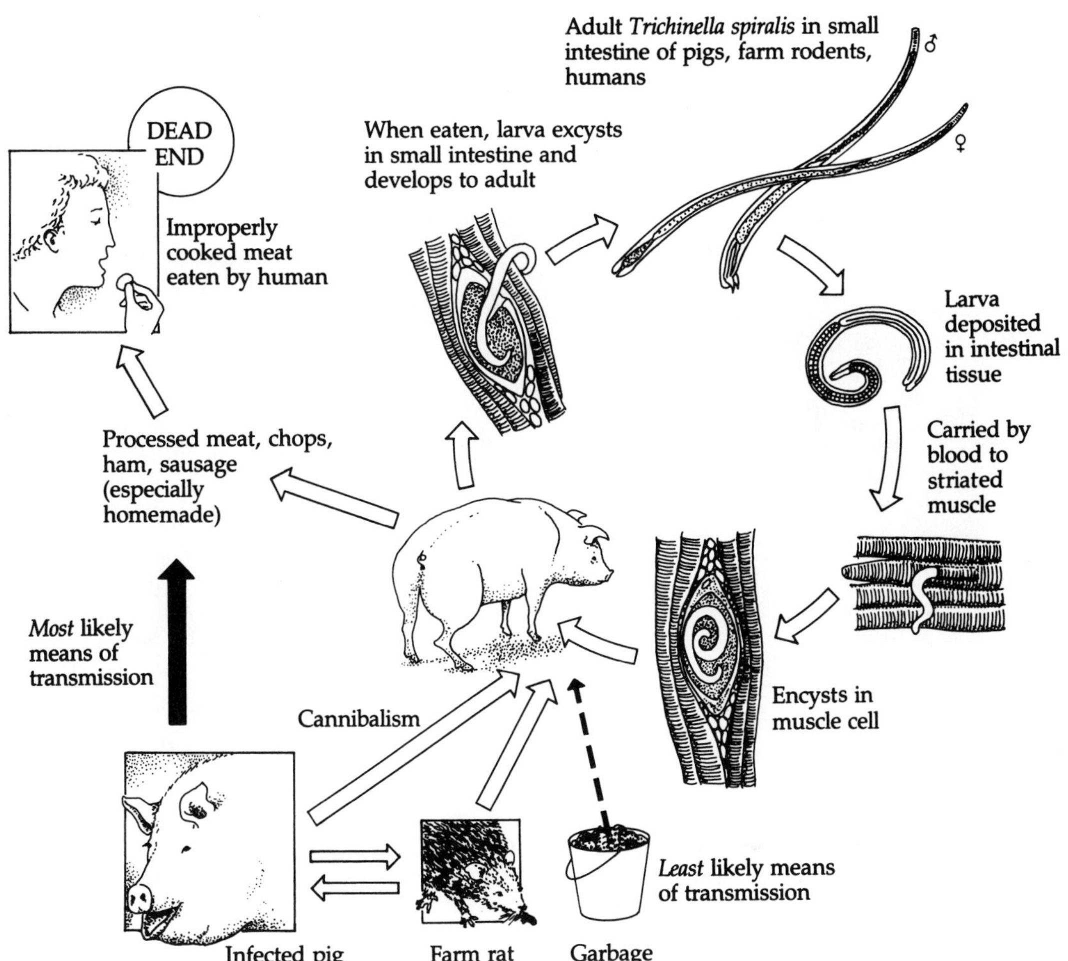
Adult *Trichinella spiralis* in small intestine of pigs, farm rodents, humans
♂
♀
DEAD END
When eaten, larva excysts in small intestine and develops to adult
Improperly cooked meat eaten by human
Larva deposited in intestinal tissue
Carried by blood to striated muscle
Processed meat, chops, ham, sausage (especially homemade)
Most likely means of transmission
Encysts in muscle cell
Cannibalism
Least likely means of transmission
Infected pig
Farm rat
Garbage

FIGURE 16-4
Life cycle of *Trichinella spiralis*.

the infective larvae by the host, the adult ovoviviparous female begins depositing first-stage larvae. It is estimated that one female produces about 1500 larvae in a period of 5–10 days. Eventually, the female dies, and the first-stage larvae, about 0.1 mm long, are carried by the lymphatic and blood vessels to the right side of the heart in venous blood.

From the heart, the larvae enter the peripheral circulation and are carried to various tissues of the body. It is only in striated muscles, especially those of the diaphragm, jaws, tongue, larynx, and eyes, that larvae develop into the infective stage. Penetration of

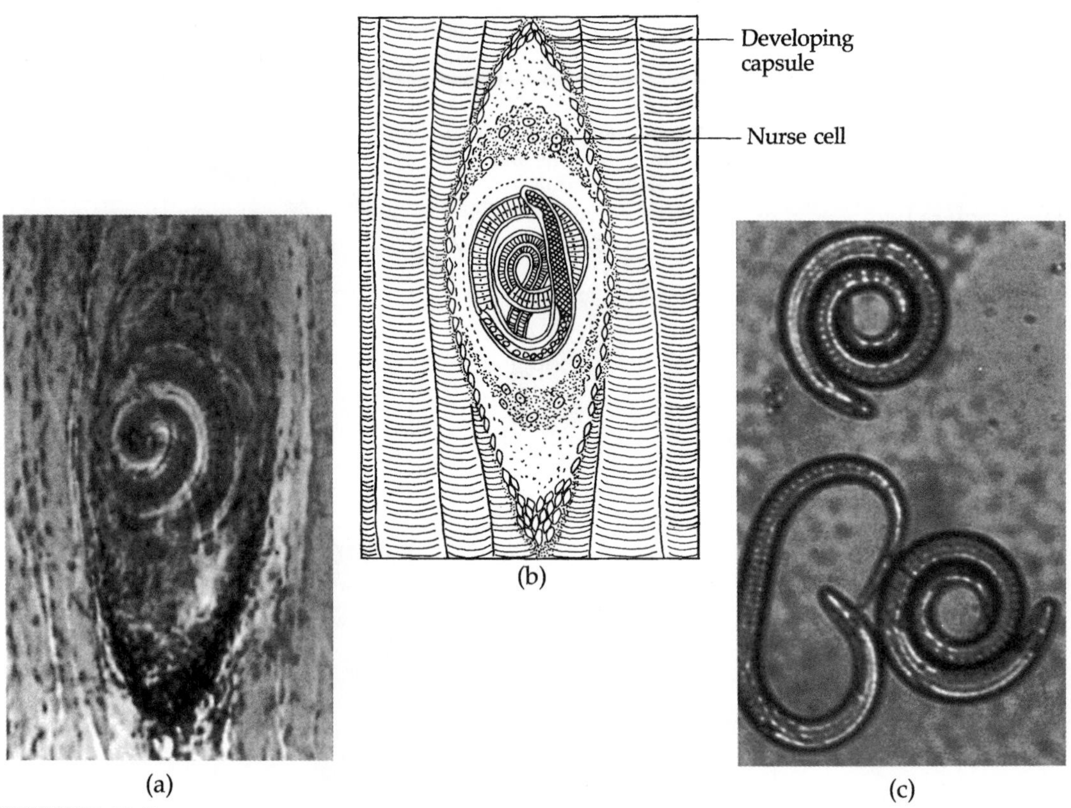

FIGURE 16-5
Trichinella spiralis **larvae encysted in skeletal muscle.**
(a) Larva-nurse cell complex. (b) Schematic representation of larva-nurse cell complex. (c) Unstained, living larvae freed from nurse cells by pepsin-HCl digestion.

muscle cells and establishment as intracellular parasites within myofibers occurs about 6 days after initial infection. Usually only one larva occupies a muscle fiber (Fig. 16-5). On or about the 17th day, the larva begins to coil. It absorbs nutrients from the host muscle sarcoplasm and becomes surrounded by a nucleated mass known as a **nurse cell.** Growth is rapid, the larva reaching a length of about 1 mm in approximately 8 weeks, at which time it becomes infective. Encapsulation begins at about the 21st day as the larva is gradually enveloped by a double, ellipsoidal capsule (0.25–0.5 mm long) of host origin. The outer capsule membrane is derived from the sarcolemma, while the inner membrane is a combination of degenerating myofibers and other cells such as fibroblasts. Capsule formation is complete in about 3 months.

Eventually, the capsule becomes calcified, a process that may begin as early as 6 months after initial infection and requires about 18 months for completion. If calcification is delayed, a *T. spiralis* larva can remain viable for several years. During capsule formation, the enclosed larva enters developmental arrest, a state in which it can survive indefinitely. When muscle harboring the encapsulated larva is eaten by a carnivorous mammal, the larva excysts and reinitiates the life cycle.

Epidemiology

The term **sylvatic trichinellosis** denotes the cycling of the disease between wild carnivores and their prey or carrion. **Urban trichinellosis**, on the other hand, is the term used to designate the cycling of the disease among humans, rats, and pigs. Rats and pigs feeding on garbage that includes infected pork waste become infected in turn. Dead or dying infected rats are themselves eaten by the pigs. Raw or poorly cooked pork, usually in sausage, harboring infective larvae then becomes the vehicle for human infections. In nature, the cycle is also maintained by cannibalistic rats.

In Alaska, where polar and black bears are common sources of human infection, there is an overlapping of sylvatic and urban trichinellosis. The disastrous 1897 Andre hydrogen balloon expedition to the Arctic provides dramatic evidence of trichinellosis in polar bears. A book and a movie, both titled *The Flight of the Eagle*, recount the story of these ill-fated Swedish explorers who, having lost most of their supplies, perished after they resorted to eating the meat of a polar bear they had killed. Lacking any means of kindling fires, they were forced to eat the meat raw. Unfortunately, the meat was infected, and the explorers died, not from exposure but from trichinellosis. Evidence of the cause of the tragedy was discovered 33 years later in the frozen, stored carcass of the bear.

Trichinellosis is a cosmopolitan disease that occurs most commonly in Europe and the United States, where there are estimated to be about 150,000–300,000 cases a year. However, the number of clinical cases reported is less than 150. The disease is rare in parts of the tropics and subtropics for the opposite reason that it is found in the United States: low consumption of pork by peoples whose diet consists primarily of fish. Ironically, in parts of the tropics where people do derive much of their protein from pork, the disease is still rare. Religious bans keep other peoples, such as Jews, Hindus, and Moslems, free of the disease, and, obviously, vegetarians are not exposed to infection.

Symptomatology and Diagnosis

The primary symptoms of trichinellosis result from larval invasion of muscle and other tissues and the hyperimmune reaction of the host to the metabolic by-products and secretions of the larvae. Although relatively few victims have infections heavy enough to produce clinical symptoms, those symptoms that do occur appear during three clinical phases: (1) mild, following penetration of adult females into the mucosa and submucosa; (2) severe, during migration of larvae; and (3) moderate, after penetration and encapsulation of larvae in muscle cells. Symptoms usually abate after 30 days.

Symptoms resulting from the first phase appear 12 hours to 2 days following ingestion of infective larvae. The microscopic lesions formed as a result of penetration become inflamed from host reactions against concomitant bacterial invasion and the worms' excreta. Nausea, fever, profuse perspiration, and diarrhea commonly occur. Some facial edema may also be present, accompanied by a slight rash. These symptoms subside within 5–7 days following onset.

The second phase may last for 3 weeks and is characterized by symptoms resembling those of diseases such as rheumatism, pneumonia, encephalitis, pleurisy, meningitis, myocarditis, and peritonitis.

During the third phase, there may be intense muscle pain, difficulty in breathing, swelling of facial muscles, weakening of blood pressure and pulse, heart damage, and nervous disorders, including hallucinations. Death may result from heart failure, respiratory complications, peritonitis, or cerebral involvement.

Most cases of trichinellosis are asymptomatic and go undetected. In suspected cases, several diagnostic laboratory procedures are available. Positive results from skin and serological tests are significant. Negative tests results, especially in the early stages of the disease, are inconclusive. Intradermal tests using a suspension prepared from larvae are sensitive enough to give positive results within an hour, provided the suspected infection is at least 2–3 weeks old. The appearance of a wheal about 5 mm in diameter indicates exposure to the worm. Several other serological procedures, such as flocculation and agglutination tests, are available and are similar in their degree of sensitivity. ELISA can detect antibodies in the serum as early as 12 days postinfection.

The definitive diagnostic procedure is the demonstration of live larvae in a specimen of biopsied muscle. In such a procedure, usually performed during about the third or fourth week of infection, a muscle section is typically taken from the deltoid or gastrocnemius muscle, placed between two slides or in a muscle press, and examined microscopically. The muscle section may be digested with pepsin before it is examined.

Treatment

No satisfactory chemotherapeutic regimen for trichinellosis has been devised. The therapeutic value of albendazole and mebendazole remains inconclusive. Bed rest and supportive treatment, such as administration of analgesics to relieve symptoms, are beneficial. In selected cases involving the heart or the central nervous system, steroid therapy has been used successfully to relieve inflammation.

Prevention

Education of the public is the most effective way to control the disease in the human population. Additionally, laws governing pork production must be strengthened. For instance, there should be widespread legislation, as there is in California, requiring the sterilization of garbage containing raw meat scraps intended for use as hog feed. Also, although costly, microscopical examination of pork should be reinstituted and updated. Finally, the public should be informed of the need to cook pork products thoroughly (at temperatures higher than 70°C), to the point at which none of the meat is pink, in order to kill the infective larvae. Microwave cooking of pork, especially roasts, should be monitored with a meat thermometer, and the temperature should reach at least 77°C.

THE SECERNENTEA

The second group of nematodes infective to humans belongs to the class Secernentea. Although species in this class exhibit morphological and life cycle differences, all possess phasmids, the minute, usually paired chemoreceptors located posterior to the anus. The adult forms of five nematodes that infect the human intestine are discussed: the thread worm, *Strongyloides stercoralis*; the two hookworms, *Ancylostoma duodenale* and *Necator americanus*; the large intestinal roundworm, *Ascaris lumbricoides*; and the pinworm, *Enterobius vermicularis*.

STRONGYLOIDES STERCORALIS

Strongyloides stercoralis and other members of this genus are unique in that they may exhibit either a **direct**, or **homogonic**, exclusively parasitic life cycle or an **indirect**, or **heterogonic**, life cycle in which free-living generations may be interrupted by parasitic generations, depending upon environmental conditions. Both the homogonic life cycle and the parasitic phase of the heterogonic life cycle involve only **protandrogonous** females, while the free-living life cycle involves both adult males and females. In protandrogonous forms, the male reproductive organs develop first and then disappear; subsequently, the female reproductive organs develop, giving the impression that the worms reproduce parthenogenetically.

Protandrogonous, parasitic females are approximately 2.0 mm long and 0.04 mm wide (Fig. 16-6a). The esophagus, lacking a posterior bulb, extends one-third the body length, and there is a shallow buccal capsule. The vulva lies in the posterior third of the body, and the didelphic uteri contain few eggs at any one time. Free-living males and females are about 1.0 mm and 2.0–2.5 mm long, respectively (Fig. 16-6b,c). The uteri of a free-living female contain far more eggs than do those of its parasitic counterpart. The free-living female is also somewhat larger and has a vulva situated in the midsection of its body.

Life Cycle

The life cycle of *S. stercoralis* (Fig. 16-7) can be divided into three phases: free living, parasitic, and autoinfectious.

Free-living Phase Free-living *S. stercoralis* dwell in moist soil in warm climates. Copulation occurs in the soil. When the sperm penetrates an oocyte, the sperm nucleus disintegrates; sperm

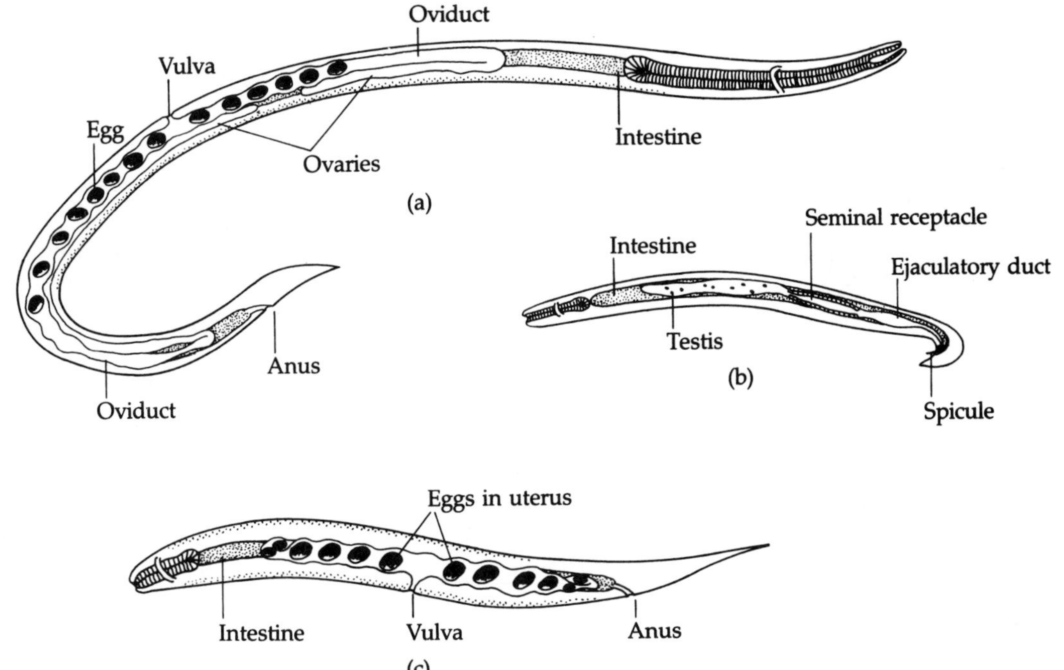

FIGURE 16-6
Morphology of *Strongyloides stercoralis*.
(a) Parasitic female. (b) Free-living male. (c) Free-living female.

penetration merely activates the oocyte to develop parthenogenetically with no contribution from the sperm's genetic material to the developing embryo. Following oviposition, the first-stage, rhabditiform larvae are well developed and require only a few hours for complete development. The eggs hatch in the soil, where the liberated larvae feed actively on organic debris, pass through four molts, and develop into sexually mature adults.

This free-living, or heterogonic, cycle may continue without interruption. However, if the environment becomes inhospitable, the rhabditiform larva molts twice to become a nonfeeding, filariform larva, the form infective to humans.

Parasitic Phase When filariform larvae encounter a human or other suitable host, they readily penetrate the skin (Fig. 16-8a) and are carried by the lymphatic vessels or the small cutaneous veins to the postcaval vein, whence they enter the right side of the heart and are carried to the lungs via the pulmonary artery. In the

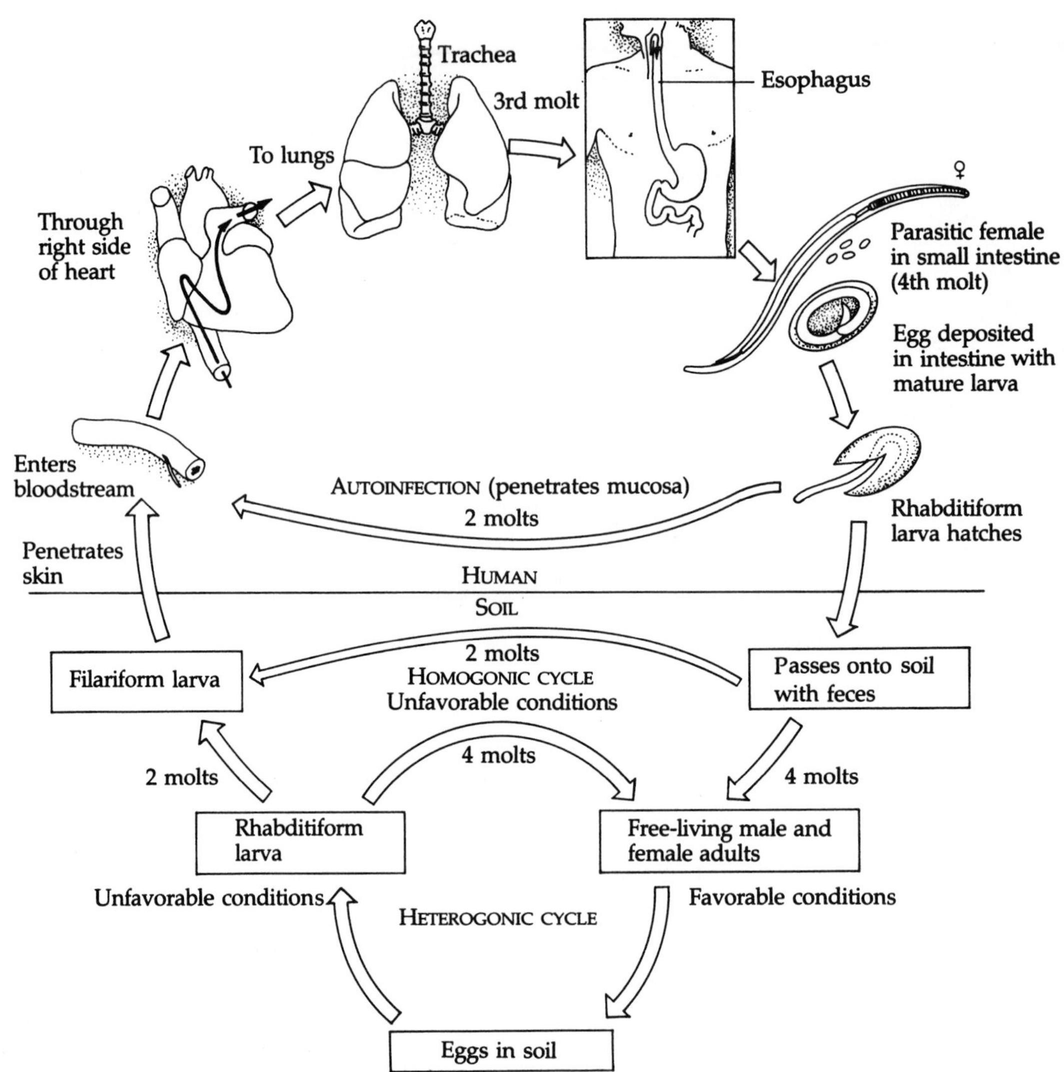

FIGURE 16-7
Life cycle of *Strongyloides stercoralis*.

lungs (Fig. 16-8b), the larvae undergo a third molt, rupture from the pulmonary capillaries, and enter the alveoli. From the alveoli, they move up the respiratory tree to the epiglottis. Abetted by coughing and subsequent swallowing by the host, the larvae migrate over the epiglottis to the esophagus and down to the small intestine. There is some laboratory evidence in experimentally in-

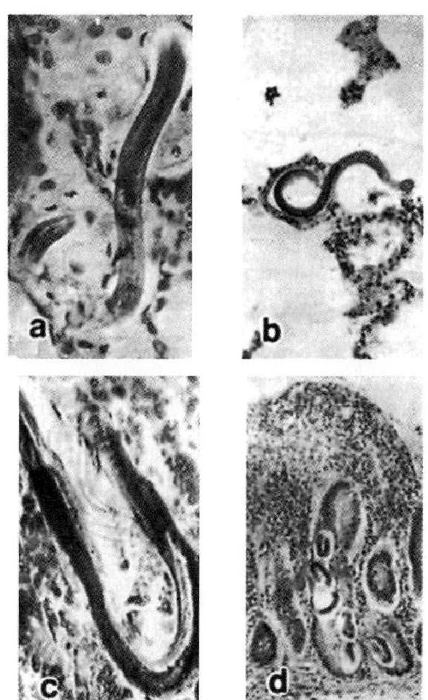

FIGURE 16-8
Strongyloides stercoralis.
(a) Filariform larva in skin. (b) Larva in lung. (c) Adult and (d) eggs in mucosa of duodenum.

fected animals that not all larvae follow the lung route to reach the intestinal tract. However, because symptoms in most infected patients involve the lungs, it appears that most larvae follow the lung route in humans.

In the small intestine, the larvae undergo a final molt and become protandrogonous worms. The worms burrow into the mucosa of the small intestine (Fig. 16-8c) and produce embryonated eggs within 25–30 days postinfection. Some investigators report that embryos are produced parthenogenetically, while others report that fertilization occurs. The eggs, averaging 54 μm by 32 μm and covered by a thin, transparent shell, hatch in the mucosa (Fig. 16-8d) into first-stage, rhabditiform larvae (Fig. 16-9a), which feed during passage through the lumen of the intestine and exit the host body with feces. Eggs are seldom found in feces. Under conditions favorable for development, the larvae become established in the soil, undergo four molts, and become free-living adults. Under adverse conditions, the rhabditiform larvae metamorphose into infective filariform larvae after two molts.

Autoinfectious Phase During passage through the host digestive tract, rhabditiform larvae may rapidly undergo two molts

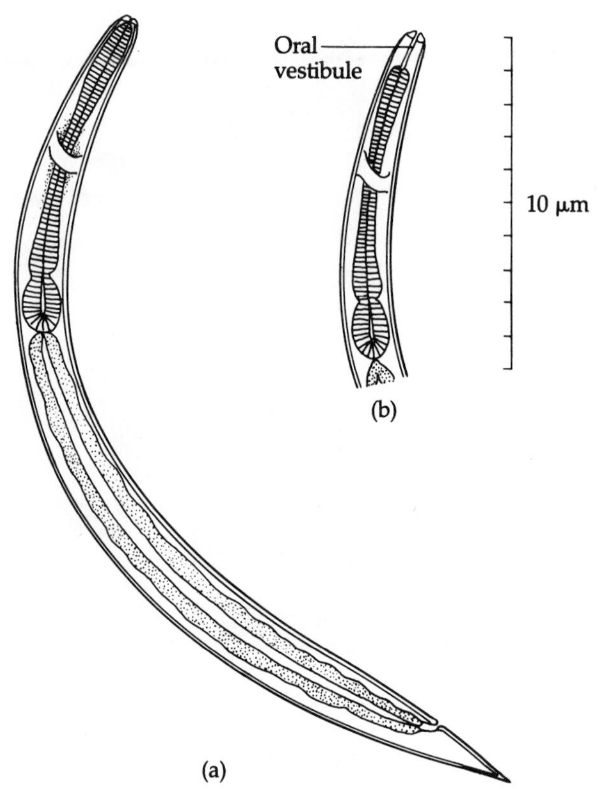

FIGURE 16-9
Rhabditiform larvae.
(a) *Strongyloides stercoralis.* (b) Anterior portion of hookworm. Note the elongated oral vestibule.

into filariform larvae. By penetrating the intestinal mucosa or perianal skin, the filariform larvae may enter the circulatory system and continue their parasitic lives without ever leaving the host. Such a cycle is not uncommon and accounts for some World War II veterans having harbored infections for more than 50 years, as well as for the development of increasingly heavy, even lethal, infections.

Epidemiology

Humans usually contract infection through contact with infective larvae in the soil; less frequently, larvae are ingested in contaminated water. It has been estimated that human cases of strongyloidiasis currently number 100–200 million worldwide. Estimated cases number 21 million in Asia, 8.6 million in Africa, 4 million in tropical America, 900,000 in the former USSR, 400,000 in North America, and 100,000 in the Pacific islands. The free-living forms thrive best in warm, moist climates where sanitation is substandard or lacking. There is a high incidence of infection among residents of mental institutions, due to the prevalence in feces of infective larvae or larvae capable of rapidly becoming infective combined with poor sanitation and/or personal hygiene. A study of 1437 mental patients in New York City institutions revealed an 18% rate of infection. Because dogs and cats also serve as sources of human infection, the disease can be considered zoonotic.

A second species causing human strongyloidiasis, *Strongyloides fuelleborni*, has been described from Papua-New Guinea and sub-Saharan Africa. This species has a predilection for young children under four years of age, in whom it often causes a fatal condition known as **swollen belly syndrome** (**SBS**). The source of the infective larva is believed to be mothers' milk.

Symptomatology and Diagnosis

Symptoms of human strongyloidiasis appear in three phases: cutaneous, pulmonary, and intestinal. The cutaneous phase is characterized by slight hemorrhaging, swelling, and intense itching (**ground itch**) at sites that have been invaded by infective filariform larvae. Occasionally, the invasion sites are secondarily invaded by infectious microbes, resulting in severe inflammation.

Larval migration through the lungs produces the pulmonary phase. Lung damage due to massive cellular reactions to the migrating larvae may delay or prevent further migration. When this happens, the larvae may develop in the lungs and commence reproducing as they would in the intestine, in which case the patient develops burning sensations in the chest, a cough, and other symptoms of bronchial pneumonia.

Intestinal symptoms appear when female worms become embedded in the mucosa and, rarely, beyond the muscularis. Moderate to heavy infections produce pain and intense burning in the abdominal region, accompanied by nausea, vomiting, and intermittent diarrhea. Long-standing infections result in chronic dysentery and weight loss. Very heavy infections may be fatal, attributable in most instances to massive invasion of tissues by filariform larvae, to secondary bacterial infections from ulceration of intestinal mucosa, or to immunosuppression (as in AIDS patients).

The surest means of diagnosis is microscopical identification of rhabditiform and sometimes filariform larvae in feces. However, children infected with *S. fuelleborni* shed eggs in their feces. Accurate diagnosis requires that larvae of *S. stercoralis* be distinguished from those of hookworms, which they resemble (Fig. 16-9). Occasionally, eggs of *S. stercoralis* are passed in the feces, in which case these eggs, as well as those of *S. fuelleborni*, also must be distinguished from hookworm eggs (see Fig. 15-13). The same is true when duodenal fluid is aspirated for examination. Sputum should also be examined for larvae.

Serological tests have proven useful. ELISA, which produces few cross-reactions, has been used successfully.

Treatment

Oral administration of 400 mg of albendazole daily for 3 consecutive days is the therapy of choice. In trials, a single oral dose of Ivermectin (200 mg/kg) has proven very successful, with a cure rate exceeding 90%. Relapses of the intestinal phase have been reported, especially in patients who are immunologically compromised (irradiated cancer patients, tissue transplant patients, AIDS patients, etc.).

Prevention

Prevention requires the sanitary disposal of human excrement, protection of skin from contact with contaminated soil, and appropriate treatment in cases of autoinfection. Screening for *S. fuelleborni* in pregnant women and for *S. stercoralis* in patients who are candidates for immunosuppressive therapy should be followed by treatment where infection is present.

NECATOR AMERICANUS AND *ANCYLOSTOMA DUODENALE*

Hookworm disease has been and remains among the most prevalent and important of human parasitic diseases. Unlike malaria, amoebiasis, and schistosomiasis, hookworm disease may not be clinically spectacular; yet, it can profoundly affect entire populations by gradually sapping the victims' strength, vitality, and overall well-being. As commonly seen in parts of the Middle East and Far East, and until several decades ago, in the Southeastern United States, victims become lethargic and nonproductive, resulting in economic losses beyond calculation. Al-

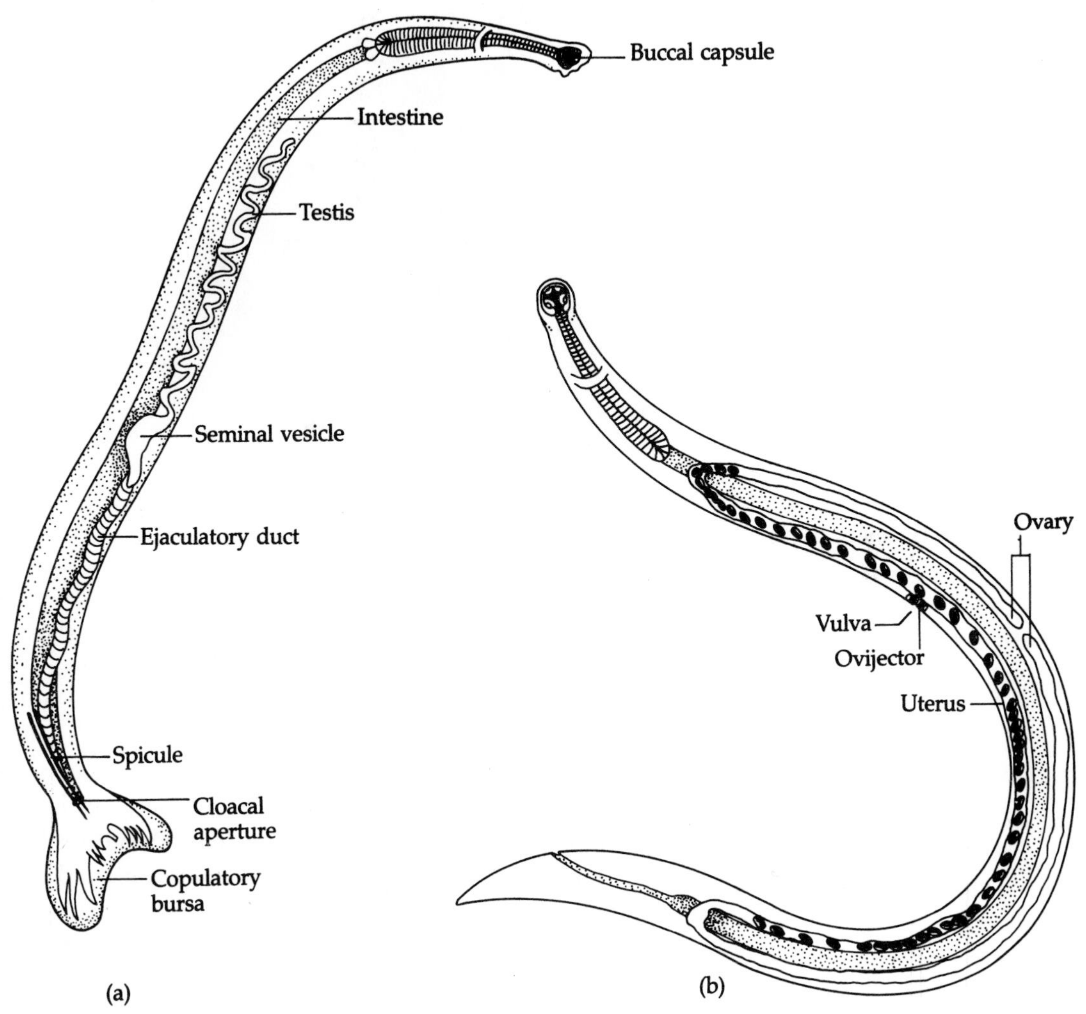

FIGURE 16-10
Morphology of adult hookworms.
(a) Male. (b) Female.

though great progress has been made in combating this scourge, hookworm disease has by no means been controlled or eradicated. It remains a major public health problem in many parts of the world, especially in developing countries.

Adults of two species of hookworms, *Ancylostoma duodenale* and *Necator americanus*, cause infection among humans. Because these worms are similar in morphology and life cycle, they will be described together, with notations on dissimilarities (Fig. 16-10).

Ancylostoma duodenale is considered the more pathogenic of

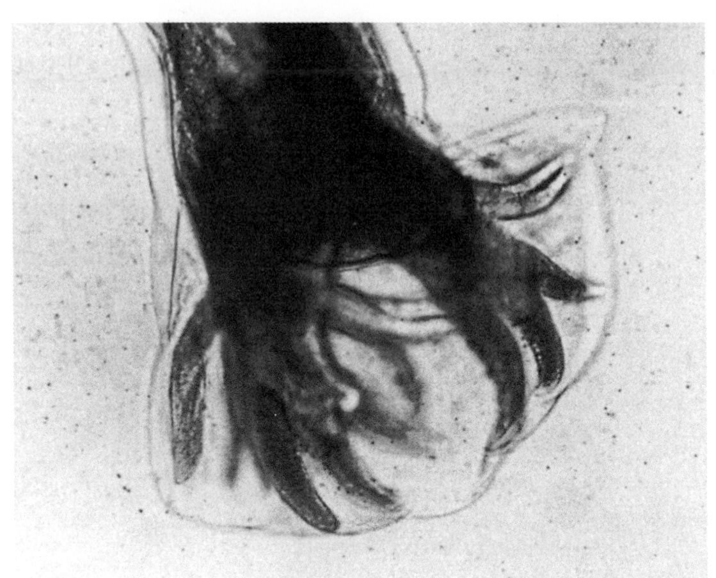

FIGURE 16-11
Copulatory bursa of male hookworm.

the two species, and its adults are somewhat larger than those of *N. americanus*. Female adults measure about 9–13 mm in length, while males are 5–11 mm long. The female reproductive system is didelphic; males have a single testis. The posterior end of the male has an umbrella-shaped bursa, with riblike rays, that expands over and envelops the vulva of the female to anchor the male during copulation (Fig. 16-11). The female's vulva is located in the anterior half of the body in *N. americanus* and in the posterior half in *A. duodenale*. There are chitinous specializations in the buccal capsules of both species (Fig. 16-12). *N. americanus*

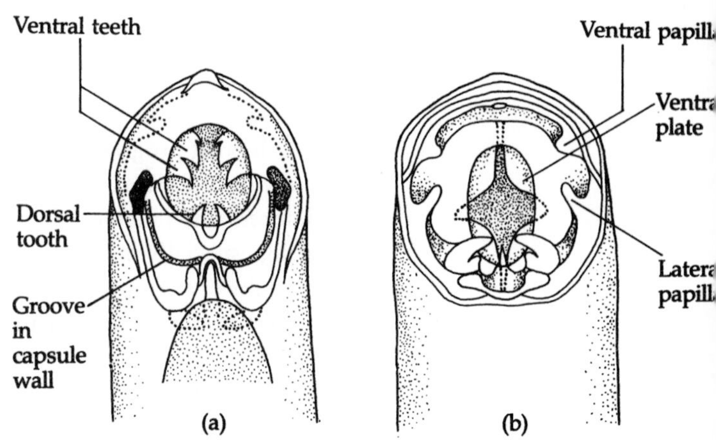

FIGURE 16-12
Hookworm buccal capsules.
(a) *Ancylostoma*. (b) *Necator*.

has a conspicuous pair of semilunar cutting plates on the dorsal wall, a concave tooth on the dorsal medial wall, and a pair of triangular lancets deeper on the ventral wall of the buccal capsule. *Ancylostoma duodenale*, in contrast, has two pairs of teeth on the ventral wall of its buccal capsule.

Eggs of the two species are nearly indistinguishable, except that those of *N. americanus* are slightly larger, measuring 64–76 μm by 36–40 μm. Eggs of both species have thin, transparent shells and bluntly rounded ends and upon oviposition enclose uncleaved embryos.

Life Cycle

Humans almost exclusively are hosts for *A. duodenale*, while dogs also are common hosts for *N. americanus*. Eggs are expelled in feces (Fig. 16-13); under optimal conditions (temperature of 23–33°C, shade, and sandy soil rich in organic materials), a rhabditiform larva matures in 1–2 days and hatches from the thin-shelled egg. The newly emerged larva, about 275 μm long, feeds on bacteria and organic materials in the soil and doubles its size in 5 days. After two molts, the rhabditiform larva becomes a nonfeeding, infective, filariform larva. During the last molt, the cuticle is retained and encloses the larva as a sheath.

The active, ensheathed, filariform larvae inhabit the upper 10 cm of soil, usually remaining within 50 cm of the initial site of oviposition, where they can live up to 6 weeks. Human infection occurs when these larvae penetrate the skin, usually of the feet and legs. Entry is most often gained through hair follicles, pores, and skin abrasions. Upon penetration, the larvae enter the host's lymphatic system, migrate to the right side of the heart, and enter the lungs via the pulmonary artery. Rupturing from lung capillaries, they enter the alveoli and migrate up the respiratory tree, molting en route, and then are coughed up and swallowed. The migratory period lasts about one week. At the third molt, each larva develops a temporary buccal capsule enabling it to develop into a feeding worm. Once the larvae reach the small intestine, they actively burrow into the intervillous spaces where, at about the 13th day, they undergo their fourth molt. They become sexually mature adults 5–6 weeks postpenetration.

Ancylostoma duodenale infection can also be acquired orally by humans and in some endemic regions this is the primary means of transmission. Following ingestion, the filariform larva is swal-

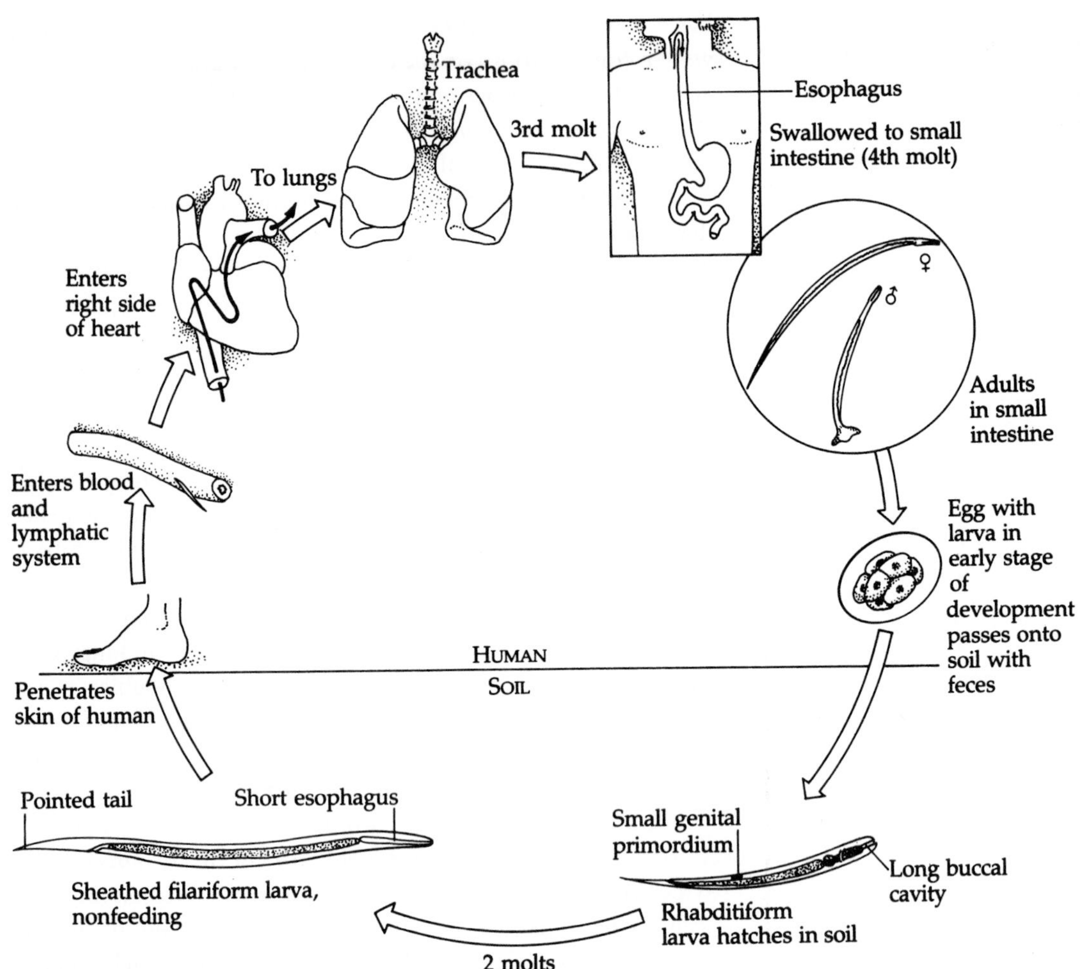

FIGURE 16-13
Life cycle of hookworm.

lowed and develops to sexual maturity in the small intestine, molting twice en route.

Epidemiology

An estimated 72.5 million humans harbor *A. duodenale*, the majority (59 million) in Asia. Some 384.3 million are infected with *N. americanus* worldwide, of which one million live in the United States.

Ancylostoma duodenale, commonly known as the Old World

hookworm, occurs in southern Europe, North Africa, India, China, Japan, and Southeast Asia. It also has been reported in the New World among Paraguayan Indians, in isolated areas of the United States, and in the Caribbean. Among coal miners in Belgium and Great Britain, the infection produces a classic form of anemia. Infected tunnel construction workers in Switzerland, Germany, and Italy are similarly affected.

Necator americanus, the New World or American hookworm, is found in the southern United States, Central and South America, and the Caribbean. This species is also indigenous to Africa, India, Southeast Asia, China, and the southwestern Pacific islands. It is believed to have been introduced into the Americas during the slave trade era or even earlier.

Four essential factors in the spread of hookworm infection are (1) shaded, sandy or loamy soil; (2) rainfall of 75–125 cm during the warm months of the year, providing sufficient moisture to assure development of eggs and larvae; (3) contamination of the soil by egg-containing feces, introduced as a result of poor sanitation and/or the use of human excrement for fertilizer; and (4) a human population that, by choice or necessity, comes in contact with contaminated soil.

Symptomatology and Diagnosis

The course of human hookworm disease can be divided into three phases: invasion, migration, and establishment in the intestine.

Invasion commences when infective larvae penetrate human skin. Although little damage is inflicted upon superficial skin layers, host cellular reactions stimulated during blood vessel penetration may isolate and kill the larvae. Local irritation from invading larvae, combined with inflammatory reaction to accompanying bacteria, evokes the urticarial condition commonly known as **ground itch**.

The migration phase is the period during which larvae escape from capillary beds in the lungs, enter the alveoli, and progress up the bronchi to the throat. This migration can produce severe hemorrhaging when large numbers of worms are involved; otherwise, a dry cough and sore throat may be the only symptoms. In areas where reinfection is continual, some filariform larvae of *A. duodenale* may invade host skeletal musculature following penetration. They remain dormant in the muscles, resuming development at a later time. While there has been no explanation for this phenomenon, it is known that dormancy can be caused by pregnancy, with development resuming at the onset of parturition. These larvae subsequently may appear in breast milk, which then becomes a vehicle for transmission to breast-feeding infants.

The most serious stage of hookworm infection arises when the parasites become established in the host's intestine. Upon reaching the small intestine, young worms use their buccal capsule and "teeth" (Fig. 16-14) to burrow through the mucosa, where they vigorously begin feeding upon blood. Salivary secretions of the worms contain anticoagulants that facilitate blood-feeding. Blood loss caused by *A. duodenale* adults is estimated to be ten times that caused by a comparable number of *N. americanus* adults. An iron-deficiency anemia develops when more than 75 *N. americanus* or 10 *A. duodenale* are present, even if 40% of the iron removed by the worms is reabsorbed by the host. The anemia is accompanied by intermittent abdominal pain, loss of appetite, and a craving to eat soil (geophagy). Heavy infections often produce severe anemia, protein deficiency, dry skin and hair, edema, a distended abdomen (especially in children), stunted growth, delayed puberty, mental dullness, cardiac failure, and even death.

Diagnosis based on clinical symptoms can be misleading, because the same symptoms may result from nutritional deficiencies

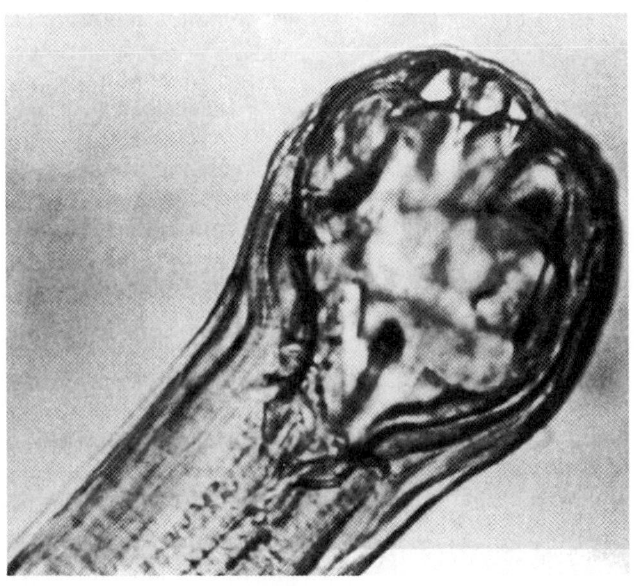

FIGURE 16-14
Light micrograph of hookworm buccal capsule.

or from a combination of infection and such deficiencies. Positive diagnosis requires identification of eggs in the feces. For light infections, concentration-type diagnostic techniques, such as zinc sulfate flotation or several modifications of the formalin–ether method, are employed.

Meticulous care in the identification of larvae is essential, especially from stools that are several days old, since the rhabditiform larvae of hookworms strongly resemble those of *Strongyloides* (Fig. 16-9) and even those of ruminant parasites such as *Trichostrongylus*, which occasionally infect humans.

Treatment

Several drugs provide effective treatment for both human hookworm species. Oral administration of mebendazole or albendazole for three consecutive days results in a very high rate of cure. Because of possible side effects, the benzimidazoles are usually contraindicated for treatment of children. Pyrantel pamoate is prescribed as an alternative drug for infantile hookworm infection. The dormant state of *A. duodenale* is not treated; treatment is deferred until the larvae leave the musculature and become established in the intestine. When severe anemia has developed due to hookworm infection, the anemia should be treated first. Although oral administration of iron prior to treatment for hookworm quickly restores hemoglobin levels, reversing the course of treatment delays for months the restoration of hemoglobin to normal levels.

Prevention

Obvious precautions to prevent the spread of hookworm infection include sanitary disposal of human excrement, treatment of infected individuals, protective measures to prevent contact with infective larvae, and correction of nutritional deficiencies to reduce susceptibility. Proper disposal of dog feces is important in programs to control *N. americanus*. Finally, education is always an important aspect of any control program.

CUTANEOUS LARVAL MIGRANS

Just as animal schistosome larvae may attack humans, filariform hookworm larvae of animals, for which humans are in-

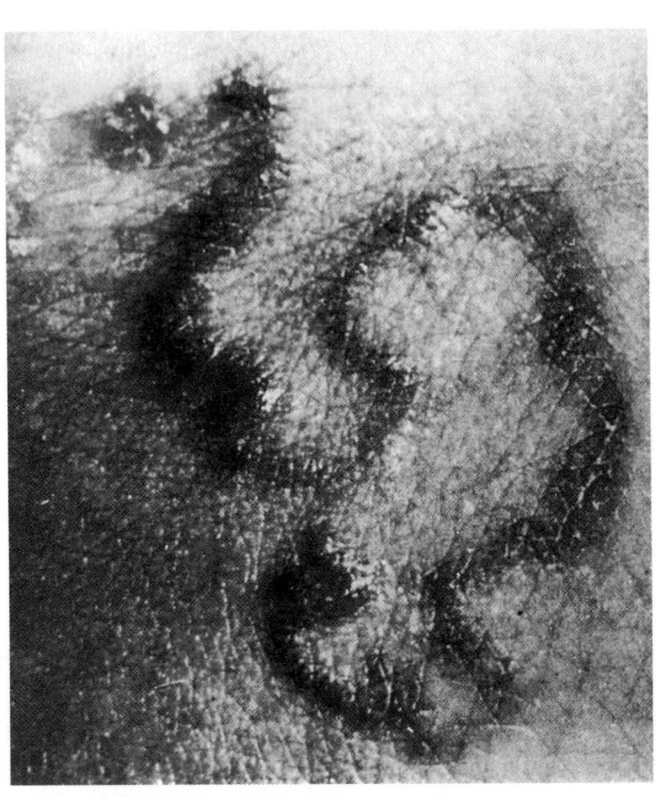

FIGURE 16-15
Cutaneous larval migrans.

compatible hosts, often penetrate human skin. Such larvae normally fail to pass beyond the stratum germinativum. Instead, they persist and migrate for some time at that level, causing a skin condition that resembles schistosome dermatitis but is called **cutaneous larval migrans**, or **creeping eruption** (Fig. 16-15). The most common agents of this condition are the dog and cat hookworms, *Ancylostoma braziliense* and *A. caninum*.

Epidemiology

Cutaneous larval migrans is prevalent in many parts of the world, particularly in tropical and subtropical regions. In the United States, the incidence is high along the Gulf Coast and in the southern Atlantic states. Humans become infected with animal hookworms by contact with soil upon which infected cats and dogs have defecated. A frequent source is children's sandboxes, which afford optimum conditions of shade, sandy soil, and warmth during summer days. Infective larvae also thrive in the soil under houses. It is not surprising, therefore, that infection rates are highest among children, plumbers, and electricians.

Symptomatology and Diagnosis

The feet, arms, and face are the most common sites of infection; however, any part of the body that comes in contact with contaminated soil is susceptible. Red, itchy papules develop at the invasion site, and the migratory paths of the larvae appear as slightly elevated ridges. These ridges represent an inflammatory response to the burrowing larvae as they make cutaneous tunnels. This tunneling, probably an attempt by the larvae to find a point of entry into the circulatory system, produces intense itching along the migratory pathways. The larval infection may persist for weeks or even months, and secondary bacterial infection is common.

Treatment

Treatment generally targets alleviation of symptoms, such as the itching, rather than destroying the larvae. A topical ointment consisting of a 10% suspension of thiabendazole has proven effective, and light infections often respond to chilling of the active portion of the lesion with ethyl chloride. The latter treatment must be administered with extreme caution, as prolonged exposure to ethyl chloride can produce second-degree burns. Any accompanying microbial infection should be treated with antibiotics and/or fungicides.

Prevention

Obviously, prevention of cutaneous larval migrans caused by hookworms depends upon avoiding contact of bare skin with soil contaminated by feces from infected cats and dogs. Toward that end, animals should be denied access to underhouse crawl spaces, sandboxes should be kept covered when not in use, and pets should be treated with appropriate anthelmintics. In addition, service personnel should always keep their extremities covered when working in areas that are suspect.

ASCARIS LUMBRICOIDES

In *Ascaris lumbricoides*, known as the large intestinal roundworm of humans, females may attain a length of 40 cm while male worms may reach 30 cm (Fig. 16-16). In both sexes, the mouth is surrounded by one dorsal and two ventrolateral lips.

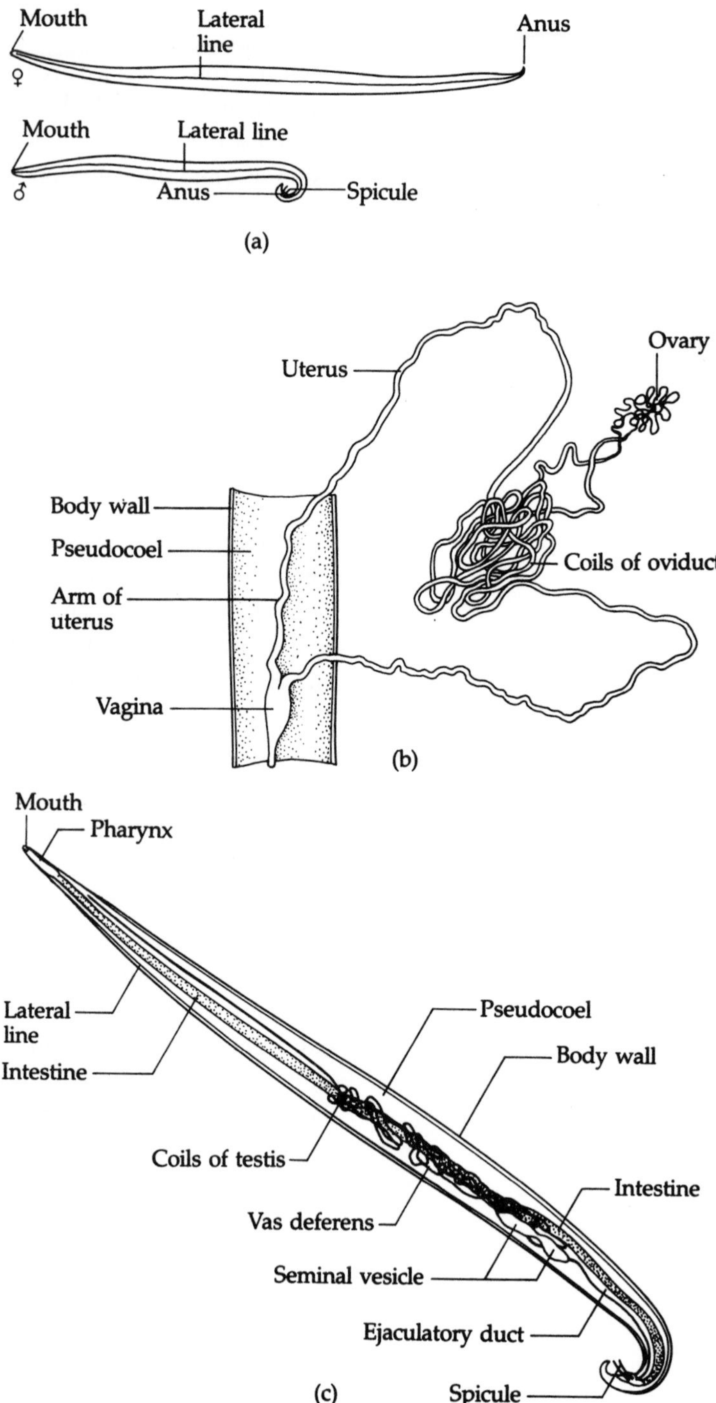

FIGURE 16-16
Ascaris lumbricoides.
(a) Male and female adults. (b) Female reproductive system teased out of body. (c) Cut-away view of adult male.

The posterior end of the female is straight while that of the male curves ventrally. The didelphic female reproductive system is located in the posterior two-thirds of the body, with the vulva about one-third of the body length from the anterior end. The female is a prodigious egg producer, depositing about 200,000 eggs daily; the uterus may contain up to 27 million eggs at a time. The fertilized egg measures 45–75 μm by 35–50 μm.

Life Cycle

Adult worms inhabit the lumen of the small intestine and draw nourishment from the semidigested food of the host (Fig. 16-17). Copulation occurs at this site, and eggs are passed with host feces. The outer, albuminous coat of the fertilized egg is golden brown due to bile pigment adsorbed from feces (see Fig. 15-13c). Among the oval, fertilized eggs are found numerous unfertilized eggs, identifiable by their elongated shape and the absence of the albuminous coat. When fertilized eggs are deposited, the zygote is uncleaved, and it remains in this state until the eggs reach soil. Eggs deposited in soil are resistant to desiccation but are very sensitive to environmental temperatures at this stage of development. The zygote within the eggshell develops at a soil temperature of about 25°C. Development ceases at temperatures below 15.5°C, and eggs cannot survive at temperatures more than slightly above 38°C.

After 2–4 weeks in moist soil at optimal temperatures and oxygen levels, the embryo molts at least once in the shell and develops to an infective second-stage larva. Eggs containing infective larvae may remain viable in the soil for two years or longer.

After being ingested by a human, eggs containing infective larvae hatch in the duodenum. The larvae actively burrow into the mucosal lining, enter the circulatory system, and are carried via the portal circulation to the liver, through the right side of the heart, and to the lungs by the pulmonary artery. This migration requires approximately one week. The larvae remain in the lungs for several days, molting twice, and eventually rupture from the pulmonary capillaries to enter the alveoli. From there, they move up the respiratory tree and trachea to the epiglottis to be coughed up, swallowed, and passed again to the small intestine. During this complex migratory process, individual worms grow from 200–300 μm in length to approximately ten times that length. A fourth molt in the small intestine is essential to the worms' sur-

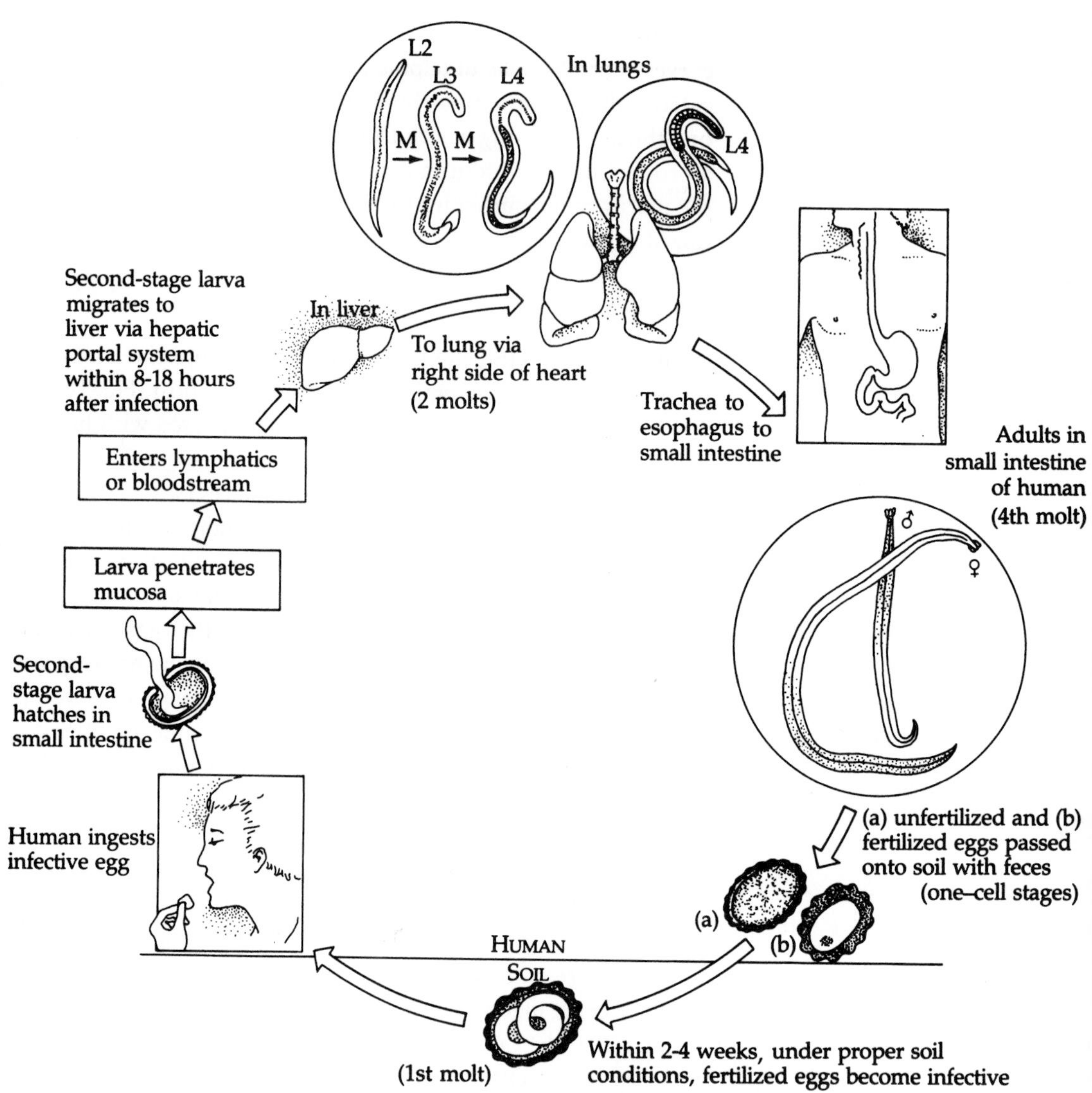

FIGURE 16-17
Life cycle of *Ascaris lumbricoides*.

vival, and only those worms that undergo this final molt develop to sexual maturity. The interval from the ingestion of infective eggs to the appearance of sexually mature worms in the small intestine is about 3 months.

Epidemiology

Distribution of *A. lumbricoides* is worldwide, but it is most prevalent in warmer climates. Dependent upon poor sanitation for its spread, human ascariasis has been described as a household and backyard infection. An estimated 1 billion people are infected, making it the most common nematode parasitizing humans. It is most prevalent in children, particularly those 5–9 years old, the group most frequently exposed to contaminated soil and least likely to observe basic sanitary practices, such as washing hands before eating and keeping hands out of the mouth. Hand-to-mouth transmission is most common; however, in countries where human excrement is used as fertilizer, contaminated vegetables are also a common source of infection. Water is rarely implicated in the transmission of *A. lumbricoides*.

Since ascariasis is more prevalent in humid climates than arid ones, its occurrence is often patchy within individual countries. For instance, prevalence ranges from 0.9% to 98.2% in Nigeria and from 0% to 76% in Ghanian villages. Generally, prevalence is highest in Africa and Asia, with 40% of the population infected. Latin America follows with 32%.

Symptomatology and Diagnosis

About 85% of ascariasis cases are symptomless; in the remaining cases, the most frequent symptom is upper abdominal discomfort of varying intensity. Symptoms such as asthma, insomnia, eye pain, and rashes represent allergic responses of the host to metabolic excretions and secretions of adult worms, as well as to dead and dying worms. Little damage results from larval penetration of the host's intestinal mucosa. However, aberrant larvae migrating to organs such as the spleen, liver, lymph nodes, and brain usually elicit an inflammatory response. Also, larvae escaping from capillaries in the lungs and entering the respiratory tree cause small, hemorrhagic foci accompanied by coughing, fever, and difficulty in breathing. Larvae in large numbers can produce numerous small blood clots, which can lead to potentially fatal pneumonitis if large areas of the lungs are affected.

Large numbers of adult worms sometimes cause mechanical blockage of the intestine and adult worms penetrating the intestinal wall or appendix may cause local hemorrhage, peritonitis, and/or appendicitis. Adult female worms may even wander up the bile duct to the liver, causing abscesses, or along the pancreatic duct, causing fatal, hemorrhagic pancreatitis. Loss of appetite and insufficient absorption of digested food also occur as a result of heavy infections. Migration of worms is sometimes abetted by high fever, chemotherapy, and administration of anesthesia.

Diagnosis is made by identification of eggs in feces (see Fig. 15-13). Because egg production per female is fairly constant, egg counts can provide reasonably accurate estimates of the number of adult worms present, provided uniform samples are used.

Treatment

For treatment of individuals in whom adult worms have been verified in the intestine but who do not require hospitalization, a single dose of pyrantel pamoate is highly effective. Mebendazole, administered over a period of 3 days, is an acceptable alternative. Piperazine citrate is highly effective in cases of intestinal obstruction. The drug paralyzes the worm, eliminating its ability to counter host intestinal peristalsis, and causes it to be passed. If the obstruction persists, surgery may be necessary.

Prevention

The most reliable preventive measure is a multipronged attack emphasizing scrupulous personal hygiene, public sanitation, health education, and environmental sanitation, especially the processing of night soil. For optimal effectiveness, such a program should be combined with treatment of the population with broad-spectrum anthelmintics two or three times annually.

VISCERAL LARVAL MIGRANS

Visceral larval migrans usually results from migration of second-stage larvae of ascaroids, the adults of which normally are found in dogs and cats, within the internal organs of accidental hosts, primarily young children. Most commonly, human visceral larval migrans develops following accidental ingestion of infective eggs of *Toxocara canis*, although several other nematode species, such as *Bayliascaris procyonis*, *Angiostrongylus cantonensis*, *A. costaricensis*, *Gnathostoma spinigerum*, and *T. cati*, can also cause the condition. Following such accidental ingestion of eggs by humans, second-stage larvae hatch, penetrate the intestinal wall, and quickly invade the liver. Although the majority of these larvae remain in the liver, some travel to the lungs and, occasionally, the central nervous system and eyes. For a period of at least several weeks, they actively migrate through tissues, leaving long trails of inflammatory and granulomatous reactive cells. Most of the larvae eventually gravitate to a single location and become encapsulated by host tissues.

While hookworms of normally nonhuman hosts are the usual suspects in cases of cutaneous larval migrans and *T. canis* is most often implicated in visceral larval migrans in humans, the location of lesions and even the presence of characteristic symptoms are not invariably reliable criteria for specific identification of the etiologic agent.

Epidemiology

As symptoms of visceral larval migrans are imprecise and inconsistent and as dog parasites were long considered noninjurious to humans, confirmed cases of this disease have been rare. However, available reports indicate that the disease occurs worldwide and probably involves several nematode species. In the United States, a high percentage of puppies and kittens are infected with *Toxocara*, perhaps as many as 98% according to some reports. The life cycle of *T. canis* appears to be completed only in puppies. In adult dogs, the second-stage larva encysts in various tissues. In pregnant bitches, these larvae can become active and migrate across the placenta, infecting the fetal pup where the life cycle is completed. The close association of young children with their pets has been cited frequently as a factor in the transmission of parasitic disease; hence, it is not surprising that this segment of the population is the most vulnerable to this disease. The ubiquitous sandbox provides an ideal medium for the survival of eggs, as do park areas and beaches where owners walk their dogs.

Angiostrongylus cantonensis infects humans in Southeast Asia, Hawaii, the Pacific Islands (Tahiti, Samoa, Cook Islands), the Philippines, Taiwan, parts of China, the Caribbean, and Madagascar; *A. costaricensis* infections are prevalent in Central and South America, notably Costa Rica, where approximately 300 cases are reported annually. The normal definitive hosts for both species are wild rats. Humans contract the disease by ingesting third-stage larvae in insufficiently cooked intermediate hosts: mollusks and crustaceans for *A. cantonensis*; the slug, *Vaginulus plebius*, for *A. costaricensis*.

Symptomatology and Diagnosis

In visceral larval migrans attributable to *Toxocara*, the degree of pathology is related to the number of infective eggs ingested and the site at which the larvae settle. Most infections are light, with symptoms including fever, pulmonary congestion, and eosinophilia. Characteristic lesions most often occur in the liver and are accompanied by concentrations of various leukocytes, especially eosinophils. The lesion is a protective response of the host, but it also protects the larva, as it isolates the parasite from further contact with host defense mechanisms.

In heavy infections, some children develop anemia from the excessive leukocyte buildup. Ocular disease may develop when larvae become entrapped in the eye. The severest consequences of infection are usually allergic reactions, especially if the patient is hypersensitive to metabolites produced by the larval nematodes. In rare instances, fatalities due to toxicariasis have been reported.

Diagnosis is complicated by the lack of a specific body of symptoms. Eosinophilia and hepatomegaly occurring in conjunction with a history of proximity to pets are clinically significant. While the only positive diagnosis is identification of the larvae, this is exceedingly difficult, as there are usually too few of them to be retrieved by needle biopsy. An effective ELISA test is currently being used to detect antibodies against the excretory–secretory antigens of *Toxocara* larvae.

Third-stage larvae of *A. cantonensis* usually migrate to the capillaries of the meninges in human patients, causing a type of eosinophilic meningoencephalitis in humans. The condition is characterized by severe headache, fever, and some central nervous system involvement. Although the disease is normally self-limiting after approximately 3 weeks, there have been instances of fatalities in humans. The larvae of *A. costaricensis*, on the other hand, lodge in mesenteric venules, causing thromboses and infarcts that lead to ulceration and even peritonitis. Most damage occurs in the large intestine, where eosinophilic granulomas sometimes mimic appendicitis symptoms.

Treatment

Most toxocariasis infections are self-limiting, and only severe cases warrant treatment. Diethylcarbamazine administered for 20 days, augmented with corticosteroids when allergic symptoms are also present, is the drug of choice. There is no reliable documentation of beneficial effects from treatment of *Angystrongylus* infections; thiabendazole and mebendazole are used merely to shorten the duration of symptoms.

Prevention

Generally, the best protection for children from exposure to *Toxocara* is routine treatment of pets for worms. Puppies and kittens should be treated every 6 months and adult pets every 2 months. Sandboxes should be covered when not in use. Education in the proper cooking of crustaceans, mollusks, and other organisms that serve as intermediate and paratenic hosts for *Angiostrongylus* is perhaps the most effective means of limiting human infection.

ANISAKIS

Anisakid nematodes include a number of ascaroid species that normally infect the stomach and intestines of various marine fishes, birds, and fish-eating mammals such as dolphins, whales, seals, and porpoises. Third-stage larvae, usually measuring about 2–3 cm by 0.5–1.0 mm, are found in the body cavities, liver, and/or musculature of a number of marine fishes that serve as intermediate or paratenic hosts in the life cycle of the worms.

Anisakis and certain other anisakid nematodes, especially *Pseudoterranova* and *Phocanema*, represent a public health concern in many parts of the United States among people who eat raw or inadequately cooked fish harboring infective larvae in their flesh. These parasites also pose a major problem in Japan and parts of Scandinavia and, at one time, did so in the Netherlands as well. Human anisakiasis has essentially disappeared from the Netherlands, due to recent laws regulating fish processing that prohibit fish being held on boats without immediate refrigeration. At ambient temperature, anisakid larvae migrate from the intestinal tract of fishes into the flesh, where they present a greater threat of being ingested by humans.

When swallowed by a human, larvae burrow into the stomach or intestinal walls and cause inflammatory responses ranging from localized granulomata to massive, eosinophilic, hemorrhagic, tumorlike growths (neoplasms with larvae at the center; Fig. 16-18). Consequent swelling of the intestinal wall may cause

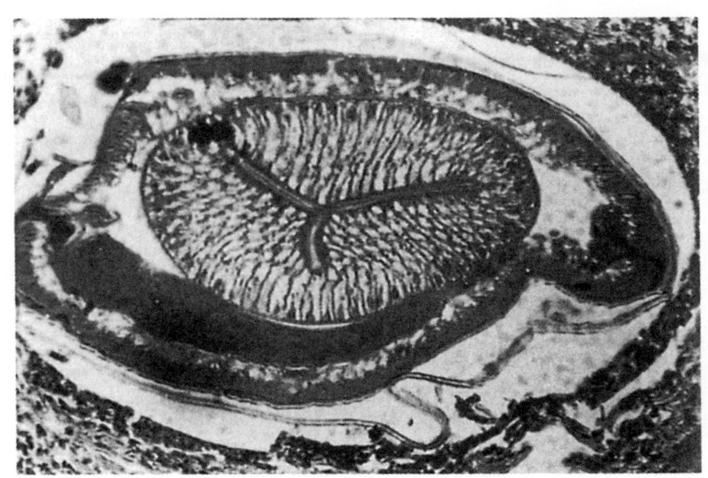

FIGURE 16-18
Light micrograph of a section through the esophagus of an *Anisakis* larva in the human intestine.

intestinal obstruction, peritonitis, and the development of abscesses. Most cases have been reported from countries where fish, such as herring in Scandinavia and sashimi in Japan, are eaten raw. With the growing popularity of sushi restaurants in the United States (especially in California and Hawaii), there has been a marked increase in anisakiasis, and a number of cases have been fatal. Definitive diagnosis is made by endoscopy or biopsy. The only treatment is surgical removal of the larva. Prevention consists of thorough cooking or proper freezing of fish.

ENTEROBIUS VERMICULARIS

This nematode, commonly known as pinworm or seatworm (Fig. 16-19), is parasitic only to humans. It is familiar to parents of young children worldwide. Female *Enterobius vermicularis*, measuring 8–13 mm by 0.4 mm, are characterized by the presence of winglike expansions (**alae**) of the body wall at the anterior end, distension of the body due to the large number of eggs in the uteri, and a pointed tail. Males are 2–5 mm long and possess a curved tail.

Life Cycle

Sexually mature worms usually inhabit the ileocaecal area of the human intestinal tract, but they can spread to adjacent regions of the small and large intestines (Fig. 16-20). Adhering to the mu-

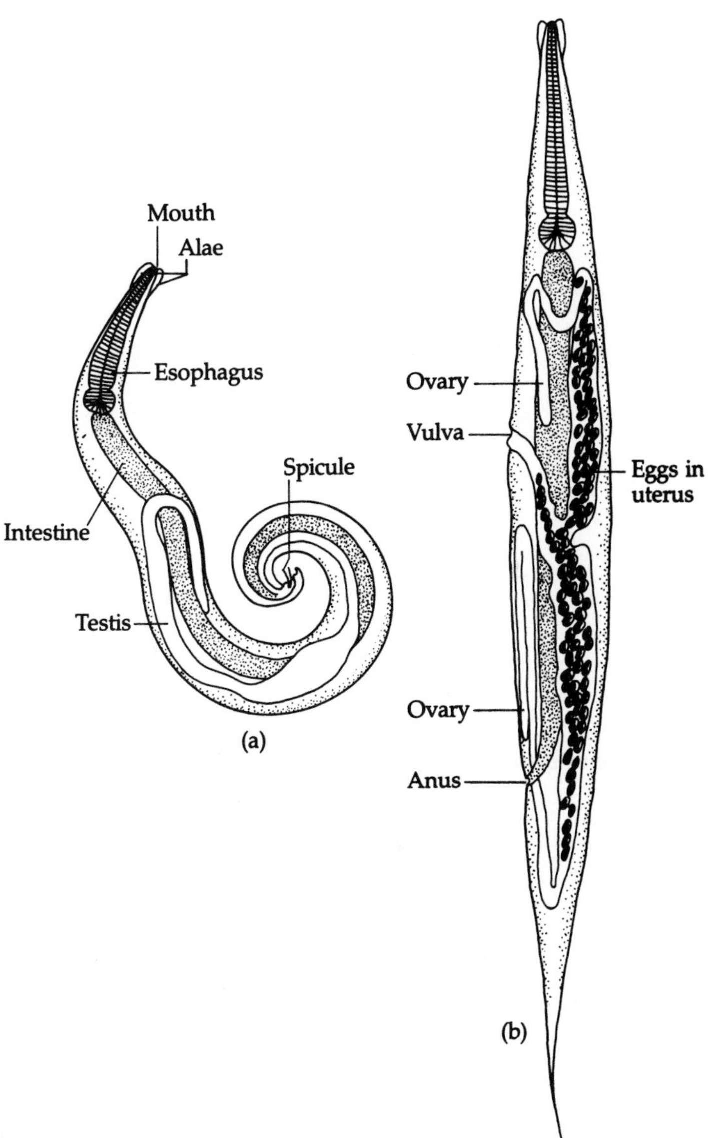

FIGURE 16-19
Morphology of adult *Enterobius vermicularis.*
(a) Male. (b) Female.

cosa, the worms feed on bacteria and epithelial cells. Males die following copulation, while egg-bearing females, with up to 15,000 eggs in their uteri, migrate to the perianal and perineal regions. There, stimulated by the lower temperature and aerobic environment, they deposit their eggs and then also die. More eggs are released when the female's body ruptures. The elongate eggs, each measuring approximately 50–60 μm by 20–30 μm, are

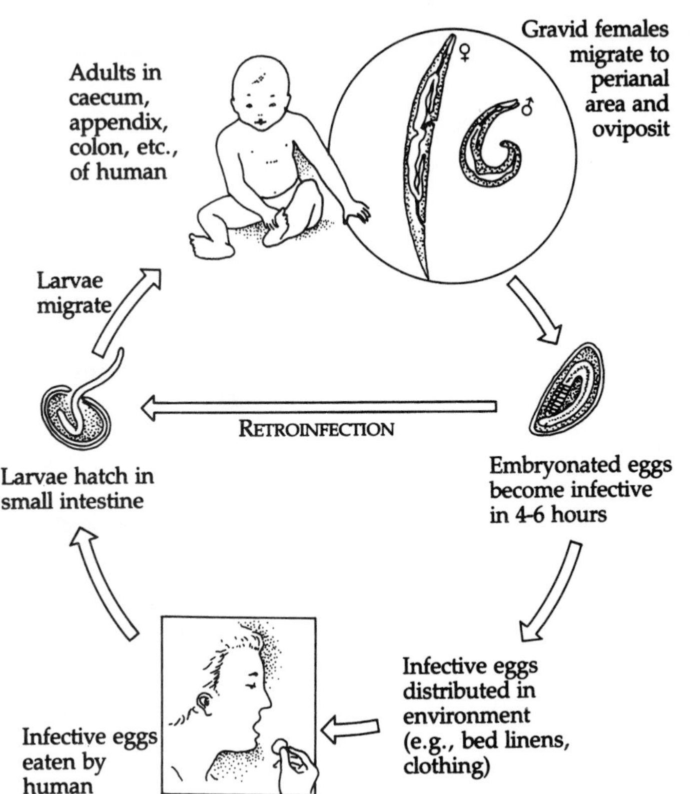

FIGURE 16-20
Life cycle of *Enterobius vermicularis.*

characteristically flattened on one side. Upon deposition, eac contains an immature larva. The infective, third-stage larva com pletes development within the egg several hours after leaving th body of the female worm. Infection and reinfection occur whe eggs containing the infective larvae are ingested by the host. Thi may happen when eggs are picked up on the hands from bed clothes or beneath fingernails contaminated when the hos scratches the perianal zone to relieve itching caused by nocturna migration of the female worms. However, the lightweight egg are sometimes airborne and, therefore, can also be inhalec Retroinfections occur when third-stage larvae hatch from per anally located eggs and enter the host's intestinal tract throug the anus.

Ingested eggs usually hatch shortly after reaching the duod num. The escaping larvae molt and develop as they migrate po teriorly, reaching sexually maturity by the time they arrive at the colon. The life cycle of *E. vermicularis* spans about 2 months. Although vulnerable to even moderately high temperatures, eggs are highly resistant to drying and remain viable for a week or more under cool, humid conditions. Some researchers claim that eggs can remain viable for years under favorable conditions.

Epidemiology

Children, especially of early school-age, are most vulnerable to *E. vermicularis* infection. The geographic distribution of the worm is global. Infections are especially prevalent in temperate zones, where an estimated 500 million persons are infected. However, prevalence varies with each locale. For instance, Alaskan Inuits display a 51% prevalence; elementary students in and around Tallahassee, Florida, 27%; preschoolers in San Francisco, 58%; Sicilian children, 77%; and children overall in the United States, 33%. *Enterobius vermicularis* is the most common nematode parasitizing humans in the United States.

Infections occur in one of four ways: (1) retroinfection, when hatched larvae migrate back into the large intestine; (2) self-infection, when the patient is reinfected by hand-to-mouth transmission; (3) cross-infection, when infective eggs are ingested, either with contaminated food or from fingers that have been in contact with a contaminated surface or body parts from infected humans; and (4) inhalation of airborne eggs. In households with heavily infected individuals, infective eggs have been found in samples of dust taken from chairs, tabletops, dresser tops, floors, baseboards, etc. In a survey to determine the distribution of airborne pollen in public places, pinworm eggs were found in theaters, not only on arm rests and baseboards but also on chandeliers high above the seats; most of these eggs, however, were no longer viable. Experiments show that at room temperature or above, fewer than 10% of such eggs survive more than 2 days, probably accounting for the less than universal infection in such public places.

Symptomatology and Diagnosis

Pinworms are not highly pathogenic. Clinical symptoms such as itching and irritation are caused by the migration of gravid females around the perianal, perineal, and vaginal areas. Heavy in-

fections in children may also produce such symptoms as slee
lessness, weight loss, hyperactivity, grinding of teeth, abdomin
pain, and vomiting. Gravid females may also migrate up the fe
male reproductive tract, become trapped in the tissues, and caus
granulomata in the uterus and fallopian tubes. They may also m
grate to the appendix, the peritoneal cavity, or even the urinar
bladder.

Diagnosis is verified when adult worms and/or eggs are d
tected. Female worms emerge at night and are frequently visib
in the perianal and perineal regions. Adult worms can often b
observed on feces as well; however, eggs are found in feces in onl
about 5% of cases. The most reliable procedure for finding egg
is to apply a strip of cellophane tape to the perianal skin, remov
the tape, and place it on a clean microscope slide for examina
tion. Negative results from this protocol for seven consecutiv
days constitute confirmation that the patient is free of infectio

Treatment

Following positive diagnosis in any individual, treatment shoul
be administered to all members of the household. Several rel
tively inexpensive and essentially nontoxic drugs are availabl
Pyrantel pamoate or mebendazole, usually administered in a sir
gle dose and repeated once after 2 weeks, is the treatment
choice. Mebendazole is contraindicated for pregnant women,
it is teratogenic in experimental animals.

Prevention

Complete eradication of pinworm infection from a population
highly unlikely. Scrupulous personal hygiene is the most effectiv
deterrent. Fingernails should be cut short, and hands should b
washed thoroughly after toilet use and before food is prepared
eaten. Because infection is most prevalent in urban areas whe
relatively large populations intermingle, education of parents h
proven most effective. Parents should be informed that it is a sel
limiting, nonfatal infection widespread among children and th
no social stigma should be attached to it. There is no evidenc
that dogs can transmit the infection. Infected children as well
other members of the household should be treated promptly. Be
clothes, towels, and washcloths from infected homes should b
carefully laundered in hot water and aired in sunlight.

SELECTED READINGS

Anderson, R. C. 1992. *Nematode Parasites of Vertebrates. Their Development and Transmission.* CAB International Publication, Oxford University Press, Oxford, England.

Bundy, D. A. P, and Cooper, E. S. 1989. *Trichuris* and trichuriasis in humans. *Advances in Parasitology* **28**, 108–173.

Cheng, T. C. 1998. Anisakiosis. In *Zoonoses.* (Palmer, S. R., Soulsby, E. J. L., and Simpson, D. I. H., Eds.), pp. 823–840. Oxford University Press, Oxford, England.

Crompton, D. W. T. 1988. The prevalence of ascariasis. *Parasitology Today* **4**, 162–169.

Grove, D. I. 1996. Human strongyloidiasis. *Advances in Parasitology* **38**, 252–309.

Miller, T. A. 1979. Hookworm infection in man. *Advances in Parasitology* **17**, 315–384.

Oshima, T. 1987. Anisakiasis—Is the sushi bar guilty? *Parasitology Today* **3**, 44–48.

SELECTED READINGS

Chapter Seventeen

BLOOD AND TISSUE NEMATODES

Seven nematodes of the superfamily Filaroidea are parasitic to humans. Generally referred to as filarial worms, these are *Wuchereria bancrofti*, *Brugia malayi*, *Onchocerca volvulus*, *Loa loa*, *Mansonella perstans*, *M. ozzardi*, and *M. streptocerca*. Because the life cycles of all seven are essentially similar, only significant variations will be noted in the discussion of each species.

One nematode of the superfamily Dracunculoidea, *Dracunculus medinensis*, is parasitic in the cutaneous tissues of humans. Its life cycle differs significantly from that of the filarial worms and is discussed separately (see p. 396).

LIFE CYCLE

The long, threadlike, adult filarial worms inhabit the lymphatic glands, tissues, and body cavities of the definitive host (Fig. 17-1). Females are ovoviviparous, the larvae hatching in the uterus. At the time of larviposition, the larvae, known as **microfilariae**, are less well developed than typical first-stage (L_1) larvae and are considered prelarvae or advanced embryos (see Figs. 15-15a–d). Once deposited by the female, microfilariae migrate into the blood vessels via the thoracic lymph duct or by penetrating the walls of the lymph vessels to invade neighboring small blood vessels. Blood-dwelling microfilariae are usually **sheathed**, retaining the flexible eggshell as a covering membrane. In tissue-dwelling species, however, the sheath is usually sloughed, and the larva is said to be **unsheathed**. Larvae can survive in blood for several years before ingestion by a suitable insect vector.

After being ingested with a blood meal by an insect vector, microfilariae develop in the digestive tract of the insect into L_1, rhabditiform larvae. The latter penetrate the midgut wall into the hemocoel and migrate to the thoracic musculature, where they undergo two molts and metamorphose within 3 weeks into in-

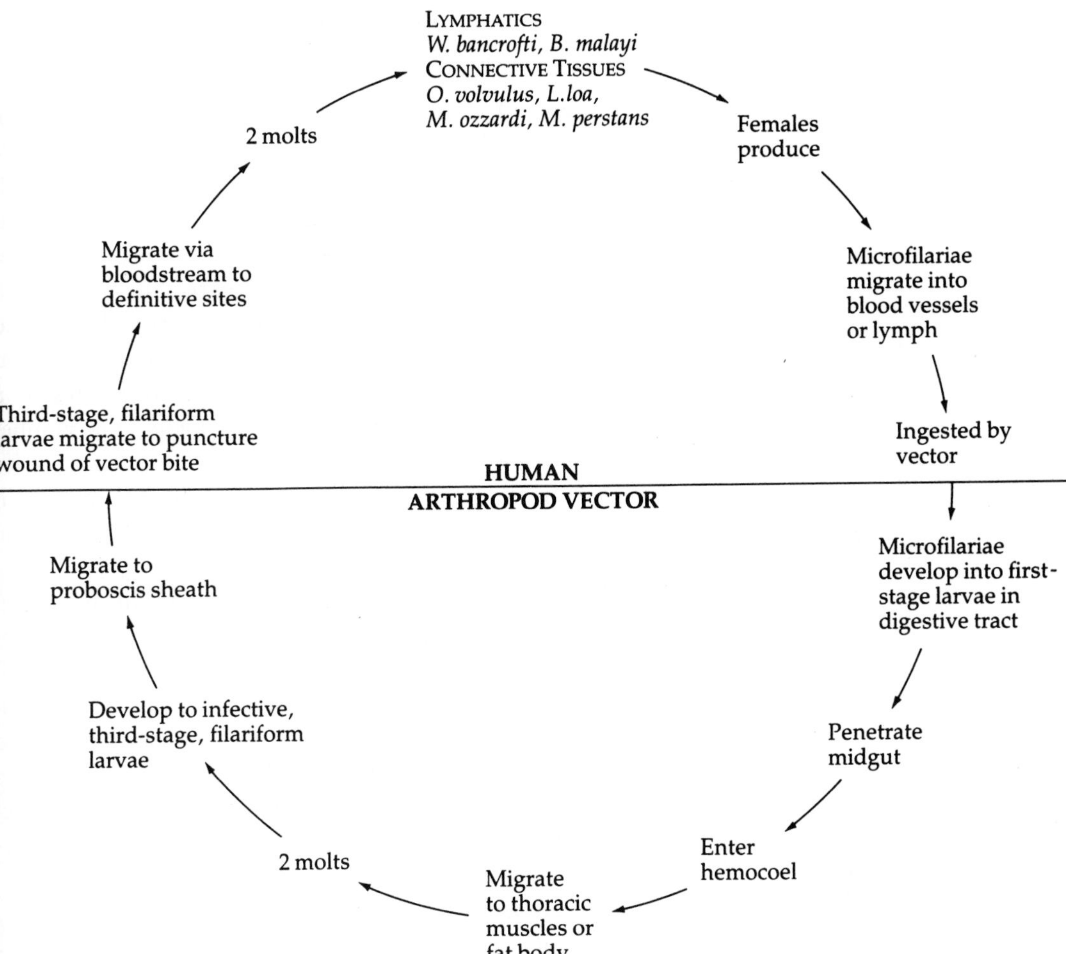

FIGURE 17-1
Generalized life cycle of filarial worms.

fective L_3, filariform larvae. These larvae then migrate to the proboscis sheath and gain access to the human circulatory system through the puncture wound made by the feeding insect. In the human host, larvae undergo two molts, metamorphosing into adult worms during migration to the definitive site of infection. Approximately 6 months later, microfilariae appear in the bloodstream.

PERIODICITY

While studying *W. bancrofti* infections among inhabitants of southern China in 1879, Patrick Manson noted a nocturnal surge in the microfilarial population in the peripheral circulation. It was later observed in a number of species of filarial worms that this periodicity varies with species (or strain) as well as with endemic area. For example, although microfilariae of *W. bancrofti* in the Caribbean, parts of North and South America, Africa, and Asia are nocturnal, those of the strain endemic to the South Pacific islands are **diurnally subperiodic**; that is, although present in the peripheral circulation at all times, they increase in number during the daytime. In the Philippines, on the other hand, twice as many larvae are present at night as during the day. When microfilariae vacate the peripheral circulation, they accumulate in the small vessels of the lungs and liver.

Microfilarial periodicity is of obvious survival value because it enhances the opportunity for microfilariae to be ingested by insect vectors at certain times. Not surprisingly, the surge of microfilariae coincides with the active feeding periods of the various insect vectors. For example, in the parasites discussed previously, the insect vector for the nocturnal *W. bancrofti* strain is the nocturnally feeding mosquito *Culex fatigans*, while the vector for the subperiodic strain is the diurnal feeder, *Aedes polynesiensis*.

Although numerous studies have been undertaken to identify the mechanism(s) responsible for microfilarial periodicity, the explanation for this phenomenon of helminth physiology remains elusive. It has been determined that this periodicity is not dependent on photoperiod or the circadian rhythm of the definitive host. For example, if the routine is altered so that the host sleeps by day and is active at night, the periodicity of microfilariae is reversed. The sleeping period of the host is characterized by physiological changes such as decreases in body temperature and oxygen tension, increases in carbon dioxide tension and body acidity, lower excretion of water and chloride by the kidneys, and lower adrenal activity. Some or all of these changes may trigger the rhythmic behavior of microfilariae. It should be emphasized, however, that different species and strains of microfilariae respond differently to similar stimuli.

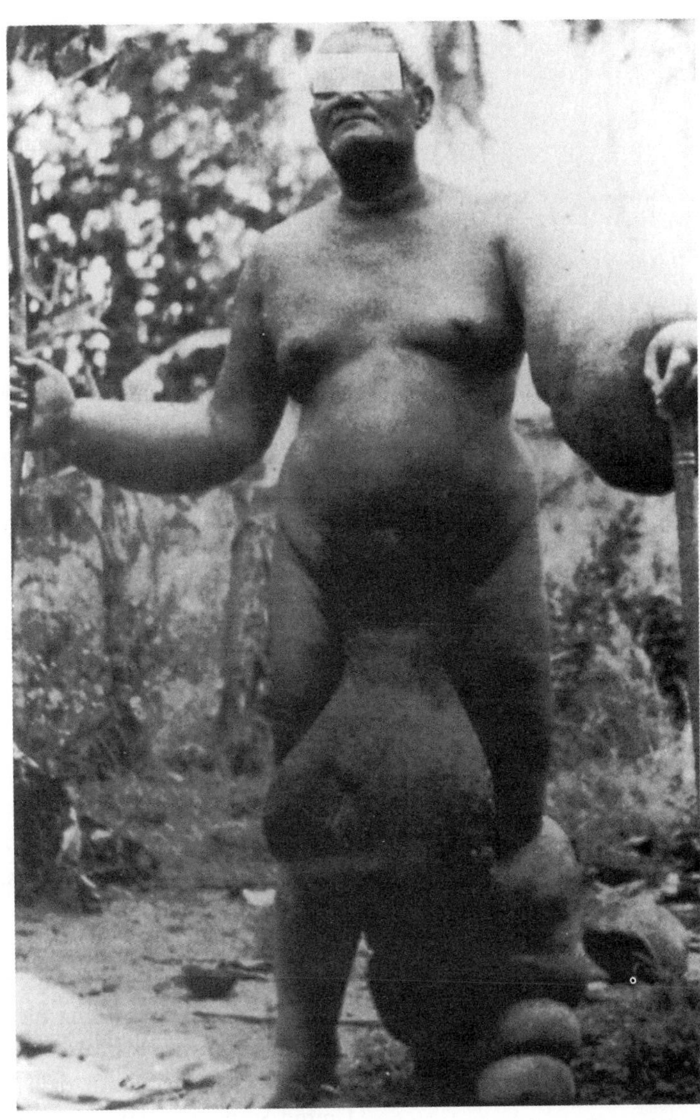

FIGURE 17-2
South Pacific native severely affected by Bancroft's filariasis.

FILARIAL WORMS

WUCHERERIA BANCROFTI

This filarial worm, parasitic only in humans, causes a lymphatic disease known as **Bancroft's filariasis**, which is characterized by extensive enlargement of extremities (Fig. 17-2). Ancients likened the thickened skin to that of elephants, giving rise to the misnomer **elephantiasis** (which literally means "caused by elephants" rather than "like elephants"). The adult female worm is 8–10 cm long, with the vulva situated anteriorly near the middle of the esophagus. Male worms are only 40 mm long and are further distinguishable by their curved posterior ends and genital spicule apparatus.

Life Cycle

Adults live intertwined with each other in the major lymphatic ducts (Fig. 17-1). Following deposition, sheathed microfilariae utilize as vectors mosquitoes of several genera, including *Culex, Aedes, Mansonia, Anopheles*, and *Psorophora*. Development in the mosquito requires 1–3 weeks. Once introduced into the definitive host, larvae molt twice and migrate to the varices of lymphatic glands of the groin and epididymis of males and the labia and mammary glands of females, where they require 6 months or more to develop to maturity.

Epidemiology

More than 120 million people are reported to be afflicted with lymphatic filariasis, with *W. bancrofti* the most common source of infection. The parasite is estimated to affect more than 100 miliion inhabitants of the Nile delta, Central Africa, Turkey, India, Southeast Asia, the Philippines, Pacific islands, Indonesia, Australia, the Caribbean, and parts of South and Central America (Fig. 17-3), with India having by far the largest number of cases. It was probably introduced into the New World during the slave trade. It is certain that infection was introduced into the United States via slaves brought to Charleston, South Carolina, and that it persisted in the Southeastern United States until the 1920s. The Pacific strain occurs throughout the Pacific islands except Hawaii.

Human infection is closely related to the ecology of the mosquito vectors as well as to human habits. For instance, the occurrence of periodic filariasis, found in areas of dense population and poor sanitation, parallels the distribution of its principal vector, *Culex fatigans*, which breeds in sewage-contaminated water. On the other hand, subperiodic filariasis in the Pacific islands often occurs in rural areas, and this correlates ecologically with its

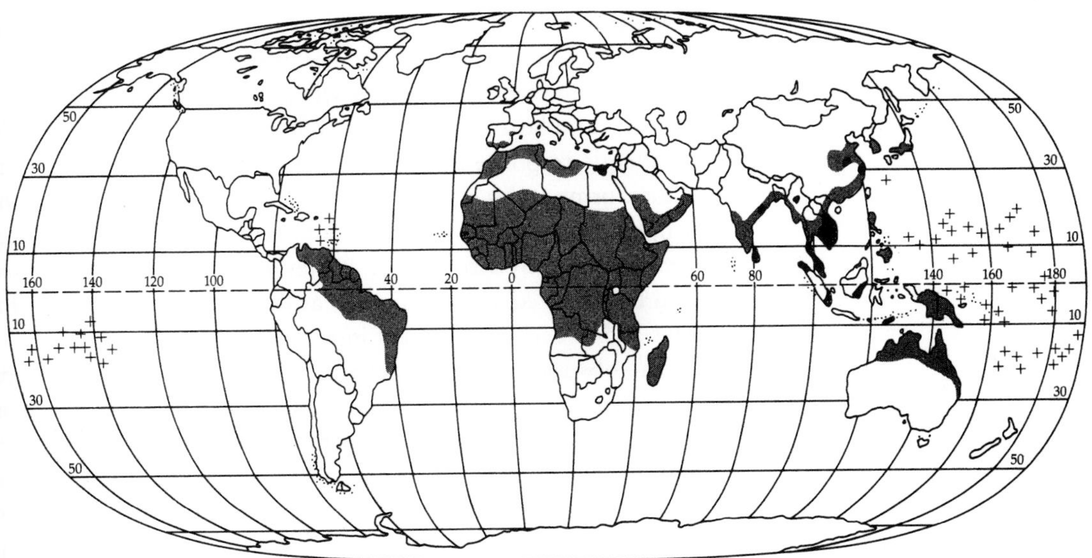

FIGURE 17-3
Distribution of *Wuchereria bancrofti*.
(+, Islands; black areas, concurrent *Brugia malayi*.)

principal vector, *Aedes polynesiensis*, a mosquito that breeds in the brush.

Symptomatology and Diagnosis

Pathology in *W. bancrofti* infection is due largely to living, dead, and degenerating adult worms. As lymph vessels and glands become blocked by the worms, edema develops; in time, the accumulation of connective tissue cells and fibers contributes to the enlargement of limbs, scrotum, and other structures.

Clinically, the disease can be divided into **incubation, acute** (inflammatory), and **obstructive** phases. The incubation phase is largely asymptomatic and may last for a year or more. Symptoms that do appear are usually mild and may include low-grade fever caused by lymphatic inflammation. In time, the adult worms die, microfilariae disappear, and the patient is often unaware of having been infected. In endemic areas, children frequently harbor microfilariae in their blood while exhibiting few symptoms. During World War II, United States armed forces in the South Pacific were constantly exposed to infection, but surprisingly few showed any microfilariae in the peripheral circulation.

The acute phase commences when the female parasites reach maturity and begin releasing microfilariae. This phase is actually an allergic response to the products of dying and degenerating adult worms and is characterized by intense inflammation of the lymph areas of the lower body of the patient. In males, the scrotum is frequently affected. Chills, fever, and toxemia, accompanied by localized swellings in the arms and legs, may persist for days and/or recur at frequent intervals.

The obstructive phase is characterized by blockage of lymph flow resulting from acute granulomatous response in the lymphatic system to dead and degenerating adult worms. This phase may eventually lead to the condition known as elephantiasis; however, only about 10% of the infected population manifests this chronic condition, and in them it develops only after many years of continual filarial reinfection. Elephantiasis is rarely seen in people less than 25 years old and is most prevalent in humans older than 40.

Diagnosis requires demonstration and accurate identification of microfilariae in the blood. The time of day (or night) at which blood should be collected and examined for motile microfilariae depends upon the strain involved. Stained thick and thin blood smears are used for species identification. Features such as the presence or absence of a sheath and the distribution of internal nuclei and organ primordia are discernible after staining. In early infections, before microfilariae are present in the blood, intradermal tests using antigen prepared from *Dirofilaria immitis* (the dog heartworm) yield almost 100% accuracy. Diagnostic procedures should be supplemented with a complete history of patient exposure in endemic areas.

Treatment

Annual or semiannual treatment with diethylcarbamazine typically reduces microfilaremia by 90%. Administered with care, it may also kill adult worms. The drug is commonly administered in combination with diethylcarbamazine-fortified salt. Daily consumption of fortified salt for a period of one year has resulted in the total elimination of lymphatic filariasis in a number of tested populations in tropical Africa. This regimen is contraindicated in regions where onchocerciasis or loaiasis is endemic. A single-dose treatment of ivermectin plus diethylcarbamazine has also proven highly effective, producing a 99% reduction in the number of microfilariae.

Edema may be alleviated by pressure bandaging of the affected region to force excess lymph from the area. Granulomatous tissue can sometimes be removed surgically, but such treatment is rarely attempted in advanced cases of elephantiasis.

Prevention

Control of and protection from mosquitoes in endemic areas should accompany mass chemotherapy of the indigenous population. The mosquito population, however, has proven difficult to control because of increased resistance to insecticides. Also hindering control efforts is the spread of urbanization in tropical regions, which has resulted in an increase in the prevalence of the disease and a concomitant increase in the number of nonsylvatic breeding sites. Mass treatment coupled with the use of screens, insect repellents, and insecticides has proven effective in controlling Bancroft's filariasis in the U.S. Virgin Islands, Puerto Rico, and Tahiti.

BRUGIA MALAYI

Until 1960, several species of filarial worms with similar microfilariae were assigned to the genus *Wuchereria.* In that year, the genus *Brugia* was established to designate the "malayi" group. Included in the genus is *B. malayi*, which infects humans. Adults of *B. malayi* closely resemble those of *W. bancrofti* but are only about half as large. Females are about 55 mm long and males about 23 mm long. The sheathed microfilariae usually appear nocturnally in the peripheral circulation, but there is also a subperiodic strain. The nocturnal strain infects humans exclusively, while the subperiodic strain infects humans, cats, macaque monkeys, and leaf monkeys.

Life Cycle

The life cycle of *B. malayi* closely parallels that of *W. bancrofti.* The principal mosquito vectors are members of the genus *Mansonia*; however, members of the genera *Aedes*, *Culex*, and, occasionally, *Anopheles* also serve in this capacity.

Epidemiology

The Pacific geographic range of *B. malayi* overlaps that of *W. bancrofti*, extending from India to China, Japan, Taiwan, Malaysia, and Indonesia (Fig. 17-3). *B. malayi* is found most often in low-lying regions, which provide optimal breeding conditions for the vectors.

Symptomatology and Diagnosis

Although *B. malayi* rarely affects the genitalia, adult worms live in the lymphatics and otherwise cause the same symptoms as *W. bancrofti*, culminating in elephantiasis. Diagnosis is identical to that for *W. bancrofti*.

Treatment and Prevention

Treatment and prevention are also the same as for *W. bancrofti*. *B. malayi* has been virtually eliminated in Japan, Taiwan, and South Korea due to strict compliance with control programs.

ONCHOCERCA VOLVULUS

Female worms measure about 50 cm by 300 μm, while males are about 42 cm by 105 μm. The male has a transversely striated cuticle reinforced externally with spiral thickenings.

Life Cycle

Adult worms are found in fibrous nodules called **onchocercomas** in the subcutaneous connective tissues and viscera of humans (Fig. 17-4), who are the only known hosts for this species. The nodules are produced by a host inflammatory response to proteins made by the worms. Usually a male and a female are coiled in each nodule, but occasionally several worms are coiled within a single onchocercoma. Immediately upon deposition within the nodules, eggs rupture and the unsheathed microfilariae migrate to the lymphatics or, more often, to the connective tissues of the skin and eyes. An adult female worm can produce millions of microfilariae. The microfilariae are positively phototactic, but because they do not live in the blood, they do not display periodicity. Blackflies, *Simulium* spp., become infected with microfilariae while taking a blood meal. The average developmental time for

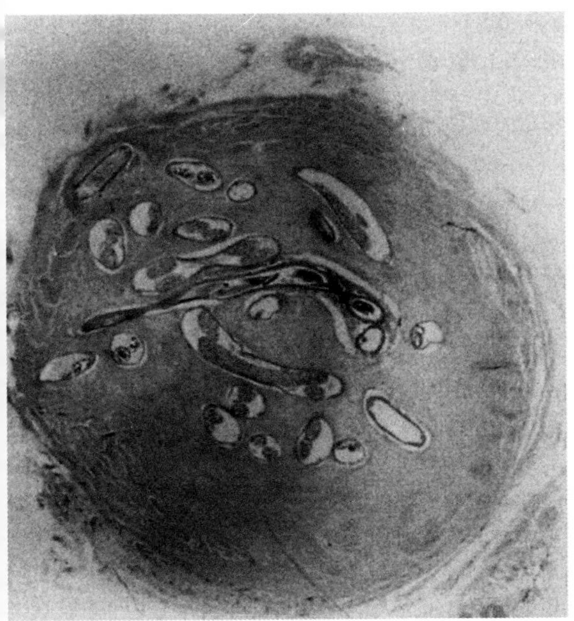

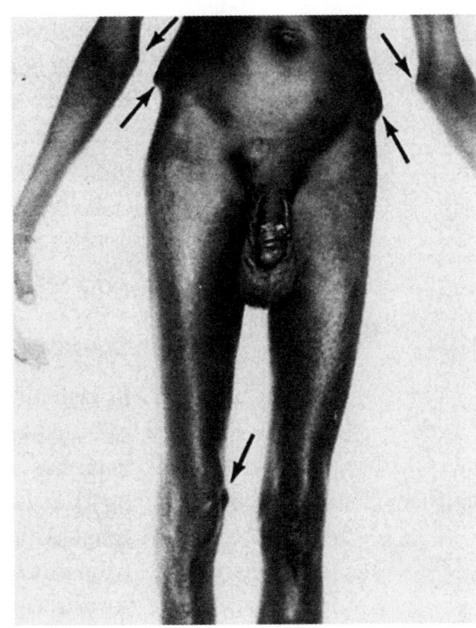

FIGURE 17-4
Onchocerca volvulus.
(Left) Section through a nodule showing adult worms with microfilariae. (Right) Onchocercomas on a native in the Democratic Republic of the Congo. Arrows point to onchocercomas on elbows, hips, and knee.

infective larvae in the vector is 2 weeks, during which time they molt twice, migrate from the hemocoel and wing musculature to the proboscis, and are deposited on human skin when the fly feeds. Infective L_3 larvae migrate into the subcutaneous tissue through the puncture site. Development to sexual maturity takes approximately a year; the life span of the worms can be as long as 14 years.

Epidemiology

The World Health Organization considers onchocerciasis the world's second leading infectious cause of human blindness. Worldwide, there are estimated to be 20 million cases of onchocerciasis, with another 120 million people at risk for the disease. Approximately 96% of the cases are in tropical Africa, although there are significant numbers in the highlands of western Guatemala, Colombia, and northeastern Venezuela as well. The disease also occurs in Mexico and the Near East. In endemic areas in Central America, infected flies abound and breed in the high mountain streams, usually 300–1200 m above sea level. Infection is common among workers on highland coffee plantations. Recent estimates show that, although the disease is being controlled to some extent in Central and South America, its prevalence is increasing in Africa, where the introduction and increasing use of irrigation techniques and the construction of hydroelectric dams and attendant lakes have led to the spread of *Simulium* breeding sites.

Symptomatology and Diagnosis

In general, onchocerciasis is a disease that manifests itself in a cell-mediated, inflammatory host response to foreign proteins from live, dead, and/or dying worms. One of the diseases caused by *O. volvulus* is commonly known as "river blindness." It is estimated that more than one-quarter of a million people suffer from this affliction. *Onchocerca volvulus* microfilariae invade the cornea, causing inflammation of the sclera, cornea, iris, and retina. Formation of fibrous tissue usually follows, leading to impaired vision or total blindness. Such ophthalmic changes require 7–9 years to develop fully.

In addition to the dramatic condition described previously, the presence of microfilariae in the connective tissues of the skin often produces severe dermatitis due to either allergic responses or toxicity. Affected areas of the skin become thickened, depigmented, wrinkled, and cracked. Because the symptoms resemble those accompanying vitamin A deficiency, it has been suggested that they reflect the parasite's competition for vitamin A or interference with its metabolism in the host.

Adult worms may also cause minor pathological alterations, including subcutaneous nodules, especially over bony prominences (Fig. 17-4). Onchocercomas caused by the Venezuelan and African strains of *O. volvulus* usually appear in the pelvic area but also occur less frequently on the chest, spine, and knees. In contrast, infection with the Central American strain more commonly produces nodules above the waist, especially on the head and neck. Although subcutaneous onchocercomas are readily excised, adult worms in deep-seated nodules continue to produce microfilariae that can migrate to the surface for transmission and continue to cause damage to the eyes.

Superficial nodules, cutaneous reactions, eosinophilia, and ocular symptoms in patients from endemic areas are strong indicators of onchocerciasis. Microscopical demonstration of microfilariae in dermal lymph or skin biopsy is proof of infection, as is the identification of adults in skin nodules.

Treatment

Ivermectin, administered in a single dose, has replaced diethylcarbamazine and suramin as the most effective treatment for onchocerciasis. The drug paralyzes the microfilariae, allowing host macrophages to remove them before they can degenerate and release allergenic materials into the circulation. Ivermectin treatment also improves the adverse skin conditions that result from the infection. However, the drug does not affect adult worms enclosed in onchocercomas or the release of microfilariae. Ivermectin treatment is contraindicated in patients who are concurrently infected with the eye worm, *Loa loa*, as it precipitates severe reactions.

Prevention

Preventive measures are threefold: surgical and chemical treatment of patients to prevent further spread of the disease, control of the insect vector population, and protection of potential victims. Patient treatment has already been discussed. Control of *Simulium* requires judicious use of insecticides on aquatic larvae, especially during the dry seasons, and on vegetation along the banks of swift-moving streams and rivers. Protective netting and screening and use of insect repellents effectively shield individuals from biting by infected flies.

LOA LOA

Adult female *Loa loa* measure 50–70 mm by 0.5 mm, with the vulva located at the extreme anterior end; adult males measure 30–35 mm by 0.4 mm. The adults live in the subcutaneous tissues of the body, where they migrate freely. Because they are often seen moving beneath the conjunctiva, these parasites are known as African eye worms.

Life Cycle

Humans and baboons are the only definitive hosts of *Loa loa*. The sheathed microfilariae display diurnal periodicity, retreating to the pulmonary capillaries at night. Various members of the mango fly genus *Chrysops* serve as vectors in which the developmental period to infective third-stage larvae lasts approximately 10–12 days. Within an hour after introduction into the definitive host as the vector takes a blood meal, the L_3 larvae penetrate to the subcutaneous and muscle tissues. There, over the next 12 months, they molt twice and metamorphose into adult worms. The life span of adult worms is estimated to be 4–17 years.

Epidemiology

An estimated 20 million patients suffer from loaiasis. Although the parasite was introduced into the Caribbean during the slave trade era, it did not persist there, and the disease is now limited to the African equatorial rain forest and southern Sudan. Infection rates are highest in regions with muddy ponds and swamps, where the vector breeds.

Symptomatology and Diagnosis

Loa loa is only mildly pathogenic. Adult worms wander throughout the body, moving through the tissues at a maximum rate of about 1.5 cm per minute. The most troublesome infection sites are the conjunctiva (Fig. 17-5) and the bridge of the nose, where impaired vision, irritation, and pain may result. Most symptoms are general inflammatory reactions to adult worms and microfilariae. Symptoms are often transient, appearing and disappearing at irregular intervals. A typical manifestation takes the form of transient, painful, subcutaneous swellings, commonly termed **fugitive** or **Calabar swellings**, which are most often seen on the hands and forearms or near the eyes and may grow to the size of a hen's egg.

Sheathed microfilariae in the spleen can cause eosinophilia and fibrosis. Victims of the infection commonly exhibit a wide range of symptoms attributable to the wandering worms, such as low-grade fever, dermatitis, pain in the limbs, edema, and eosinophilia.

Diagnosis is usually based on sightings of the wandering worm in the conjunctiva, the presence of Calabar swellings, eosinophilia, and/or diurnal demonstration of microfilariae in blood. Antigens prepared from the dog heartworm, *Dirofilaria immitis*, are useful diagnostic tools when other techniques are inconclusive.

Treatment

Surgical removal of wandering adult worms from the conjunctiva is advisable. Diethylcarbamazine is the drug of choice to kill

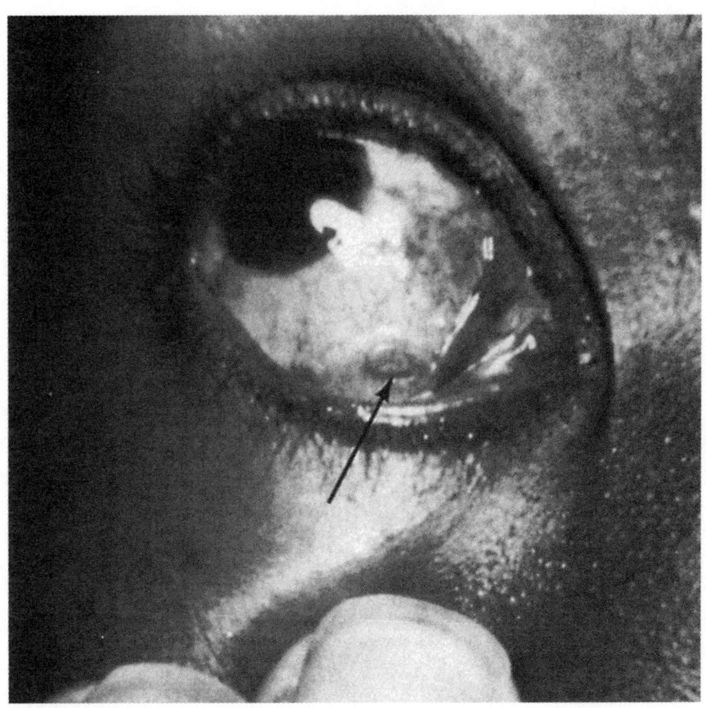

FIGURE 17-5
Adult female *Loa loa* under conjunctiva.

microfilariae; however, it can produce serious side effects ranging from encephalitis to death. Ivermectin has been used effectively, but in mixed infection with *O. volvulus*, this drug, too, can have severe side effects; this fact takes on special significance in view of the overlap in the distribution of onchocerciasis and loaiasis in West and Central Africa. Neither drug affects adult worms.

Prevention

The protocol recommended for control and prevention of infection with *O. volvulus* and other filarial worms applies for *Loa loa* infection as well.

MANSONELLA OZZARDI, MANSONELLA PERSTANS, AND *MANSONELLA STREPTOCERCA*

The precise number of *Mansonella* species infective to humans has not been firmly established. There are striking similarities among all of the infective species, and the validity of assigning them to separate species may warrant challenge. In all instances, members of the midge genus *Culicoides* serve as vectors, and adult worms reside in the body cavities and neighboring associated tissues of the definitive hosts. *Mansonella ozzardi* favors visceral adipose tissue; *M. perstans* prefers the peritoneal cavity and, occasionally, the pericardial cavity; and *M. streptocerca* adults and microfilariae favor the subcutaneous tissue. The unsheathed microfilariae of the three species display no periodicity and are readily visible in blood and other host tissues. *Mansonella ozzardi* is endemic in northern Argentina, the northern coast of South America, and Central America. *Mansonella perstans* is found primarily in tropical Africa and to a lesser degree in South America and the Caribbean. *Mansonella streptocerca* is common in East Africa, including Uganda, Kenya, and southern Sudan.

Other than local tissue reaction in the form of hydrocoels, no dramatic symptoms are associated with infection by these parasites.

THE GUINEA WORM

DRACUNCULUS MEDINENSIS

Awareness of *Dracunculus medinensis* dates back to antiquity. The "fiery serpent" of the biblical Israelites (Numbers 21:6), *D. medinensis* is today commonly called the guinea worm or Medina worm. Long and thin, the adult female measures 500–1200 mm by 0.9–1.7 mm and the adult male 12–29 mm by 0.4 mm.

Life Cycle

Adult worms inhabit the body cavity, its surrounding membranes, and the connective tissue of the human host. Male worms are rarely observed. The vulva, positioned equatorially in young females, is atrophied and nonfunctional in adults. The branched, gravid uterus, filled with thousands of larvae, compresses the intestine of the female and renders it nonfunctional. Gravid females migrate to the subcutaneous tissues of infected humans.

In the subcutaneous tissues, gravid worms direct their heads toward the skin and secrete an irritant that causes papules to form in the host dermis, most frequently on the ankles and wrists (Fig.

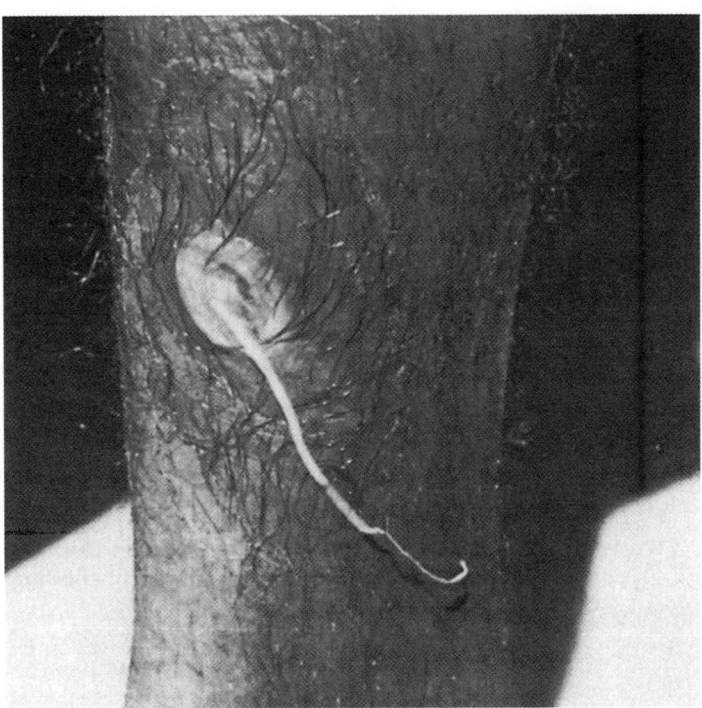

FIGURE 17-6
Female *Dracunculus medinensis* partially protruding from blister on leg.

17-6). As each papule grows, it assumes the external appearance of a blister, eventually rupturing and leaving a cup-shaped ulcer in the skin. When the open ulcer comes in contact with water, a loop of the worm's uterus prolapses, either through the broken anterior end of the body or through the mouth, and ruptures, releasing numerous first-stage, rhabditiform larvae into the water. The larvae can survive in the aquatic environment for several days. Cold water stimulates contraction of the female body wall, causing larvae to be ejected in spurts. As the larvae are ejected, the body wall continually eases out of the ulcer and atrophies, and the remaining portion of the worm shortens proportionately. Larvae ingested by a suitable species of the copepod genera *Cyclops*, *Mesocyclops*, and *Thermocyclops* burrow through the midgut and enter the hemocoel. The presence of more than five or six larvae is fatal to the arthropod.

Within the hemocoel of the copepod, the rhabditiform larvae undergo two molts, metamorphosing into infective, sheathed, L_3 larvae in approximately 20 days. When drinking water contaminated with infected copepods is consumed by a human, the larvae, freed from the crustacean during digestion, exsheath in the duodenum of the human host. The larvae then burrow through the mucosa, undergo two additional molts, and lodge in the liver, body cavity, or subcutaneous tissues, where they mature in 8–12 months. The adult female is fertilized about 3 months postinfection; males usually die and degenerate 3–7 months after infection. A period of 10–14 months elapses between the initial infection of the human host and the eruption of skin blisters.

Epidemiology

Human infection occurs throughout Africa except for the southern regions, in southwestern Asia (including southern India and Nepal), and, to a lesser extent, in northeastern South America and the West Indies. It is estimated that the number of guinea worm cases worldwide was 3.5 million until recently. Recent estimates indicate that only 160,000 cases persist, approximately one-third of them in the Sudan. Two criteria are requisite for completion of the life cycle: (1) ingestion of infected copepods and (2) contact of the infected human host with water. In drought-stricken areas of Africa, pools of stagnant water abundant with copepods provide ready sources of infection for natives in search of drinking water. In southern India, the step-well is a prime source of infection. The practice of standing ankle or knee deep in the well to fill water containers allows gravid female worms in open ulcers of infected persons to release their larvae. Copepods, previously infected by larvae released in a similar fashion, are drawn with the drinking water, providing a source of new infections.

A number of animals, including canines, felines, horses, and raccoons, have been implicated as possible reservoir hosts for the infection. However, because there are a number of other species of *Dracunculus* with which *D. medinensis* can be confused, the importance of these animals as reservoirs is not known.

Symptomatology and Diagnosis

Dracunculus medinensis infection causes a broad spectrum of nonspecific symptoms, including eosinophilia, nausea, diarrhea, asthma, and fainting; these symptoms are believed to result from the absorption of metabolic wastes produced by female worms during papule formation. In addition, cutaneous ulcers caused by female worms are common sites for secondary bacterial and fungal infections that often produce permanent scars and muscle damage.

Female worms that fail to reach host skin sometimes cause reactions in deeper tissues of the body. Commonly, they degenerate or become calcified; degeneration stimulates the release of strongly antigenic molecules that can cause fluid-filled abscesses, while calcification near a joint may produce a type of chronic arthritis.

The appearance of localized blisters or ulcers or the microscopical identification of larvae or an adult female, especially the protruded head, constitute diagnosis. X-ray examination may reveal calcified worms. An ELISA test is available, but its use to date has been limited.

Treatment

Both chemotherapeutic and mechanical techniques, including surgery, are employed for the removal of adult worms. The drug of choice is metronidazole administered over a 7–10 day period. Metronidazole acts not only on the worm itself but also as an anti-inflammatory agent. Mechanical withdrawal of the gravid female from the ulcerated area requires painstaking care, and the worm must be extracted slowly. If the worm breaks during the extraction process, larvae escape into the subcutaneous tissues, causing severe and painful inflammatory reactions. The ancient method, dating back to biblical days, of winding the worm on a stick is still used in parts of Africa and Asia (Fig. 17-7). During the procedure, the worm is wound around a stick which is slowly turned, withdrawing the worm a few centimeters a day. Applying cold water to the area hastens the process by causing expulsion of more larvae to the exterior and allowing exposure of an additional 5 cm or so of the worm. The caduceus, the official emblem of the medical profession, includes a pair of serpents wrapped around a staff. It is not inconceivable that it may have been derived from this ancient method of *D. medinensis* removal.

Prevention

As with other parasitic diseases, prevention and control require interruption of the life cycle. It is essential that the practice of

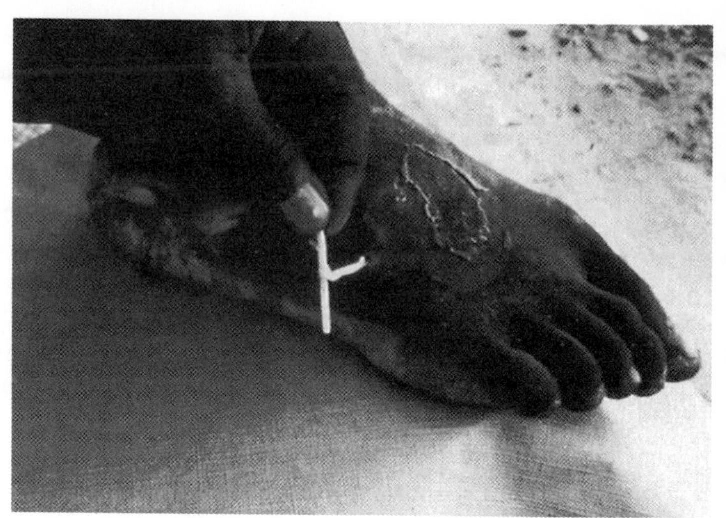

FIGURE 17-7
Female *Dracunculus medinensis* slowly being withdrawn from ulcer on foot with twig.

bathing and washing in sources of drinking water be discontinued. Water suspected of being contaminated should be boiled or filtered before use, and whenever possible, drinking water should be obtained from swift-running waterways, which are usually free of copepods. Chemical treatment of water with chlorine or copper sulfate to destroy copepods is an alternative. These measures have already proven so successsful that an end to guinea worm disease is predicted for the very near future.

SELECTED READINGS

Cheng, T. C. 1983. Cutaneous lesions due to nonarthropod parasites. In *Cutaneous Infestations of Man and Animal* (Parish, L. C., Nutting, W. B., and Schwartzman, R. M., Eds.), pp. 237–254. Prager, New York.

Chernin, E. 1983. Sir Patrick Manson's studies on the transmission and biology of filariasis. *Reviews of Infectious Diseases* **5**, 148–166.

Denham, D. A. 1998. Zoonotic infections with filarial nematodes. In *Zoonoses* (Palmer, S. R., Soulsby, E. J. L., and Simpson, D. I. H., Eds.), pp. 783–788. Oxford University Press, Oxford, England.

Duke, B. O. L. 1984. Filtering out the guinea worm. *World Health* **3**, 29.

Duke, B. O. L. 1990. Onchocerciasis (river blindness)—Can it be eradicated? *Parasitology Today* **6**, 82–84.

Molyneux, D. H., and Davies, J. B. 1997. Onchocerciasis control: Moving towards the millennium. *Parasitology Today* **13,** 418–425.

Periès, H., and Cairncross, S. 1997. Global eradication of Guinea worm. *Parasitology Today* **13,** 431–437.

Pinder, M. 1988. *Loa loa*—a neglected filaria. *Parasitology Today* **4,** 279–284.

Turner, P., and Michael, E. 1997. Recent advances in the control of lymphatic filariasis. *Parasitology Today* **13,** 410–411.

PART FIVE

ARTHROPODA

Chapter Eighteen

ARTHROPODS AS VECTORS

Members of the phylum Arthropoda probably constitute the largest number of individuals and species of any phylum in the animal kingdom. There are at least 760,000 known species of arthropods. According to current classification systems, the phylum is divided into four subphyla: Trilobitomorpha, Chelicerata, Crustacea, and Uniramia. This chapter deals with the role of Chelicerata (ticks and mites) and Uniramia (insects) as vectors of human disease-producing organisms (Fig. 18-1).

Although most arthropods generally are of little if any medical importance, they are of considerable biological interest, particularly to parasitologists. Furthermore, parasitic arthropods, such as ticks, mites, and certain insects, are of considerable medical and veterinary importance not only because they inflict direct injury upon their hosts but also because many serve as vectors for various pathogenic microorganisms and viruses.

SIGNIFICANCE OF ARTHROPODS AS VECTORS

Disease-producing organisms transmitted to humans by arthropods have significantly influenced human history and demography. The plague, or Black Death, that so tragically decimated the population of Europe in the fourteenth century is vivid documentation of the toll such a disease can exact. Trench fever, the scourge of World War I, also attests to the gravity of vector-borne diseases. Other such diseases that have had dramatic impact upon historic events and eras include trachoma during Napoleon's invasion of Egypt, malaria and yellow fever during the construction of the Suez and Panama canals, and African trypanosomiasis and malaria during the European explorations of Africa in the nineteenth century.

The disease agents transmitted by various arthropods vary widely in size and degree of pathogenicity. The smallest are submicroscopic viruses no larger than a large protein molecule and

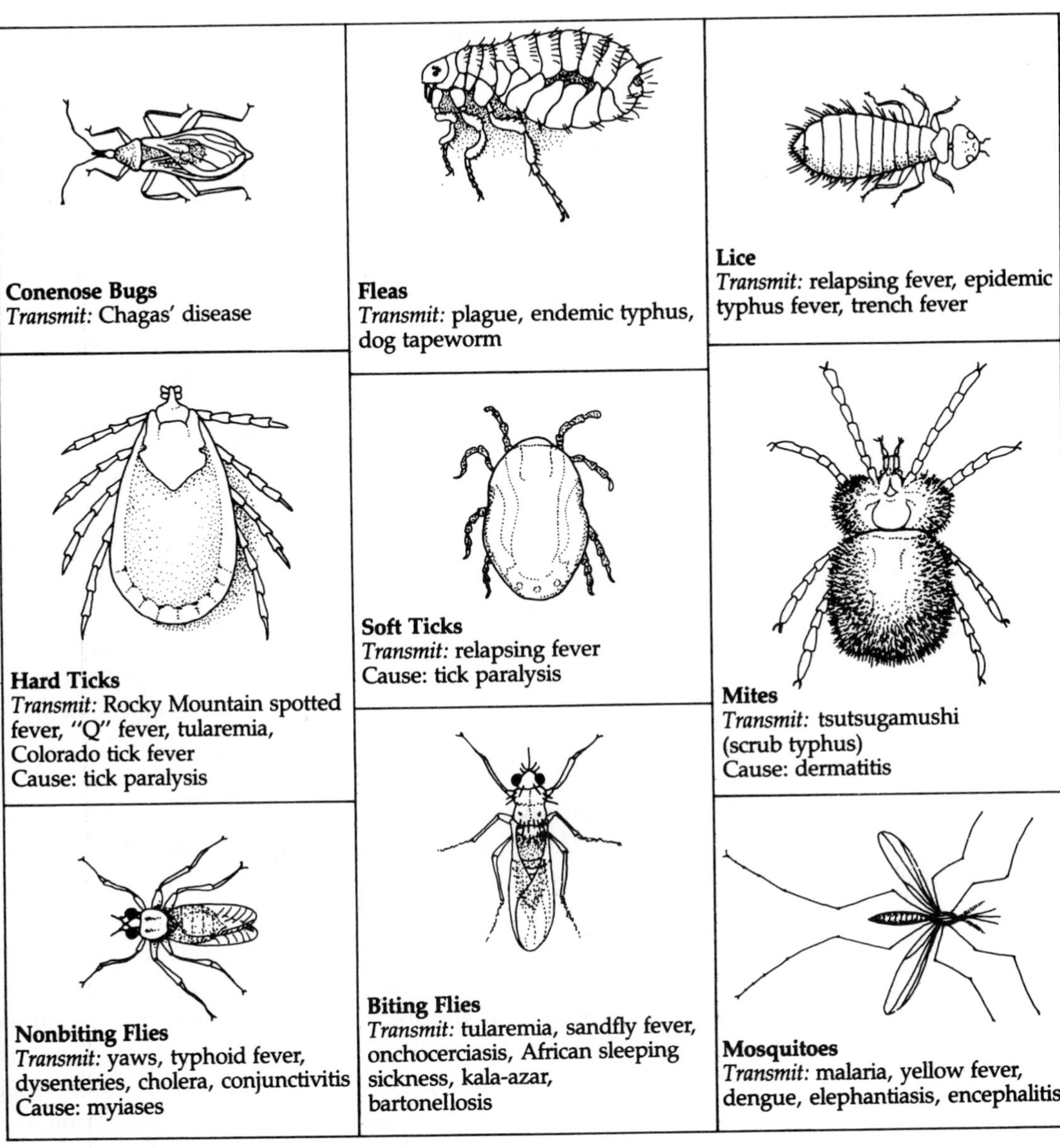

Conenose Bugs
Transmit: Chagas' disease
Fleas
Transmit: plague, endemic typhus, dog tapeworm
Lice
Transmit: relapsing fever, epidemic typhus fever, trench fever
Hard Ticks
Transmit: Rocky Mountain spotted fever, "Q" fever, tularemia, Colorado tick fever
Cause: tick paralysis
Soft Ticks
Transmit: relapsing fever
Cause: tick paralysis
Mites
Transmit: tsutsugamushi (scrub typhus)
Cause: dermatitis
Nonbiting Flies
Transmit: yaws, typhoid fever, dysenteries, cholera, conjunctivitis
Cause: myiases
Biting Flies
Transmit: tularemia, sandfly fever, onchocerciasis, African sleeping sickness, kala-azar, bartonellosis
Mosquitoes
Transmit: malaria, yellow fever, dengue, elephantiasis, encephalitis

FIGURE 18-1
Some arthropods that transmit pathogens of human disease.

are obligate parasites of cells. Rickettsiae, currently considered a highly specialized form of bacterium, are somewhat larger than most viruses, although their size range overlaps that of the larger viruses and smaller bacteria. Like viruses, rickettsiae are obligate parasites, and they are at some point dependent upon arthropods for transmission. Unlike viruses but like many bacteria, rickettsiae are vulnerable to antibiotics. Next in order of size, bacteria thrive in a wide range of environments and display equally diverse metabolic patterns and host relationships. Although many bacteria are free living, many others form symbiotic relationships of commensalistic, mutualistic, or parasitic nature. The role of insects in the transmission of protozoans such as *Plasmodium, Leishmania*, and *Trypanosoma* and of nematodes such as *Wuchereria*, *Onchocerca*, and *Brugia* has already been discussed. A number of tapeworm infections are also arthropod-transmitted. For instance, *Dipylidium caninum* is transmitted by fleas, *Diphyllobothrium latum* by copepod crustaceans, and *Hymenolepis diminuta* by beetles. The lung fluke *Paragonimus westermani* uses a crustacean as the second intermediate host in its life cycle.

The manner in which the various organisms parasitic to humans are transmitted dictates the type of association the arthropods establish with the parasites. The simplest relationship is one in which the arthropod is a **mechanical vector**, functioning merely as a passive carrier of the etiologic agent. Examples of this type include typhoid organisms and *Entamoeba histolytica* cysts from contaminated excreta, which adhere to body parts or pass through the digestive tracts of the common housefly and cockroach and are subsequently transferred to food and drink touched by the insects. As a **biological vector**, the arthropod is used by the disease-producing organism not only as a vehicle of transmission but also as an environment for development and/or reproduction prior to its infective stage.

Biological transmission is of four types. In **propagative biological transmission**, the disease-producing organism reproduces in the arthropod but undergoes no further development; examples are the plague bacillus in the flea and the yellow fever virus in the mosquito. In **cyclopropagative biological transmission**, the disease-producing organism not only reproduces but undergoes cyclical changes in the arthropod as well. *Plasmodium* spp. and trypanosomes transmitted by mosquitoes and by tsetse flies, respectively, are examples of this type. In **cyclodevelopmental biological transmission**, the disease-producing organism undergoes vital cyclical changes in the arthropod vector but does not multiply there. For example, filarial worms must spend a portion of their life cycle in their mosquito vectors although they reproduce elsewhere. Finally, in **transovarial transmission**, certain disease-producing organisms, such as rickettsiae that cause Rocky Mountain spotted fever and scrub typhus, are transmitted from infected parent arthropods (i.e., ticks and mites) to their offspring.

Once the etiologic agent has reached the stage infective to humans, there are several means by which it moves from arthropod to human host. Infective forms of parasites carried by certain blood-sucking flies exit the insect's mouthparts during the blood meal and enter human skin through the puncture. The malarial parasite uses a more efficient mechanism to reach its human victim: the infective form reaches the salivary gland of the mosquito and enters the human bloodstream via saliva secreted by the insect into the human skin while feeding. Other insect-transmitted infections, such as viral encephalitis, yellow fever, dengue, and sleeping sickness, are transmitted in a similar fashion. In some nonblood-feeding arthropods, the feeding larva (e.g., maggot) ingests the agent, retaining it in the digestive tract during metamorphosis; later, the resulting adult arthropod transmits the agent to the human via vomit or excreta on food and drink.

GENERAL STRUCTURAL FEATURES

In the early phases of their evolution, primitive arthropods were conspicuously multisegmented, each segment equipped with a pair of appendages; in present forms, some segments are fused, the number of appendages is reduced, and (among insects) most species have evolved wings, all of which markedly enhances the mobility of arthropods. In insects, the most successful of terrestrial animals, the body is divided into three regions (Fig. 18-2): the **head**, with a variety of mouthparts and sense organs; the more or less rigid **thorax**, bearing three pairs of walking appendages and usually wings; and the segmented **abdomen**, lacking appendages. Acarines, the ticks and mites, represent the second-most successful group of terrestrial arthropods. They have two major body regions but are wingless and possess four pairs of walking appendages (Fig. 18-3). Segmentation in ticks and mites is so indistinct that they appear to be unsegmented.

Arthropods have a chitinous exoskeleton, the **cuticle**, that extends to all external openings. The rigid cuticle limits growth; therefore, periodic molting is required. The **open circulatory sys-**

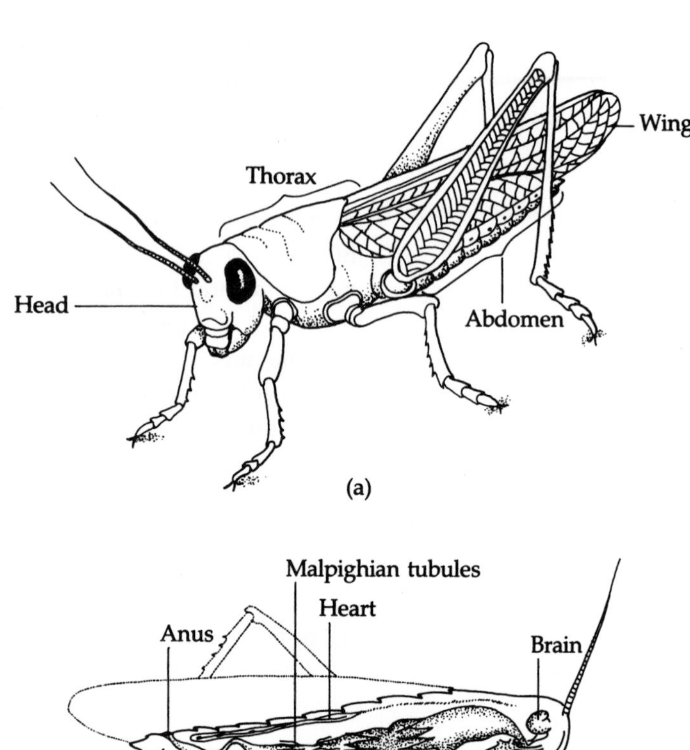

FIGURE 18-2
Anatomy of a typical insect.
(a) External. (b) Internal.

tem consists of a dorsal tubular heart that slowly pumps hemolymph through large sinuses that make up the major body cavity, or **hemocoel.** Hemolymph is not always involved in oxygen transport; in many terrestrial forms, gaseous exchange between cells and environment is accomplished through a system of branched tubules, or **tracheae.** The nervous system consists of a pair of ventral nerve cords with segmentally arranged ganglia; the typical "brain" is a major ganglion located dorsally in the head region and linked to the nerve cords by circumesophageal connectives from the anteriormost ventral ganglion. Nitrogenous wastes are excreted by terrestrial insects and most acarines in the

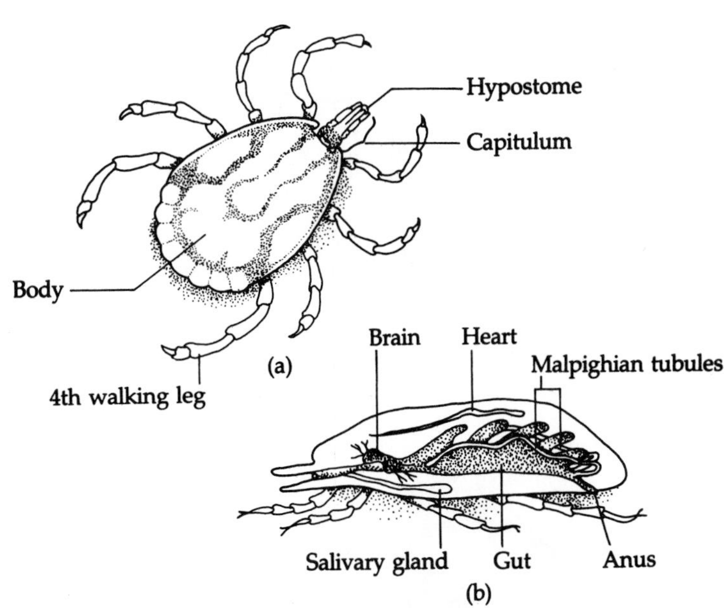

FIGURE 18-3
Anatomy of a typical acarine.
(a) External. (b) Internal.

form of uric acid produced in **Malpighian tubules** that empty into the hindgut.

Arthropods acquire disease-producing organisms primarily during feeding. Because their food sources are so varied, the mouthparts of arthropods likewise vary widely. The mouthparts of early insects were adapted for chewing, and many extant species, including grasshoppers, bees, ants, wasps, cockroaches, and termites, retain that adaptation. Although chewing insects are ineffective as biological transmitters of pathogenic organisms, knowledge of their basic mouthparts is essential for understanding the evolutionary modifications that have produced the more specialized feeding apparatuses.

Lying directly behind the "upper lip," or **labrum**, are the first of the true mouthparts, the paired **mandibles**, which are heavily sclerotinized and bear jagged teeth along their medial margins. Behind them are the paired, jointed **maxillae**. The **hypopharynx** is not a true mouthpart but an unsegmented, tubular outgrowth of the body wall arising from the ventral, membranous floor of the head. The "lower lip" of insects is the heavily sclerotinized, segmented **labium**. The mandibles masticate the food, and the maxillae and labium push the pulverized food into the mouth.

In more advanced insects, the major modification of the feed-

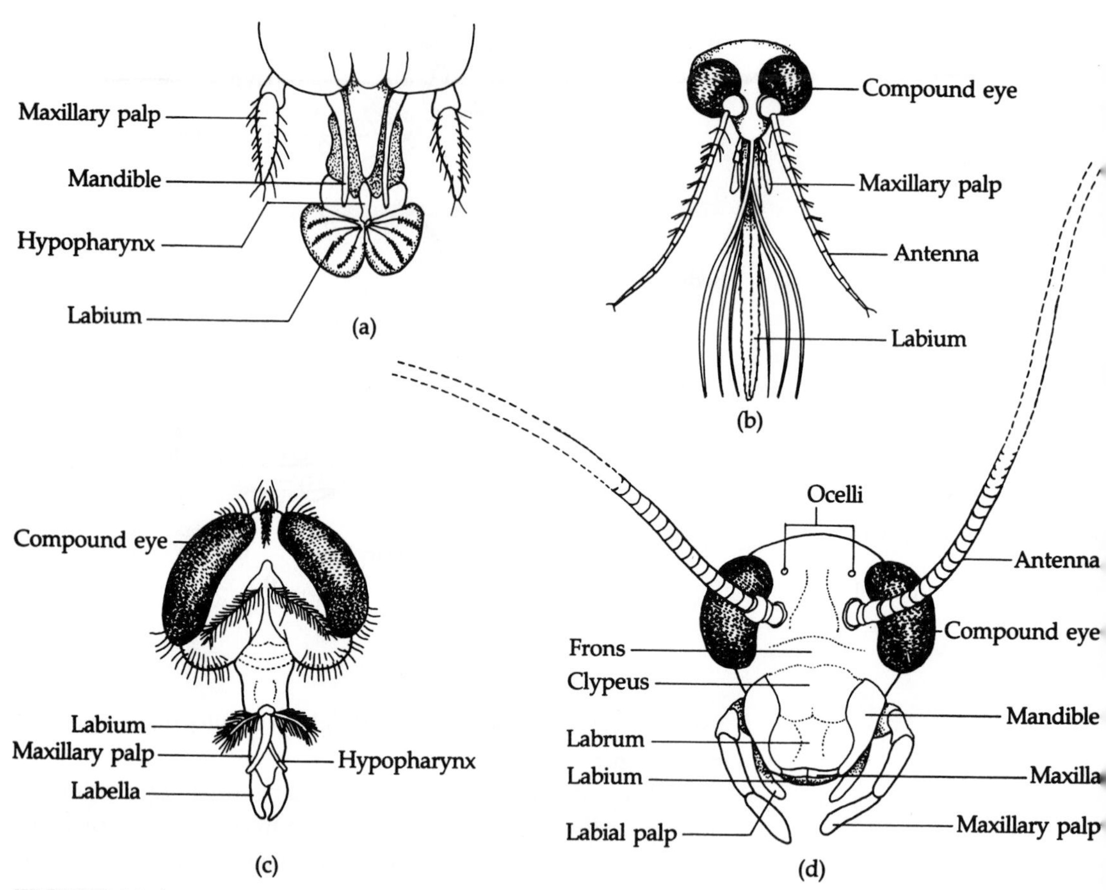

FIGURE 18-4
Types of some insect mouthparts.
(a) Cutting–sponging. (b) Piercing–sucking. (c) Sponging. (d) Chewing.

ing apparatus is the evolution from the chewing type to one of several cutting and/or piercing types (Fig. 18-4).

The **cutting–sponging type**, characteristic of horseflies, features sharp-bladed mandibles and long, styletlike maxillae. The mandibles cut and tear the skin of the host, and the spongelike labium collects the blood and conveys it to the esophagus by means of a tube formed partially by the hypopharynx.

The mouthparts of most nonbiting dipterans, such as the common housefly, are of the **sponging type**, similar to the cutting–sponging type except that the mandibles and maxillae are nonfunctional. The remaining parts form a proboscis with a spongelike apex called the **labella.** Liquid food is conducted to the mouth through minute capillary channels on the labella. Solid food is ingested only after being dissolved or suspended in deposited saliva.

The **piercing–sucking type**, characteristic of mosquitoes, flies, lice, and bedbugs, features mandibles, maxillae, and hypopharynx modified into a long, thin, tubular, sharp-tipped stylet for piercing skin. This narrow tube is enclosed by the labrum to form a **stylet bundle** that is held in a groove on the labium. Together, the stylet bundle and labium make up the **proboscis.** While not itself penetrating the skin, the labium guides the bundle into the wound site. During insect feeding, the stylet bundle pierces the skin of the host like a hypodermic needle, and blood is withdrawn through it. The hypopharynx usually contains the salivary gland duct.

Among acarines, mites are more versatile in their feeding habits than ticks. Although mites may feed on decaying animal matter, feces, plants, animal secretions, and blood, ticks feed only on the blood of reptiles, birds, and mammals. Since the mouthparts of ticks and mites are similar, those of the former will serve to illustrate both groups (Fig. 18-5).

The **capitulum** is a small anterior projection bearing three structures that constitute the acarine mouthparts: the elongate **hypostome,** a pair of segmented **chelicerae,** and a pair of segmented **pedipalps.** The hypostome, usually toothed, is medially located, ventral to the mouth with its free end projecting anteriorly. Bilateral chelicerae are located on the dorsolateral surfaces of the hypostome, flanking the mouth. The free end of each chelicera is forked, one branch forming a fixed, dorsal, toothed digit, the **digitus externus,** the other a lateral, movable **digitus internus.** With these appendages, acarines pierce and/or tear the host's skin and insert the toothed hypostome or the entire capitulum into the opening. The appendages also serve as anchors when the parasite is attached. Paired pedipalps arise from the base of the capitulum at its antero-lateral margin. During feeding, the pedipalps either bend outward (in "soft ticks") as the chelicerae and hypostome penetrate the flesh, or they remain rigidly and intimately associated with the hypostome (in "hard ticks") during skin penetration. In either instance, the pedipalps serve as counteranchors while the tick is attached to the host.

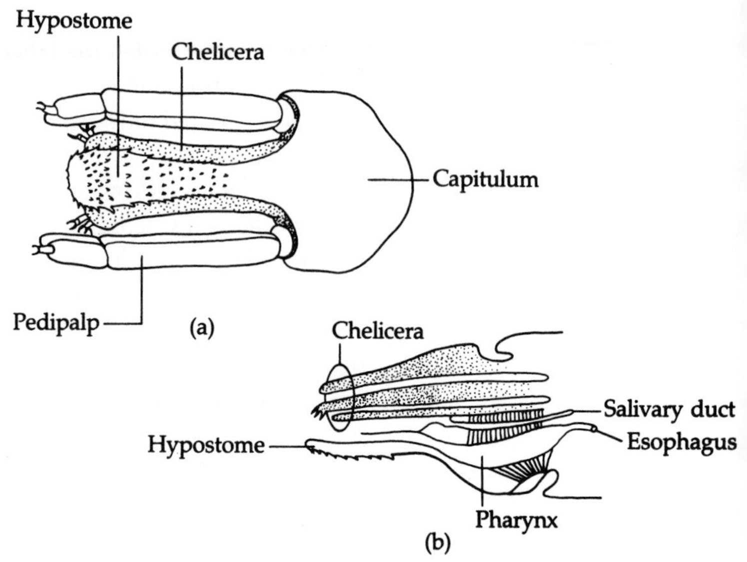

FIGURE 18-5
Mouthparts of ticks.
(a) Ventral aspect of capitulum.
(b) Longitudinal section through tick head.

THE DIPTERANS

While the previous sections dealt with structural modifications in arthropod vectors and some of the means by which they transmit pathogens, the remainder of the chapter focuses upon specific arthropods and some of the human pathogens they transmit. Numerous arthropod-transmitted pathogens have been discussed in preceding chapters devoted to protozoans and helminths, and appropriate references are made to those earlier chapters.

Because of their overwhelming numerical preponderance among arthropod vectors and the medical importance of the pathogens they transmit, dipterans are treated separately from other insects. Alone they may transmit as many disease organisms as all other insects combined.

The development of dipterans is typical of insects with **holometabolous**, or **complete, metamorphosis**. The phases of the life cycle include the **egg**, a fixed number of **larval** stages, a single **pupal** stage, and the **imago** or **adult** stage. More primitive insects, in contrast, are characterized by **hemimetabolous**, or **incomplete, metamorphosis**. In these insects, life cycle phases include the egg and a fixed number of **nymphal** stages, which gradually metamorphose serially to the adult stage. The body form of the nymphs resembles that of the adult. All of the insects discussed in this chapter, with the exception of reduviid bugs and lice, display holometabolous life cycles.

BITING DIPTERANS

Mosquitoes

A number of species of the mosquito family Culicidae are active transmitters of organisms responsible for human disease. Two groups in this family, the anophelines and the culicines, are quite distinct biologically. The cigar-shaped anopheline eggs, for example, are equipped with side floats and are normally deposited diffusely over water. Culicine eggs, on the other hand, possess no side floats and are often deposited in raftlike arrays on the surface of water (*Culex*), in cushionlike arrangements under water plants (*Mansonia*), or on damp surfaces to await heavy rains (*Aedes*; Fig. 18-6).

Although anopheline larvae appear immediately under and parallel to the surface of the water, culicine larvae hang from breathing tubes anchored either to the water surface (*Culex* and

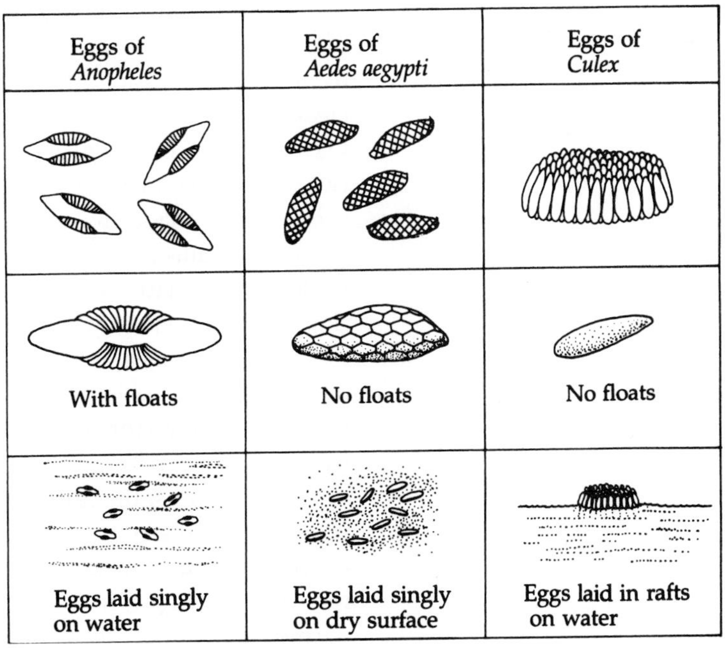

Eggs of *Anopheles*	Eggs of *Aedes aegypti*	Eggs of *Culex*
With floats	No floats	No floats
Eggs laid singly on water	Eggs laid singly on dry surface	Eggs laid in rafts on water

FIGURE 18-6
Mosquito eggs.

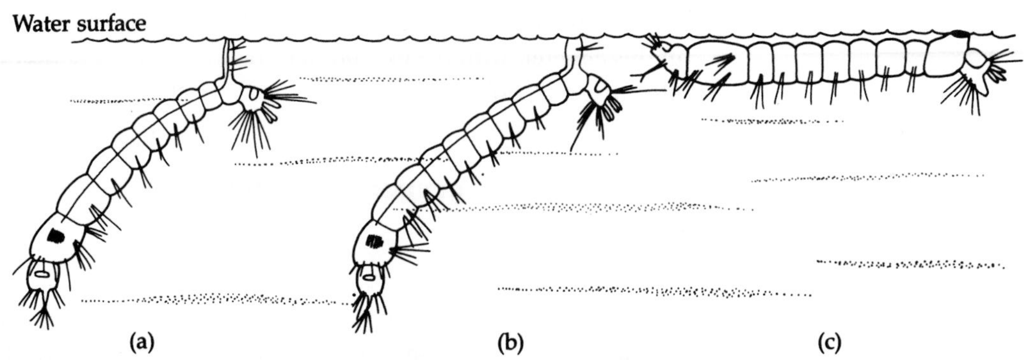

FIGURE 18-7
Mosquito larvae.
(a) *Culex* adhering to water by its breathing tube. (b) *Aedes*. (c) *Anopheles*.

Aedes) (Fig. 18-7) or to the stems of aquatic vegetation (*Mansonia*). Adults are distinguishable by the configuration and angle of their body parts (Fig. 18-8). Anopheline body parts are arranged in a straight line, inclined at an angle to the surface upon which they alight, while those of culicine adults are bent into a humpbacked posture.

Three groups of pathogenic organisms are transmitted to humans by mosquitoes. One group consists of the causative agents of malaria, *Plasmodium* spp. The role of the anopheline mosquito in the transmission of human malaria has already been discussed (see p. 130). Although there are approximately 350 known species of *Anopheles* throughout the world, only about two dozen are major transmitters of human malaria. Many species are genetically or ecologically incompatible with the malarial organism. For example, differences in susceptibility of mosquito populations to *Plasmodium* sometimes reflect variations in gene frequency in different geographic areas. Also, ecological hazards such as storms and droughts influence the mosquitoes' feeding habits and oviposition and, therefore, affect the life span of the vector and its ability to harbor the parasite effectively.

Filarial worms, the causative agents of human filariasis, constitute a second group of mosquito-borne pathogens. Numerous anopheline and culicine species serve as vectors for these organisms. It has been previously noted (see p. 384) that the ecology of the mosquito, especially its feeding cycle, is inextricably linked to

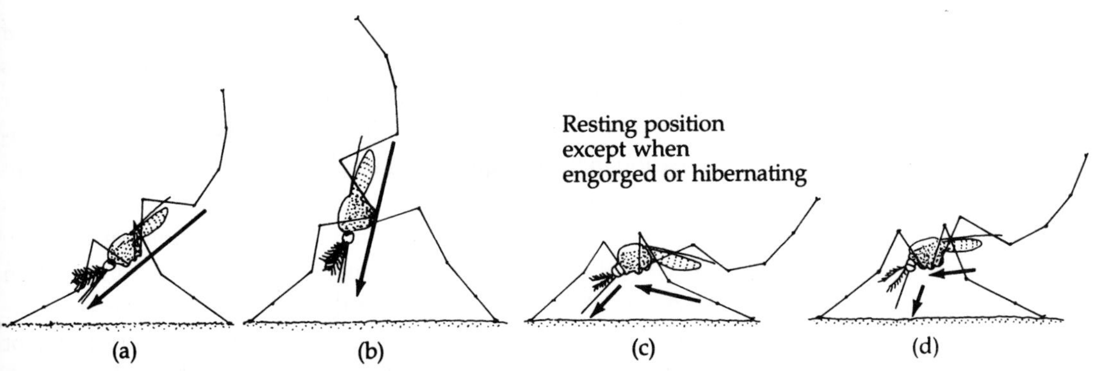

FIGURE 18-8
Resting positions of common mosquitoes.
(a, b) *Anopheles*. (c) *Aedes*. (d) *Culex*.

the periodicity of microfilarial surge in the human host. For instance, the principal vector of the nocturnally surging *Wuchereria bancrofti* is the nocturnally feeding mosquito *Culex fatigans*, while the subperiodic variety of *W. bancrofti* employs the diurnal feeder *Aedes polynesiensis*.

The third group of pathogens are the arboviruses, arthropod-borne viruses transmitted from one person to another by insects or acarines. More than 200 diseases are transmitted in this manner, approximately three-quarters of them by mosquitoes, a few by biting flies, and the rest by ticks. The most serious of the arboviral diseases are the hemorrhagic fevers and the encephalitides. In hemorrhagic fever, increased permeability of capillary walls caused by the viruses precipitates bleeding from kidneys, lungs, gums, nose, etc. In viral encephalitis, viral attacks upon the central nervous system cause symptoms ranging from minor back pain to temporary paralysis, with sometimes lingering spastic effects.

Yellow fever was at one time the most prevalent of the hemorrhagic diseases. It has now lost this undesirable distinction to dengue hemmorhagic fever. During construction of the Panama Canal, yellow fever caused such widespread illness among the workers that the project came to a halt. It was then that the Yellow Fever Commission, under the leadership of Walter Reed and his associates James Carroll, Jesse W. Lazear, and A. Agramonte, won acclaim by proving Carlos Finlay's hypothesis that the pathogen is transmitted by *Aedes aegypti*.

Female mosquitoes acquire the virus while feeding on blood of yellow fever victims. A single female ingests thousands of viruses at one feeding and usually remains infective for the rest of her normal life, 200–240 days. Under field conditions, the normal incubation in the mosquito is 12 days; however, fluctuations in temperature can alter incubation times. For instance, in mosquitoes exposed to temperatures of 36.8°C, the incubation period is reduced to 4 days; at 21°C, it is lengthened to 18 days. In addition to *A. aegypti*, other members of the genus *Aedes* serve as natural vectors for yellow fever; among these are *A. vittatus* in Egypt and *A. simpsoni* and *A. africanus* in eastern Africa. Jungle animals, especially monkeys, serve as natural reservoirs for the yellow fever virus.

Currently, the World Health Organization reports that world incidence of this disease fluctuates from one hundred to several thousand cases annually. Vector control and mass inoculation have virtually eliminated endemicity in the Americas and greatly reduced the incidence in Africa.

Two hemorrhagic fevers, **dengue hemorrhagic fever** and **breakbone fever**, are transmitted by several species of *Aedes*. The former is endemic in Southeast Asia; most recently, it has assumed epidemic proportions in 14 countries in the Americas and in several countries in Asia, the Pacific islands, and Africa. Dengue is now considered the most important mosquito-borne disease affecting humans, with 2.5 billion people at risk globally. It has a mortality rate of about 5%, with most fatal cases among children. Breakbone fever is nonlethal and is characterized by a rash, high fever, and pain in the joints. It has been reported in Japan, New Guinea, northern Australia, the Philippines, Hawaii, and most recently Mexico and the southwestern United States.

In the United States and parts of Latin America, viral encephalitides, such as **Western** and **Eastern equine encephalitis, St. Louis encephalitis**, and **Venezuelan equine encephalitis**, are usually nonlethal. Culicine mosquitoes are the principal vectors, and transmission is from birds to horses or humans, both of which are dead ends in the transmission sequence. A similar but more serious disease, **Japanese B encephalitis**, occurs in Japan.

Blackflies

Onchocerca volvulus, the causative agent of human onchocerciasis (see pp. 390–392), is transmitted by the blackflies *Simulium*

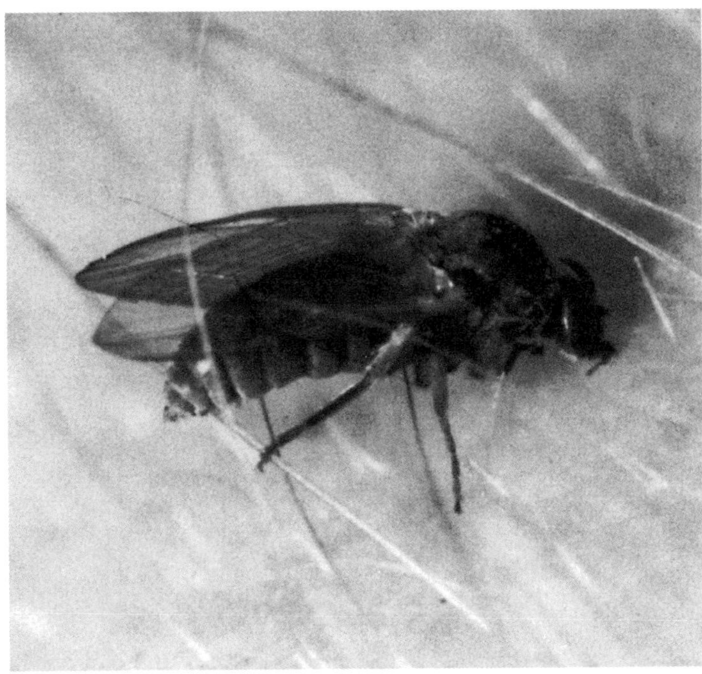

FIGURE 18-9
Blackfly, *Simulium damnosum*, taking a blood meal from a human.

damnosum (Fig. 18-9) and *S. neavei* in Africa and *S. ochraceum*, *S. callidum*, and *S. metallicum* in Mexico, Central America, and South America. Females of *Simulium* spp. deposit eggs in fast-flowing water ranging from streams to large rivers; in the latter, eggs are deposited most abundantly where there are rapids and in areas below dams. The hatched larvae and resulting pupae remain in the aquatic habitat. Adult female flies feed on the blood of a variety of mammals, including humans. In addition to transmitting onchocerciasis to humans, the bites of blackflies can themselves be troublesome, frequently producing severe reactions.

Sandflies

Phlebotomine sandflies (Fig. 18-10) transmit three different types of organisms pathogenic to humans. The viral disease, **sandfly fever**, occurs in the Mediterranean region, central Asia, southern China, parts of India, Sri Lanka, and parts of South America. Of short duration, it is not considered serious. In the northwestern regions of South America, sandflies transmit the bacterium *Bar-*

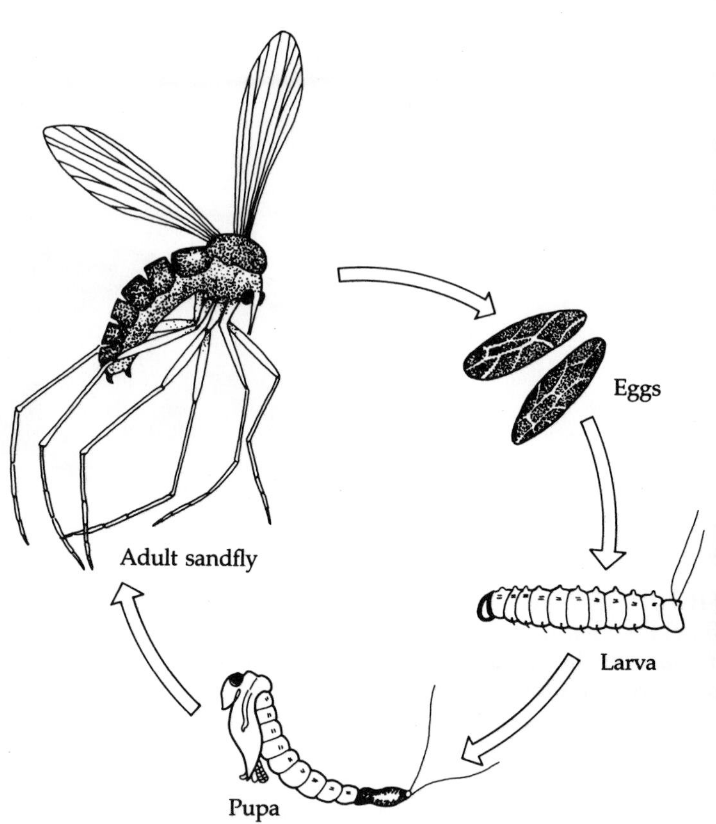

FIGURE 18-10
Stages in the life cycle of the sandfly *Phlebotomus* sp.

tonella bacilliformis, the causative agent of **Corrion's Disease** (**bartonellosis**), a severe, often fatal illness. The third group of pathogens transmitted by sandflies consists of protozoans that cause the various types of **leishmaniasis** (see pp. 101–112).

The phlebotomine sandflies that serve as vectors for these pathogens generally belong to two genera: *Phlebotomus* in the Eastern Hemisphere and *Lutzomyia* in the Western Hemisphere. A small insect, measuring 1.25–2.5 mm long, the sandfly has long, slender legs and short setae covering most of its body parts and wings. The females use piercing–sucking mouthparts to extract juices from plants and blood from various vertebrates, including humans. Sandflies are not strong fliers, usually remaining close to their breeding sites in damp areas rich in organic debris, e.g., under logs and dead leaves, inside hollow trees, and in animal burrows.

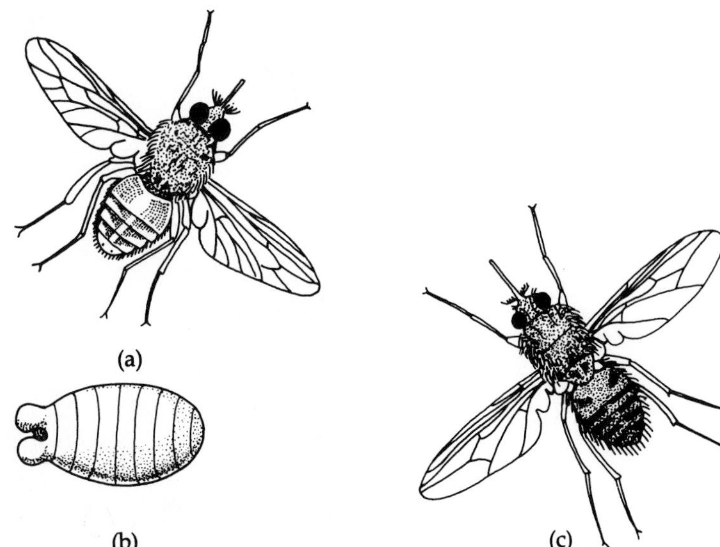

'IGURE 18-11
'setse fly, *Glossina.*
a) *G. palpalis.* (b) Pupa. (c) *G.
ıorsitans.*

Tsetse Flies

Members of the genus *Glossina* (Fig. 18-11) are a menace not only because they are vectors for **African trypanosomiasis** (see pp. 112–120) but also because both male and female flies feed on blood and their bites inflict large, painful welts on their victims (Fig. 18-12). Although *Glossina* was once widespread, it is now limited to continental Africa south of the Tropic of Cancer. During the life cycle of this important vector, the female harbors in her body a supply of fertilized eggs that hatch at intervals into larvae that feed from specialized "milk glands." The developing fourth-stage larva is deposited in a shady spot, usually at the base of a tree or shrub, and immediately burrows into the soil and pupates. A single female tsetse fly deposits 8–10 larvae, one at a time, at intervals of 10–12 days each. The adult fly emerges in 3–4 weeks.

Although several species will feed on human blood, they appear to prefer that of wild game. The various species of *Glossina* are ecologically adapted to different locales according to feeding preferences and site choices for larviposition. For instance, the two species that transmit trypanosomiasis breed either under trees near rivers and lakes, taking their blood meals from people at drifts or watering places (West African sleeping sickness), or in

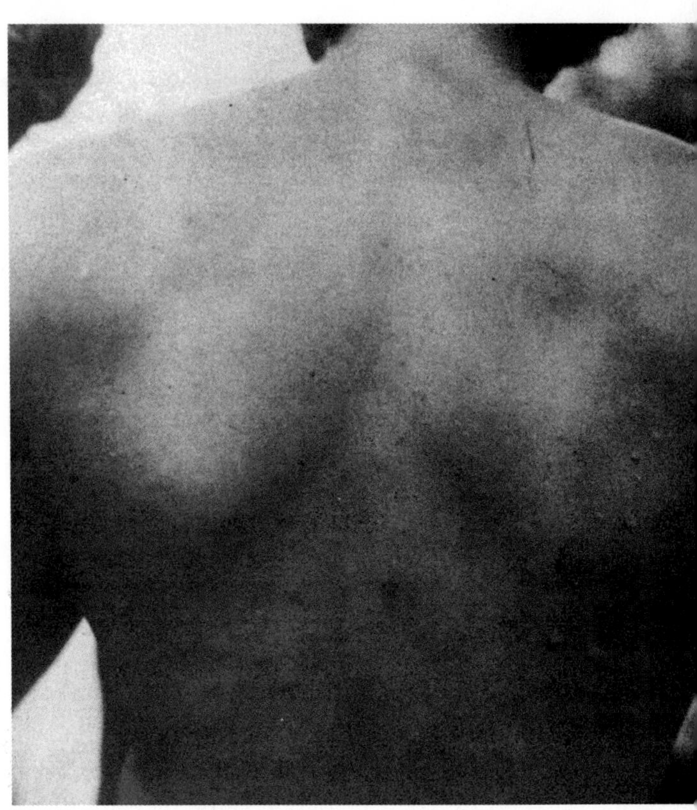

FIGURE 18-12
Tsetse fly welts on human skin.

open woodland, feeding mainly on large game (East Africa sleeping sickness).

Tabanid Flies

Tabanid flies (Fig. 18-13) are large, stoutly built, and oft brightly colored. Strong fliers, they viciously attack a variety mammals, including humans. Only adult females are blood fee ers and, hence, have mouthparts adapted for cutting and pier ing. Members of two genera, *Chrysops* (deerflies) and *Taban* (horseflies) serve as major transmitters of human pathogens.

Tabanid flies are prominent among the arthropod vectors such bacterial diseases of humans and/or animals as **tularem** and **anthrax**. Tularemia, a disease of humans in the United State Canada, northern Europe, the former USSR, Turkey, and Japa is caused by *Francisella tularensis*, for which wild rabbits oft serve as sylvatic reservoir hosts. One of the vectors for *F. t*

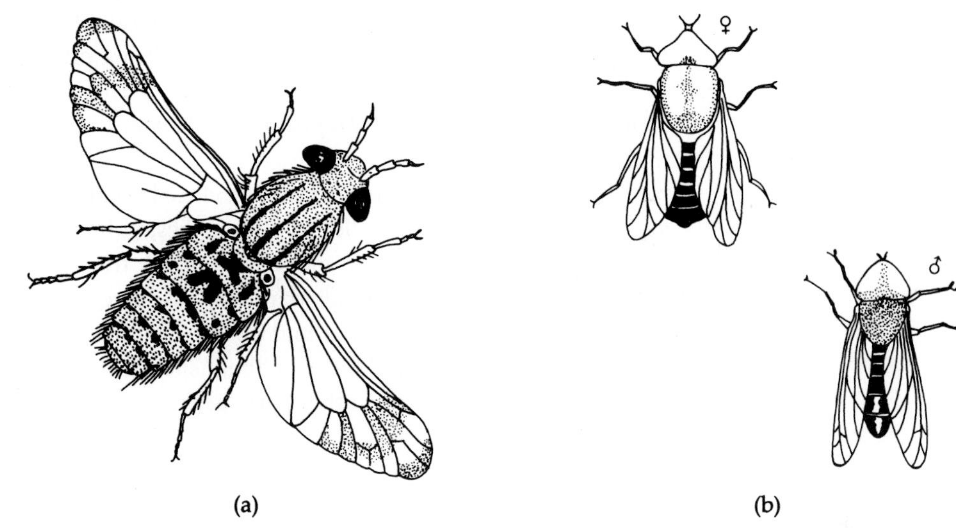

FIGURE 18-13
Tabanid flies.
(a) *Chrysops.* (b) *Tabanus* (male and female).

larensis is *Chrysops discalis*. Anthrax, a much-dreaded disease of cattle caused by *Bacillus anthracis*, is also a serious disease among humans. *Tabanus striatus* and other tabanid flies are common vectors. **Loaiasis**, caused by the African eye worm *Loa loa* (see pp. 393–395) is transmitted to humans by several diurnally feeding species of *Chrysops*, including *C. dimidiata* and *C. silacea*.

NONBITING DIPTERANS

The common housefly (*Musca*), the bluebottle fly, and a number of blowflies (*Calliphora*) are examples of nonbiting dipterans. Adults are nonparasitic and are primarily considered household and farm pests. Nevertheless, they are capable of mechanically transmitting via contaminated appendages a variety of human pathogens, including the bacteria that cause **typhoid fever** (*Salmonella typhi*) and **bacillary dysentery** (*Shigella dysenteriae* and certain strains of *Escherichia coli*). In addition, the causative agents of two eye diseases, **trachoma** and **conjunctivitis**, are transmitted by this group of dipterans. The etiology of the latter two diseases has not been established conclusively. Trachoma is probably caused by a virus of the psittacosis–lymphogranuloma group, while conjunctivitis is attributable to several different bacteria. These flies are also suspected of transmitting other agents of human diseases, such as *Vibrio comma*, the bacterium responsible for **cholera**, and *Treponema pertenue*, the spirochete that causes **yaws**.

A number of other organisms that produce human disease are also commonly associated with nonbiting flies, although there is no direct evidence that these flies act as major transmitters. In fact, one body of opinion holds that only two categories of disease, namely, certain intestinal and ocular disorders, are transmitted by flies and that, like the bedbug, such flies are unjustly maligned as transmitters of other pathogens.

OTHER INSECTS

A significant factor in the epidemiology of diseases transmitted by nondipteran insects is the vastly limited mobility of the three groups in this category (reduviid bugs, fleas, and lice) compared to dipterans. Although reduviid bugs possess functional wings, they are poor fliers. Fleas and lice are wingless.

REDUVIID BUGS

There are about 2500 known species of reduviid, or assassin, bugs (Fig. 18-14). Characteristically, a short, three-jointed proboscis protrudes from the tip of the head. The insects feed primarily on body fluids of other insects, although some attack humans and other animals. They are comparatively large insects, measuring 1.5–2 cm long, and some are brightly colored. Members of three genera, *Triatoma*, *Panstrongylus*, and *Rhodnius*, are the major vectors for **Chagas' disease** (see pp. 120–125). Although several dozen species belonging to these genera occur in various countries of North and South America (Fig. 18-15), relatively few actually serve as significant vectors for Chagas' disease. Most species are arboreal and feed on the blood of wild animals, and their importance lies in their role in maintaining the infection in sylvatic reservoirs. Species that commonly inhabit or occasionally intrude into human dwellings are the major trans-

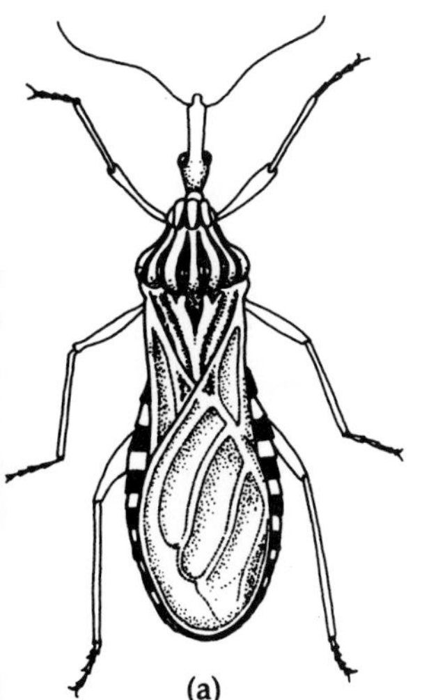

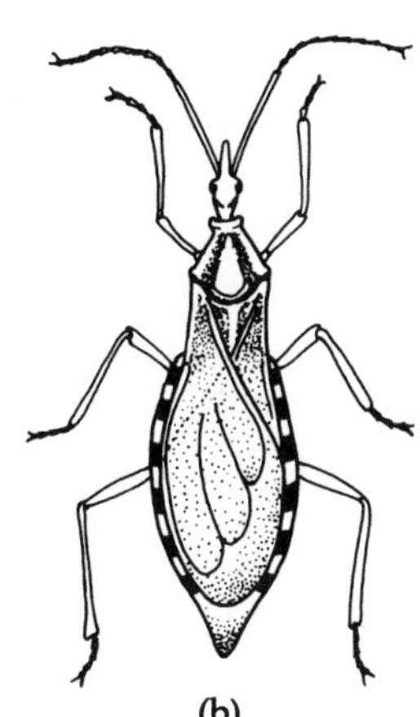

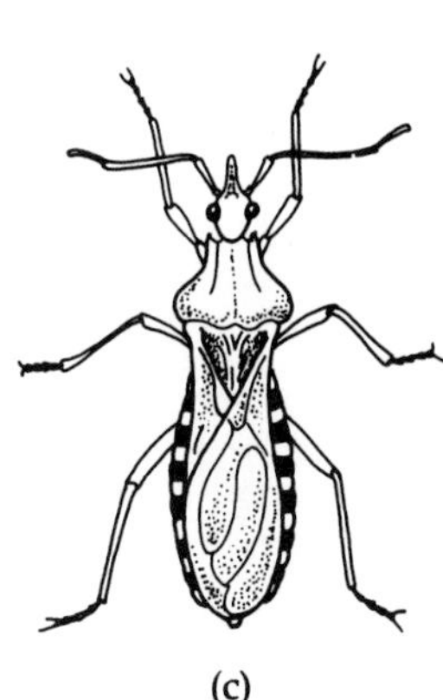

FIGURE 18-14
Some bloodsucking reduviids.
(a) *Triatoma*. (b) *Rhodnius*. (c) *Panstrongylus*.

mitters to humans. Such insects, unlike transient mosquitoes, actually invade the homes and establish stable colonies in cracks and crevices of walls and in thatched roofs. The adults emerge at night for a blood meal once or twice a week. Their bites are painful, often resulting in itchy swellings from toxins injected during feedings. The life cycle is of the hemimetabolous type. The female deposits eggs in wall crevices, furniture, and roofs, and wingless nymphs hatch in 8–30 days. Development to adulthood generally progresses through five nymphal instars to sexual maturity. The cycle is temperature dependent and may require from 6 months to 2 years for completion.

FLEAS

Although the parasitologist's interest in fleas (Fig. 18-16) usually focuses on their blood-sucking habits and their role as intermediate hosts for helminth parasites, the primary concern here is with their role as vectors for pathogenic organisms.

Fleas constitute a small, highly specialized order of insects of obscure origin and evolution. Eggs are deposited by females a few

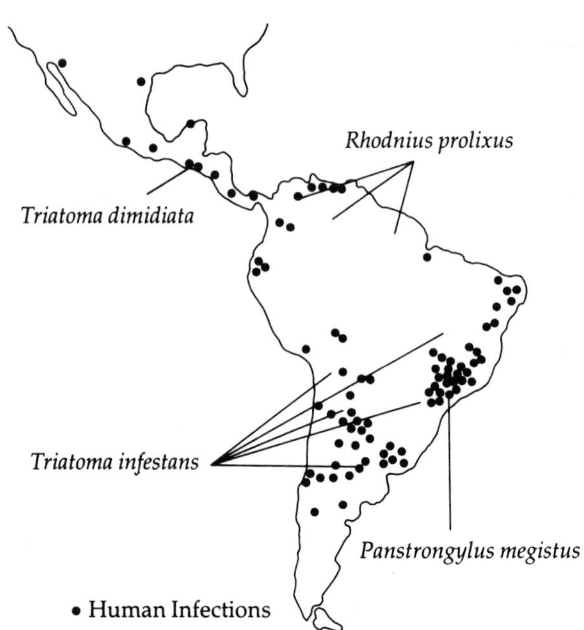

FIGURE 18-15
Distribution of reduviids and Chagas' disease.

at a time, usually 3–20, either on or off the host. When deposited on the host, they soon fall off because they are not adhesive; therefore, they are commonly found in the host's abode. A cephalic spine expedites the hatching of a whitish, legless, vermiform larva with a distinct head; at this stage, the larva resembles those of certain dipterans. The mouthparts of the larva are of the chewing type, and nourishment is derived from decaying vegetable and animal matter. The larval growth period varies from 9 to 200 days, depending on such environmental conditions as humidity, temperature, and oxygen tension. Flea larvae usually undergo two molts, which alternate with growth periods prior to pupation. The duration of the pupation period also depends upon environmental conditions, varying from 7 days to a year.

The adult flea is flattened laterally, wingless, and equipped with muscular hind legs for jumping. The body is covered with backwardly directed spurs and bristles that facilitate the animal's movement through the fur or feathers of the host. Although many fleas are host specific in their blood-feeding habits, others display little specificity.

A notorious organism transmitted by fleas is the bacillus *Yersinia pestis*, which causes **bubonic plague**. During the fourteenth century, the Black Death, as it was commonly called, killed

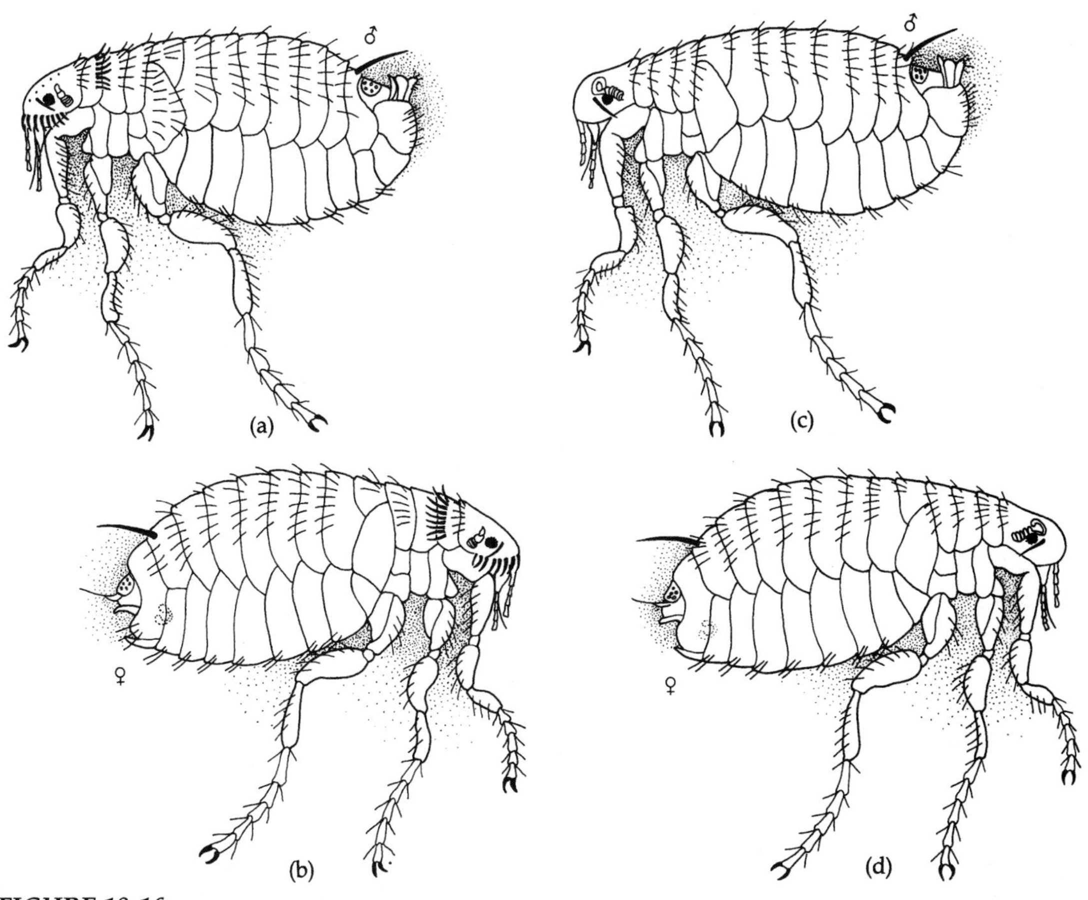

FIGURE 18-16
Fleas.
(a) Male of the cat flea *Ctenocephalides felis*. (b) Female *C. felis*. (c) Male of the Oriental rat flea *Xenopsylla cheopis*. (d) Female *X. cheopis*.

a quarter of the population of Europe. Epidemics in the sixth century and the **Great Plague of London** in 1665 likewise took heavy tolls in human lives. These epidemics probably originated in central Asia and spread via caravans and, later, international shipping. Epidemics recurred as late as the nineteenth century. According to WHO statistics, there are now about 1000–6000 cases of plague annually, and the use of antibiotics and other medications has reduced the annual mortality rate to 100–200. Presently, in the sparsely populated regions of the western and southwestern United States, large numbers of wildlife serve as sylvatic

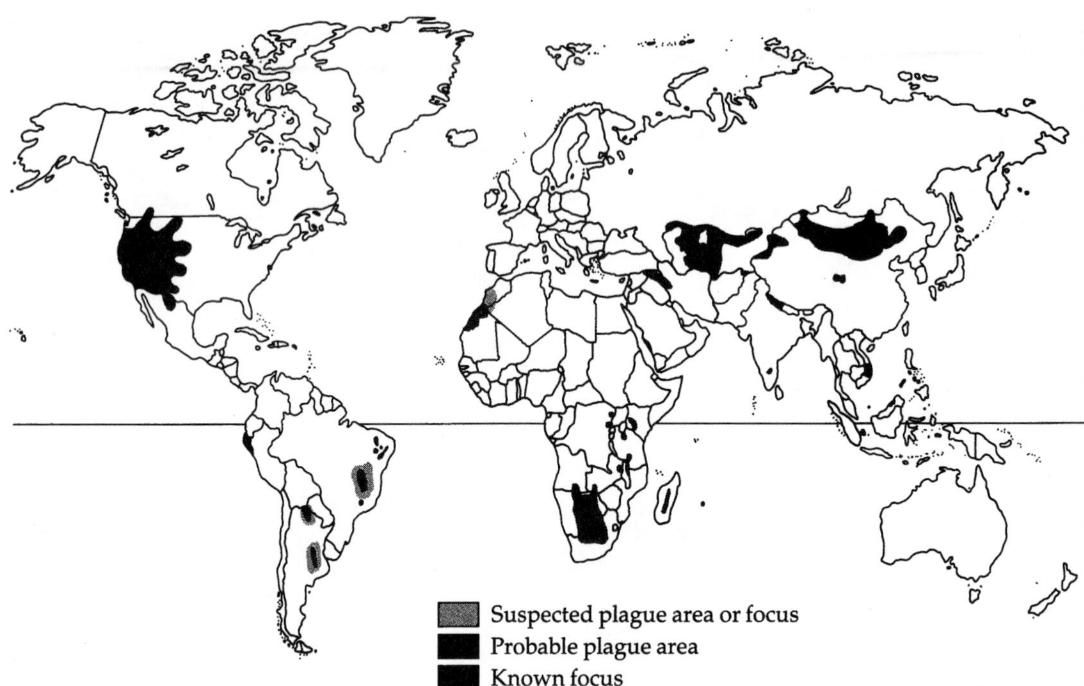

FIGURE 18-17
Distribution of plague throughout the world as of 1969.

reservoirs, harboring the disease-producing bacterium and representing a continual threat of infection to humans who encroach on these environs (Fig. 18-17).

In the usual course of a *Y. pestis* infection, there is an interchange of fleas between wild, infected rodents and domestic rats. The disease spreads rapidly among the domestic rat population, killing a high percentage. Transfer of the infection from rats to humans requires that the flea feed upon both. The common human flea *Pulex irritans*, although capable of parasitizing both humans and domestic animals, rarely feeds on rats and, therefore, is not an important vector of the plague bacillus. However, several species of the genus *Xenopsylla* do feed on both humans and other animal hosts, including rats. *Xenopsylla cheopis*, the Asiatic rat flea, is the most commonly encountered species in this genus and is the major vector for plague bacilli. Presumed to have originated in the Nile Valley, it has spread throughout the world on rat hosts. Male and female fleas acquire the bacilli while feeding on infected rats. The ingested bacilli proliferate in the flea's

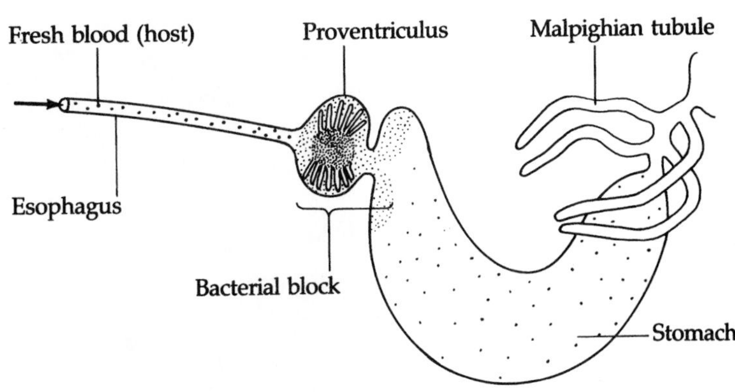

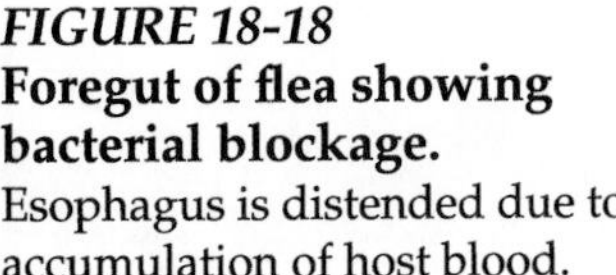
FIGURE 18-18
Foregut of flea showing bacterial blockage.
Esophagus is distended due to accumulation of host blood.

digestive tract and form a semisolid plug, blocking the gut and rendering the flea unable to completely ingest food (Fig. 18-18). In spite of increasing hunger, the flea's repeated attempts to take in blood are futile; during each attempt, extracted blood is regurgitated into the host bloodstream along with portions of the bacterial plug, resulting in the introduction of large numbers of bacilli into the host.

In humans, plague bacilli proliferate in the blood, causing highly lethal **septicemic plague**. Bacilli localize in swellings called **buboes** (Fig. 18-19) in the groin and armpits. The bacterial count

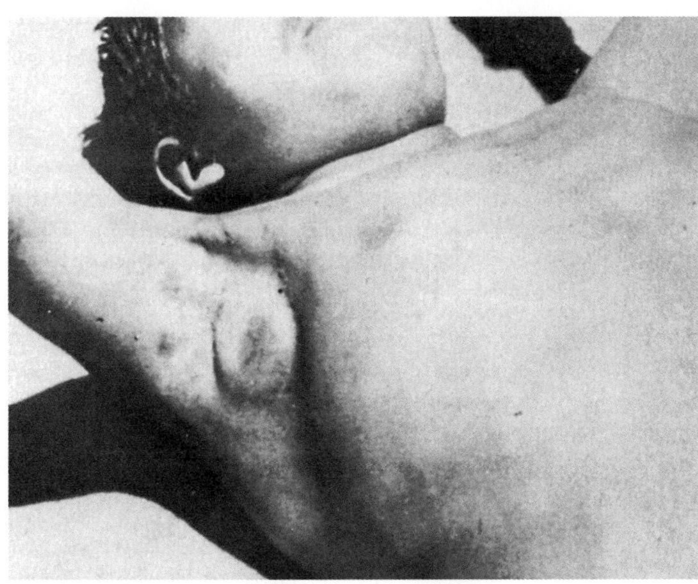
FIGURE 18-19
Plague buboes on human patient.

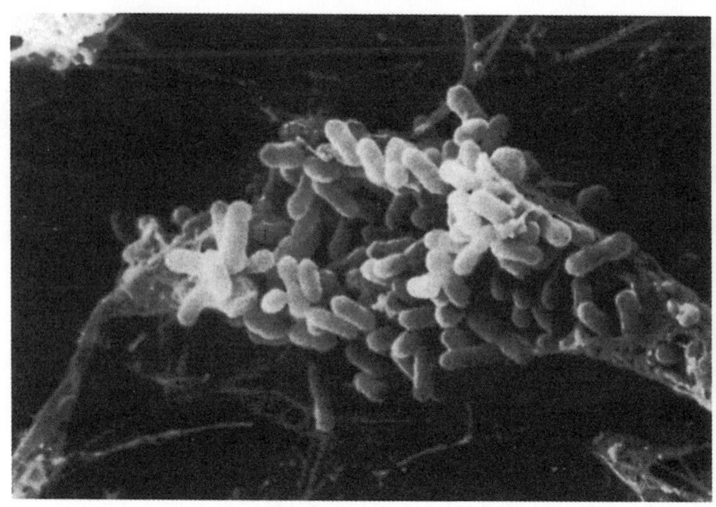

FIGURE 18-20
Scanning electron micrograph of *Rickettsia prowazecki*, the causative agent of epidemic typhus.

in the blood is low, rendering bubonic patients virtually noninfectious to fleas or other humans. This is not the case, however, with the highly contagious and lethal **pneumonic plague**, the form of the disease that affects the lungs. Interhuman transmission of bacilli can result from airborne, contaminated sputum expelled during patients' coughing attacks. In rare instances, transmission to humans results from direct contact with the pelts of infected animals.

In addition to carrying plague, fleas serve as vectors for the **murine** or **endemic typhus** organism *Rickettsia typhi* (Fig. 18–20), transmitted when contaminated flea feces is rubbed into the bite wound. Fleas acquire the rickettsia during feeding from a wide variety of infected animals, including humans, rats, and mice. *Xenopsylla cheopis* is the principal vector for this rickettsia, which causes a mild disease found throughout much of the temperate regions of the world.

Pasteurella tularensis, the tularemia-causing organism, and *Salmonella enteritidis*, the salmonellosis-causing bacterium, are also transmitted to humans by fleas, and fleas serve as intermediate hosts for two tapeworms that infect humans: *Dipylidium caninum* (see pp. 288–289) and *Hymenolepis nana* (see pp. 283–287).

LICE

There are two orders of lice (Fig. 18-21): Mallophaga, the biting lice; and Anoplura, the sucking lice. Mouthparts of the biting

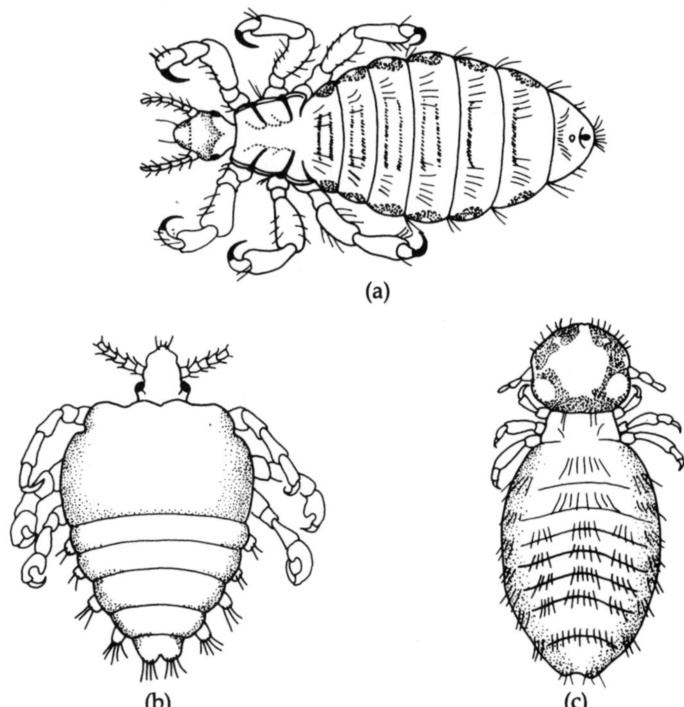

FIGURE 18-21
Lice.
(a) *Pediculus humanus.* (b) *Phthirus pubis.* (c) *Trichodectes canis* of dogs.

louse are of the chewing type but are greatly reduced in size and number and are difficult to analyze without intensive study. Mouthparts of the sucking louse consist of an eversible set of five stylets through which the louse can suck host blood.

One of the mallophagans, *Trichodectes latus*, merits attention as a transmitter of a potential human pathogen. It serves as an intermediate host for the dog tapeworm *Dipylidium caninum,* an occasional parasite of humans (see pp. 288–289).

The anopluran, *Pediculus humanus*, or body louse, is an ectoparasite of several animals, including humans, and the major vector for three important human diseases: **relapsing fever, louse-borne** or **epidemic typhus,** and **trench fever.** A second anopluran species of medical importance is *Phthirus pubis,* the crab louse, which has been induced to transmit typhus-producing rickettsiae to laboratory animals. However, the body louse is the chief vehicle for transmission of this disease in nature.

Lice live in intimate contact with their human hosts. Because lice are wingless and sluggish in movement, new infestations usually occur only through direct physical contact between humans. Low standards of personal hygiene, especially when exacerbated by warfare or disaster, create a favorable climate for louse infestation and, therefore, the spread of louse-borne diseases.

Relapsing fever is a cosmopolitan disease caused by the spirochaete *Borrelia recurrentis*. The body louse ingests the spirochaete while feeding upon an infected host. *Borrelia recurrentis* lives and reproduces in the hemocoel of the louse, where it apparently can survive for the life of the vector with no adverse effect upon the insect. Because the spirochaete has no available egress from the louse, transmission occurs when the louse's body is crushed and its contaminated body fluids enter the human host through mucus membranes or breaks in the skin. Louse-borne relapsing fever, an exclusively human disease, is characterized by intermittent high fever and rash and has a mortality rate of under 10%. The symptoms resemble those of typhus; consequently, the two were not recognized as distinct diseases until 1840.

Louse-borne, or epidemic, typhus is an ancient disease; once much dreaded, it is now limited to Asia, North Africa, and Central and South America. Caused by the rickettsia *Rickettsia prowazeki,* the last great typhus epidemic occurred in Europe immediately after World War I, with an estimated death toll of more than 3 million people. Unlike the spirochaete responsible for relapsing fever, the typhus organism is transmitted from the feces of the louse. When ingested by the louse in a blood meal from an infected human, rickettsiae invade the epithelial cells of the insect's stomach, where they multiply. The cells eventually burst, releasing large numbers of the infective organism into the louse's gut, whence they exit with feces. Damage to the louse's intestinal tract is so extensive that ingested blood diffuses into the hemocoel in such quantities that the insect turns red and usually dies. The contaminated feces quickly dries into a fine powder that remains infective for several months. Rickettsiae are inhaled by human hosts, penetrate the mucus membranes of the eyes, or are rubbed into breaks in the skin along with contaminated louse feces. The disease is characterized by high fever accompanied by headache, nausea, delirium, and stupor, usually followed by the appearance of a dull, mottled rash on the body. Untreated victims either recover spontaneously or die in about two weeks, with a higher mortality rate among elderly victims than among children. Those who survive the disease may harbor infective organisms for many years.

Similar to but milder than typhus, trench fever is caused by a rickettsia, *Rochalimaea quintana*, and transmitted by contaminated louse feces. Unlike *R. prowazeki*, *R. quintana* is an extracellular pathogen in humans, causing typhuslike symptoms that culminate in a rash that disappears within 24 hours. The disease is debilitating but rarely fatal and, except for a few isolated outbreaks, rarely occurs today. However, it was one of the most common diseases during World Wars I and II.

THE ACARINES

Ticks are the major acarine vectors of human disease-producing organisms, with mites playing a far lesser role. The acarine life cycle is similar to that of a number of other blood-feeding arthropods. Females lay clusters of eggs, from which hexapod larvae emerge in 1–4 weeks. The larvae and all subsequent stages are blood-feeders. Larvae metamorphose through four or five 8-legged nymphal stages, the final molt culminating in the adult stage. In some tick species, such as *Ixodes dammini*, the life cycle may extend over a period of up to 2 years.

TICKS

These acarines (Fig. 18-22) are classified into two groups: soft ticks and hard ticks. One distinguishing characteristic is the relationship of the mouthparts to the rest of the body. In soft ticks, the mouthparts are completely concealed by the soft body; in hard ticks, they project from the body. Hard ticks also possess hard, shiny shields that cover the dorsal surface completely in the male but do so only partially in the female.

The two tick groups are also ecologically distinct. Soft ticks hide in cracks and crevices of houses, animal burrows, and similar areas during daylight hours, emerging at night to feed on host blood and to lay eggs. Hard ticks, on the other hand, spend most of their lives on their hosts, the major portion of that time gorging on blood. Female hard ticks produce far more eggs than their soft-bodied counterparts and usually die following oviposition. Some species of hard ticks spend their entire lives on one host; other species utilize two or even three hosts. In multihost species, the ticks drop off the host animals indiscriminately, thereby infesting large areas of land.

Ornithodoros spp., soft-bodied ticks, transmit to humans sev-

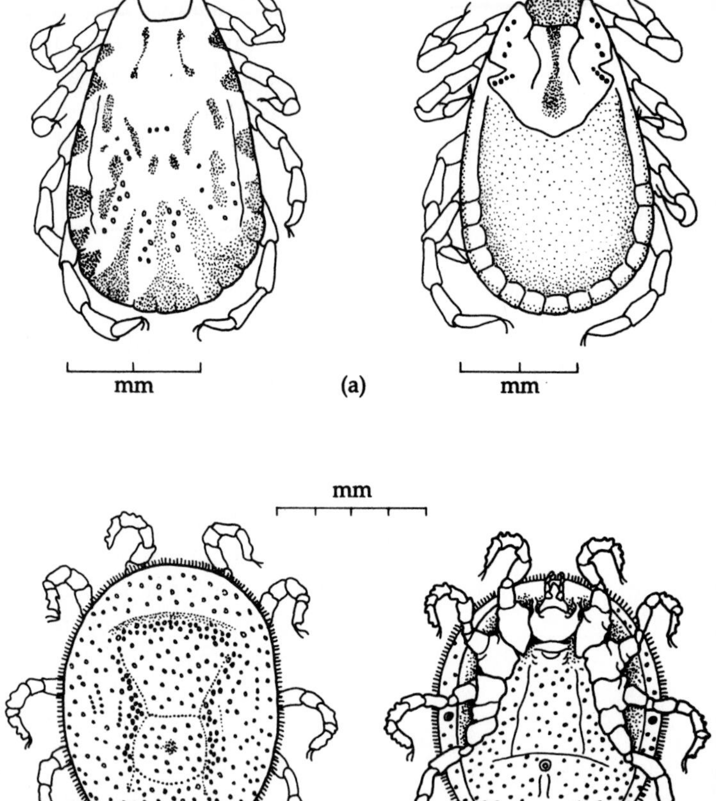

FIGURE 18-22
Ticks.
(a) Hard tick, *Dermacentor andersoni* (male left, female right). (b) Soft tick; *Ornithodoros moubata* (dorsal aspect left, ventral aspect right).

eral species of the spirochaete genera *Spirochaeta* and *Borrelia.* These bacteria cause **tick-borne relapsing fever,** a disease often endemic in tropical and subtropical regions of the world. Because of this endemicity, visitors, such as campers and hunters, are apt to suffer more acutely than natives, whose symptoms tend to be mild as a result of an aquired tolerance.

Like most tick-borne diseases, relapsing fever is zoonotic, being transmitted from wild rodents and other small mammals to humans. Spirochaetes, ingested by a tick during a blood meal, gradually spread throughout the body of the arthropod, with those invading the salivary glands most likely to be transmitted to a vertebrate host during subsequent feeding.

Symptoms of the disease are similar to those of the louse-borne variety. The primary attack, characterized by severe headache and high fever, lasts a few days and, if left untreated, is usually followed by several relapses occurring at short intervals. The patient usually recovers after 3–6 relapses, although in the African variety there may be as many as 11 relapses.

A group of closely related rickettsial diseases are transmitted by hard ticks. **Rocky Mountain spotted fever**, caused by *Rickettsia rickettsia*, is indigenous to North America, and **tick-borne typhus**, caused by *Rickettsia conorii*, is found throughout the world. Although Rocky Mountain spotted fever is considered a dangerous disease if left untreated, most tick-borne rickettsial diseases are not particularly serious. They are usually zoonotic, with humans rarely being sources of the organisms.

Dermacentor andersoni is the principal vector for *R. rickettsia* in the Rocky Mountain states, and *D. variabilis*, the American dog tick, is the principal vector in the central and eastern states. Several species of *Rhipicephalus* serve as vectors for *R. conorii* in Africa and the Mediterranean area. The rickettsiae, acquired when the tick feeds on an infected vertebrate, spread throughout the body of the arthropod, causing no apparent harm. The microorganisms penetrate both the egg cells in the ovaries and the cells of the salivary glands, allowing transmission of the rickettsiae to progeny as well as to other animals. Numerous wild animals serve as reservoirs for *R. rickettsia*, while *R. conorii* is harbored only by canines.

Symptoms of Rocky Mountain spotted fever are high fever accompanied by chills, headache, and, at times, a typhuslike stupor. These symptoms are followed in 4–5 days by the appearance of a rash over the entire body. The disease, sometimes fatal to older patients, is far more pernicious than tick-borne typhus, which is rarely fatal.

Another hard tick, *Ixodes scapularis* (Fig. 18-23), is the principal vector for the spirochaete *Borrelia burgdorferi*, the causative agent of **Lyme disease** or **Lyme borreleosis** in the United States. Lyme disease is currently considered the most frequently diagnosed tick-transmitted disease of humans in the United States and possibly the world. It was estimated in 1993 that Lyme disease represented 81% of all tick-borne diseases, with more than 40,000 human cases of the disease reported worldwide.

First reported in 1975 in Lyme, Connecticut, Lyme disease has now been found in Europe, Australia, the former USSR, China, Japan, and Africa. The disease, which produces symptoms similar to those of rheumatoid arthritis, begins as a rash at the site where the tick takes a blood meal. Fatigue, fever, chills, and headache may

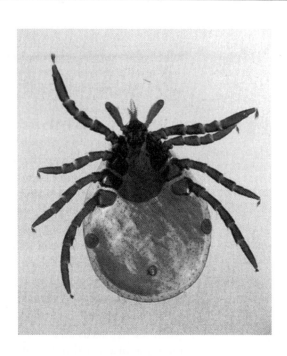

FIGURE 18-23
Light microscope view of *Ixodes* spp.

also occur during this stage, which may last up to 30 days. Neurological complications with muscular pains may then become evident. A small percentage of patients (5%) may also show transitory cardiac malfunctions lasting from 3 days to 6 weeks. Several months after the appearance of the rash, rheumatoid arthritis affecting the knees and other large joints ensues. These symptoms persist indefinitely unless treated. Treatment with any of several broad-spectrum antibiotics has proven effective.

Although ticks are second only to mosquitoes as vectors for viruses, diseases ascribed to such arboviruses are confined mainly to Europe and Asia. Among such diseases are several types of encephalitis, with mortality rates varying from virtually 0% to as high as 25–30%, depending upon the type of virus. Almost all of these diseases are zoonotic, with small mammals and birds serving as sylvatic reservoirs and hard ticks serving as the usual vectors.

MITES

The larvae of harvest mites and allied forms (Fig. 18-24) often remain on hosts for long periods of time, dropping off at random. Like hard ticks, they infest entire, large areas frequented by their hosts and are not limited to nests, dens, or other abodes.

Mites are responsible for the transmission of *Rickettsia tsutsugamushi*, the causative agent for **scrub typhus**, also known as

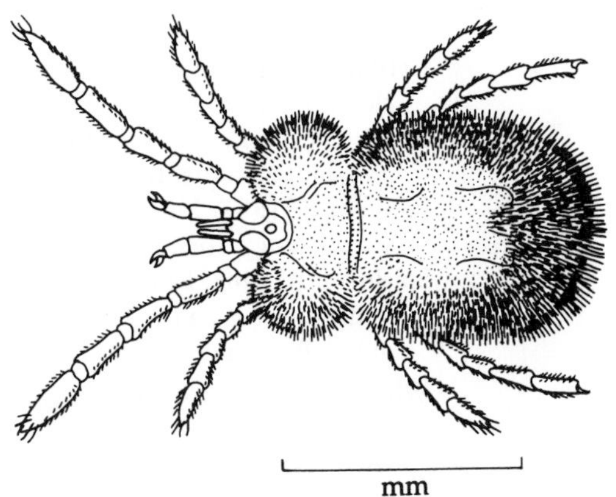

FIGURE 18-24
***Trombicula*, a mite vector of scrub typhus.**

"mite disease" or tsutsugamushi fever. Scrub typhus occurs over large areas of Asia, including Japan and the southern part of the former USSR. Humans become infected from the bite of larval chigger mites of the genus *Leptotrombidium*. The larval mites that serve as vectors acquire the rickettsiae from natural reservoir hosts such as voles, rats, and other small mammals. The rickettsiae are then harbored in the mites' salivary glands, whence they are transmitted to human hosts. The infected mite carries the rickettsial population throughout its entire development from nymph to adult, and even though the adult mite is free living and feeds on insect eggs and minute arthropods, it passes the rickettsiae on, via the egg, to the next generation.

The pathology of the disease ranges from mild to grave. Symptoms usually appear after an incubation period of 4–10 days following the bite of an infected larval mite. An ulcer commonly forms at the site of the bite, and symptoms such as high fever and headache are common.

SELECTED READINGS

Beati, L., and Raoult, D. 1998. Mediterranean spotted fever and other spotted fever group rickettsiae. In *Zoonoses* (Palmer, S. R., Soulsby, E. J. L., and Simpson, D. I. H., Eds.), pp. 217–240, Oxford University Press, Oxford, England.

Bennett, C. E. 1996. Ticks and Lyme disease. *Advances in Parasitology* **36**, 344–405.

Busvine, J. R. 1979. Arthropods: Vectors of disease. In *Studies in Biology*. Edward Arnold, London.

Jonas, G. 1978. Africa: Taming of the tsetse. *RF Illustrated* **4**, 1–4.
Kettle, D. S. 1995. *Medical and Veterinary Entomology* (CAB International Publication). Oxford University Press, Oxford, England.
McDaniel, B. 1979. *How to Know the Ticks and Mites.* William C. Brown, Dubuque, IA.
Piesman, J. 1987. Emerging tick-borne diseases in temperate climates. *Parasitology Today* **3**, 197–199.
Spielman, A. 1988. Lyme disease and human babesiosis: Evidence incriminating vector and reservoir hosts. In *The Biology of Parasitism* (Englund, P. T., and Sher, A., Eds.), pp. 147–165. Alan R. Liss, New York.
White, D. J. 1998. Lyme disease. In *Zoonoses* (Palmer, S. R., Soulsby, E. J. L., and Simpson, D. I. H., Eds.), pp. 144–153. Oxford University Press, Oxford, England.

CLASSIFICATION OF THE ARTHROPODA*

PHYLUM ARTHROPODA

Subphylum Uniramia

CLASS INSECTA

ORDER DIPTERA

With functional forewings and reduced, knoblike hindwings (halteres); mouthparts variable (piercing–sucking or rasping–lapping) as is body form; complete metamorphosis.

Family Simulidae

Bodies short and stout. Thorax much arched, giving humpbacked appearance; legs comparatively short; antennae 10- or 11-jointed, slightly longer than head; ocelli absent; compound eyes on males large and contiguous, those on females widely separated; proboscis not elongate; palpi 4-jointed. (Genus mentioned in text: *Simulium.*)

Family Psychodidae

Bodies mothlike; antennae slender, clothed with whorls of hair, long in males; wings with 9–11 mm long, parallel veins, with no cross-veins except at base. (Genera mentioned in text: *Phlebotomus, Lutzomyia.*)

*Only those taxa that include organisms mentioned in the text are included.

Family Culicidae

Bodies slight; abdomen long and slender; wings narrow; antennae with 15 segments, plumose in males; proboscis long and slender; wings with fringe of scale-like setae on margins; compound eyes large, occupying a large portion of surface of head; ocelli lacking. (Genera mentioned in text: *Aedes*, *Anopheles*, *Culex*, *Mansonia*.)

SUPERFAMILY BRACHYCERA

Family Tabanidae

Bodies comparatively large, 7–30 mm long; wings well developed with veins evenly distributed; eyes large and widely separated (dichoptic) in females, contiguous in males (holoptic); antennae usually short and three-jointed, third joint with 4–8 annuli. (Genera mentioned in text: *Chrysops*, *Tabanus*.)

Suborder Cyclorrapha

SUPERFAMILY (OR GROUP) SCHIZOPHORA

Family Muscidae

Typical flies; hypopleural or pteropleural bristles present; basal abdominal bristles reduced, antennae plumose. (Genera mentioned in text: *Musca*, *Glossina*.)

Family Calliphoridae

Bodies, especially abdomens, metallic green or blue, less frequently violet or copper colored; large; antennae plumose; hypo- and pteropleural bristles present; posteriormost posthumeral bristle present and more ventral than presutural bristle; second ventral abdominal sclerite with edges overlying or in contact with ventral edges of corresponding dorsal sclerites. (Genus mentioned in text: *Calliphora*.)

ORDER HEMIPTERA

Primarily ectoparasitic; bodies medium sized; with piercing–sucking mouthparts forming a beak; antennae 6- to 10-segmented; eyes compound and large; with two pairs of wings; **corium** (thickened portion) present at base of outer wing; thinner extremities of outer wing overlapping on dorsum when insect is at rest; wing venation reduced; abdomen without cerci; holometabolous metamorphosis.

Family Reduviidae

Beak short, three-jointed, attached to tip of head; distal end of beak resting on prosternum in groove when not in use; ocelli present in winged species (with few exceptions); antennae four-jointed. (Genera mentioned in text: *Triatoma, Rhodnius, Panstrongylus.*)

ORDER COLEOPTERA

Few species endoparasitic in other insects; with two pairs of wings; forewings (elytra) veinless, hard, covering dorsal aspect of abdomen while in resting position, meeting along middorsal line; mouthparts of chewing type; antennae of 10–14 segments; compound eyes conspicuous; legs heavily sclerotized; holometabolous metamorphosis. (Genus mentioned in text: *Tenebrio.*)

ORDER SIPHONAPTERA

Adults small and wingless; ectoparasitic on birds and mammals; bodies laterally compressed; legs long, stout, and spinose; antennae short and clubbed, fitting in depressions along side of head when not extended; mouthparts of piercing–sucking type; holometabolous metamorphosis.

Family Pulicidae

Three thoracic tergites together longer than first abdominal tergite; head evenly rounded along margin; no vertical suture from dorsal margin of head to bases of antennae; abdominal tergites with one row of setae. (Genera mentioned in text: *Pulex, Xenopsylla.*)

ORDER MALLOPHAGA

Ectoparasitic on birds and mammals; bodies of small to medium size, usually dorsoventrally flattened and wingless; with chewing mouthparts; antennae short, with three to five segments; with reduced compound eyes and no ocelli; thorax small; legs stout and short; no cerci on abdomen; hemimetabolous metamorphosis.

Suborder Ischnocera

Antennae three- or five-segmented, filiform, not concealed; maxillary palpi absent, mandibles vertically oriented; parasitic on birds and mammals.

Family Trichodectidae

Antennae three-jointed; with one claw on tarsi; parasitic on mammals. (Genus mentioned in text: *Trichodectes.*)

ORDER ANOPLURA

Ectoparasites of mammals; bodies of small to medium size, dorsoventrally flattened, and wingless; mouthparts modified as piercing–sucking organ that is retractile; antennae short, with three to five segments; some with legs terminating as hooked claws; thorax fused; abdomen of five to eight distinct segments; hemimetabolous metamorphosis.

Family Pediculidae

Parasites of primates, including humans; bodies fairly robust, not covered with dense spines; abdomen armed with pleural plates (paratergites) and with tergal and sternal plates in most species; with well-developed eyes, comprised of pigment granules and a lens; with legs approximately equal in length or with first pair slightly smaller. (Genera mentioned in text: *Pediculus*, *Phthirus*.)

Subphylum Chelicerata

ORDER ACARINA

Highly specialized arachnids with body divided into proterosoma and hysterosoma, distinguishable as boundary between second and third pairs of legs; segments of mouth and its appendages situated on capitulum (gnathostoma), more or less sharply set off from rest of body; typically with four pairs of legs; usually six podomeres of legs but may vary from two to seven; positions of respiratory and genital openings variable.

Suborder Metastigmata (Ixodides)

Large, parasitic acarines known as ticks; mouth with recurved teeth modified for piercing; tracheal spiracle located behind third or fourth pair of coxae.

Family Ixodidae (Hard Ticks)

Body ovoid; scutum present in all stages; scutum of adult males extending to posterior margin of body; scutum of adult females, like that of larvae and nymphs, restricted to propodosomal zone; capitulum anterior and visible from dorsal view; festoons usually present; eyes, if present, situated dorsally on sides of scutum; segments of pedipalps fused, not movable; porose areas present on base of capitulum in females; stigmatal plates large, posterior to fourth coxa; only females distended when engorged with blood; with marked sexual dimorphism. (Genera mentioned in text: *Dermacentor, Ixodes, Rhipicephalus*.)

Family Argasidae (Soft Ticks)

Integument leathery in nymphal and adult stages, and wrinkled, granulated, mammillated, or having tubercles; scutum absent in all stages; capitulum either subterminal or protruding from anterior margin of body in nymphs and adults, subterminal or terminal in larvae; capitulum lying in distinctly or indistinctly marked depression (camerostome) in all stages; pedipalps freely articulate in all stages; porose area absent in both sexes; eyes usually absent (if present, on supracoxal folds); stigmata near third coxa lacking stigmal plates; both sexes distended when engorged with blood; sexual dimorphism slight. (Genus mentioned in text: *Ornithodoros*.)

Appendix A

DRUGS FOR PARASITIC INFECTIONS: PARTIAL LIST OF GENERIC AND BRAND NAMES

*__Albendazole__ Zentel (SmithKline Beecham)

Amphotericin B Fungizone (Squibb)

Antimony dimercaptosuccinate (stibocaptate) Astiban (Hoffman-LaRoche, Switzerland)

Benzyl benzoate Scabanca (Anmca Laboratories, Canada); others

**__Bithionol__ Bithin (Tanabe Seiyaku, Japan)

Chloroquine HCl and Chloroquine phosphate Aralen (Winthrop); others

Cupric oleate Cuprex (Beecham Research Laboratories)

Crotamiton Eurax (Ciba-Geigy); Crortan (Alcon Laboratories)

**__Dehydroemetine__ (Hoffman-LaRoche)

*__Diethylcarbamazine citrate__ Hetrazan (Laderle Laboratories)

Diiodohydroxyquin (iodoquinol) (Glenwood Laboratories)

**__Diloxanide furoate__ Furamide (Clin-Comar-Byla)

***__Flubendazole__ similar to Mebendazole (Janssen)

Furazolidone Furoxane (Norwich-Eaton)

***__Halofantrine__ Halfan (SmithKline Beecham)

**__Ivermectin__ Mectizan (Merck & Co.)

*Available in the United States only directly from company.
**Available from Centers for Disease Control Drug Service.
***Not available in the United States.

Lindane (gamma benzene hexachloride) Kwell (Reed & Carnrick); others
Malathion Ovide (GenDerm)
Mebendazole Vermox (Janssen)
Mefloquine Lariam (Roche)
**Melarsoprol Arsobal (Specia)
Metrifonate (trichlorfon) Bilarcil (Bayer)
Metronidazole Flagyl (Searle); others
Niclosamide Yomesan, Niclocide (Bayer)
**Nifurtimox Lampit (Bayer)
Niridazole Ambilhar (Ciba-Geigy)
***Ornidazole Tiberal (Hoffman-LaRoche)
Oxamniquine Vansil (Pfizer)
Paromomycin sulfate Humatin, Aminosidine (Parke, Davis)
Pentamidine isethionate Pentam 300, NebuPent (Rhône-Poulenc)
Permethrin Nix (Burroughs, Wellcome); Elimite (Herbert)
Piperazine citrate Antepar (Burroughs, Wellcome); others
Praziquantel Biltricide (Bayer)
Primaquine diphosphate Primaquine (Winthrop)
***Proguanil Paludrine (Ayerst)
Pyrantel pamoate Antiminth (Roerig)
Pyrethrins and Piperonyl butoxide Rid (Pfizer); others
Pyrimethamine Daraprim (Burroughs, Wellcome)
Pyrimethamine plus Sulfadoxine Fansidar (Hoffman-LaRoche)
Pyrvinium pamoate Povan (Parke, Davis)
***Quinacrine HCl Atabrine (Winthrop)
***Quinine dihydrochloride and sulfate (many companies)
**Sodium stibogluconate (antimony sodium gluconate) Pentostam (Burroughs, Wellcome)
*Spiramycin Rovamycine (Rhodia Pharma GmbH)
**Suramin sodium Germanin (Bayer)
Thiabendazole Mintezol (Merck Sharpe & Dohme)
***Tinidazole Fasigyn (Pfizer)
Trimethoprim–sulfamethoxazole Bactrim (Hoffman-LaRoche); Septra (Burroughs, Wellcome)
***Tryparsamide

Appendix B

CURRENT CHEMOTHERAPEUTIC REGIMENS

Infection	Drug	Adult Dosage	Pediatric Dosage
Amoebiasis (*Entamoeba histolytica*)			
Asymptomatic			
Drug of Choice:	Diloxanide furoate	500 mg 3 × day/10 days	20 mg/kg/day in 3 doses/10 days
Alternative(s):	Diiodohydroxyquin	650 mg 3 × day/20 days	30–40 mg/kg/day in 3 doses/20 days
	Paromomycin sulfate	25–30 mg/kg/day in 3 doses/7 days	25–30 mg/kg/day in 3 doses/7 days
Mild to Moderate Intestinal Disease			
Drugs of Choice:	Metronidazole	30 mg/kg day/8–10 days	30 mg/kg/day/8–10 days
	or Tinidazole	2 g/day/3 days	2 g/day/3 days
	or Ornidazole	2 g/day/10 days	2 g/day/10 days
	or Secnidazole	2 g in single dose	2 g in single dose
Invasive Amoebiasis			
Drugs of Choice:	Metronidazole	30 mg/kg/day/8–10 days	
	or Tinidazole	2 g/day/5 days	
	or Ornidazole	2 g in single dose	
	or Secnidazole	1.5 g/day/5 days	
Amoebic Meningoencephalitis (*Naegleria* spp., *Acanthamoeba* spp.)			
Drug of Choice:	Amphotericin B	1 mg/kg/day, uncertain duration	1 mg/kg/day, uncertain duration > 2 yrs old
Acylostomiasis (*Ancylostoma duodenale, Nectator americanus,* Hookworm)			
Drugs of Choice:	Mebendazole	100 mg/2 × day/3 days	100 mg/2 × day/3 days/>2 yrs old
	or Albendazole	100 mg/2 × day/3 days	100 mg/2 × day/3 days/>2 yrs old
	or Flubendazole	100 mg/2 × day/3 days	100 mg/2 × day/3 days/>2 yrs old
	or Pyrantel pamoate	1 dose/11 mg/kg (max 1 g)	1 dose/11 mg/kg (max 1 g)
Anisakiasis (*Anasakis* spp.)			
Treatment of Choice:	Surgical Removal		
Alternative:	Thiabendazole	25 mg/kg/day/3 days	25 mg/kg/day/3 days
Ascariasis (*Ascaris lumbricoides*)			
Drug of Choice:	Pyrantel pamoate	1 dose 11mg/kg (max 1 g)	1 dose 11 mg/kg (max 1 g)
Babesiosis (*Babesia* spp.)			
Chloroquine has been used and produces symptomatic improvement but does not reduce parasitemia. Pentamidine isethionate also has been used. A combination of quinine and clindamycin has been reported to be successful in a few patients.			
Balantidiosis (*Balantidium coli*)			
Drug of Choice:	Tetracycline	500 mg/4 × day/10 days	500 mg/4 × day/10 days
Alternative:	5-nitroimidazole	2 g/day/3 days	2 g/day/3 days
***Brugia malayi* (see Filariasis)**			
Chagas' Disease (see Trypanosomiasis)			

Cutaneous Larval Migrans (*Ancylostoma braziliense, A. caninum*)			
Drug of Choice:	Thiabendazole	25 mg/kg/2×day/2 days (topically or orally)	25 mg/kg/2×day/2 days (topically or orally)
Calamine lotion provides symptomatic relief			
Dientamoebiasis (*Dientamoeba fraqilis*)			
Drug of Choice:	Diloxanide	500 mg/3 × day/10 days	20 mg/kg/day in 3 divided doses/10 days
Dracunculiasis (*Dracunculus medinensis*)			
Drug of Choice:	Metronidazole	25 mg/kg/day/10 days	25 mg/kg/day/10 days
Alternative:	Mebendazole	1 dose/100 mg; repeat after 2 wks	1 dose/100 mg/>2 yrs old; repeat after 2 wks
Enterobiasis (*Enterobius vermicularis*)			
Drugs of Choice*:	Mebendazole	1 dose/100 mg; repeat after 2 wks	1 dose/100 mg/> 2yrs old; repeat after 2 wks
*All members of	or Albendazole	1 dose/400 mg	1 dose/400 mg/> 2 yrs old
household should	or Pyrantel	1 dose 10 mg/kg;repeat after 2–4 wks	
be treated concurrently	or Piperazine citrate	65 mg/kg/day (max 2.5 g/day)/7 days; repeat after 2 wks	65 mg/kg/day (max 2.5 g/day)/7 days; repeat after 2 wks
Filariasis (*Wuchereria bancrofti; Brugia malayi; Loa loa*)			
Drug of Choice:	Diethylcarbamazine citrate*	Day 1: 50 mg Day 2: 50 mg/3×day Day 3: 100 mg/3×day Days 4–21: 2 mg/kg/3×day	Day 1: 25–50 mg Day 2: 25–50 mg/3×day Day 3: 50–100 mg/3×day Day 4: 2 mg/kg/3×day
		*Under 10 yrs, half total adult dosage	
Giardiasis (*Giardia lamblia*)			
Drug of Choice:	Metronidazole	2 g/day/3 days	15 mg/kg/day in divided doses/5–10 days
Leishmaniasis (*Leishmania tropica; L. major*)			
Drug of Choice:	Sodium stibogluconate	Local therapy; injection of 1–3 ml into base of lesion, repeat once or twice	
Leishmaniasis mexicana (*Leishmania mexicana*, American Cutaneous Leishmaniasis)			
Drug of Choice:	Sodium stibogluconate	Inject 20 mg Sb5+/kg day intramuscularly until skin smears are negative for at least 4 wks. In case of relapse, pentamidine should be used (inject 4 mg/kg 3 times/wk/5–25 wks or longer)	
Leishmaniasis donovani (*Leishmania donovani*, Kala Azar, Visceral Leishmaniasis)			
Drug of Choice:	Sodium stibogluconate	Injection 20 mg Sb5+/kg intramuscularly/day (max. 850 mg Sb5+ for a minimum of 20 days)	
Leishmaniasis infantum (*Leishmania infantum*)			
Drug of Choice:	Meglumine antimoniate	Intralesional injection of 1–3 ml; repeat once or twice if no response is apparent at intervals of 1–2 days	

continues

Infection	Drug	Adult Dosage	Pediatric Dosage
Leishmaniasis amazonensis & L. peruviana (***Leishmania amazonensis; L. peruviana***)			
Drugs of Choice:	Meglumine antimoniate or Sodium stibogluconate	Local therapy: inject 1–3 ml into base of lesion; repeat once or twice if no response apparent at intervals of 1–2 days. Systematic therapy: inject 10–20 mg Sb5+/kg intramuscularly daily until skin smears are negative	
Leishmaniasis guyanensis (***Leishmania guyanensis***)			
Drug of Choice:	Pentamidine	Injection of 3–4 mg/kg/1×–2× wk until lesion is no longer visible	
Leishmaniasis panamensis (***Leishmania panamensis***)			
Drugs of Choice:	Meglumine antimoniate or Sodium stibogluconate	Injection of 20 mg Sb5+/kg/day intramuscularly until skin smears are negative for at least 4 wks	
Malaria (***Plasmodium falciparum; P. ovale; P. vivax; P. malariae***)			
For suppression or chemoprophylaxis of malaria while in endemic area for all *Plasmodium* except chloroquine-resistant *P. falciparum*			
Drug of Choice:	Chloroquine	Day 1: 10 mg/kg, then 5 mg/kg 6–8 hrs later Day 2–3: 5 mg/kg in single dose	<50 kg; 5 mg/kg/1× wk and continued for 6 more wks after last exposure to endemic area
For prevention of attack after departure from areas where *P. vivax* and *P. ovale* are endemic			
Drug of Choice:	Primaquine diphosphate	Gametocytocidal therapy: 0.5–0.75 mg/kg one dose	Gametocytocidal therapy: 0.5–0.75 mg/kg one dose
For treatment of *Plasmodium* spp. except chloroquine-reistant *P. falciparum*			
Drug of Choice:	Chloroquine	Total dose: 25 mg/kg over 3 days Day 1: 10 mg/kg, 5 mg/kg 6–8 hrs later Days 2 & 3: 5 mg/kg one dose	Total dose: 25 mg/kg over 3 days Day 1: 10 mg/kg, 5 mg/kg 6–8 hrs later Days 2 & 3: 5 mg/kg one dose
For treatment of severe illness, parental dosage—only if dose cannot be administered, regardless of severity (all *Plasmodium* except chloroquine-resistant *P. falciparum*)			
Drug of Choice:	Quinine	Intravenous: 16.4 mg/kg infused over 4 hrs followed by 8.2 mg/kg every 8 hrs. Initial dose should be halved if patient received quinine, quinidine, or mefloquine during previous 12–24 hrs Oral: 500 mg every 8 hrs for 3, 7, or 10 days	Intravenous: 16.4 mg/kg infused over 4 hrs followed by 8.2 mg/kg every 12 hrs. Initial dose should be halved if patient received quinine, quinidine, or mefloquine during previous 12–24 hrs. Oral: 8.2 mg/kg every 8 hrs for 3, 7, or 10 days
Onchocerciasis (***Onchocerca volvulus***)			
Drug of Choice:	Ivermectin	Annual or biannual single dose of 150 μg/kg	Annual or biannual single dose of 150 μg/kg

Schistosomiasis (***Schistosoma haematobium, S. mansoni, S. japonicum***)			
Drug of Choice:	Praziquantel	One dose 40 mg/kg*	One dose 40 mg/kg*
		*In some areas dosage may be increased to 60 mg/kg	
Alternative for *S. haematobium:*	Metrifonate	7.5 mg/kg 3 occasions at intervals of 2 wks	7.5–10 mg/kg 3 occasions at intervals of 2 wks
Strongyloidiasis (***Strongyloides stercoralis***)			
Drug of Choice:	Albendazole	400 mg for 3 consecutive days	> 2 yrs: 400 mg for 3 consecutive days
Tapeworms (Adult or Intestinal Stage)			
Diphyllobothriasis (***Diphyllobothrium latum,*** **Broadfish Tapeworm**)			
Drug of Choice:	Praziquantel	1 dose 10–25 mg/kg	1 dose 10–25 mg/kg
Alternative:	Niclosamide	1 dose 2 g	< 10 kg: 1 dose 0.5 g 10–35 kg: 1 dose 1 g
Dipylidiasis (***Dipylidium caninum,*** **Dog tapeworm**)			
Drug of Choice:	Niclosamide	One dose, 2 g chewed thoroughly	under 4 yrs: 1 dose/1 g over 4 yrs: 1 dose/1.5 g
Hymenolepiasis (***Hymenolepis nana, H. diminuta***)			
Drug of Choice:	Praziquantel	One dose, 15–25 mg/kg	one dose, 15–25 mg/kg
Alternative:	Niclosamide	one dose, 8 g chewed throughly, then 4 g for 6 days	11–34 kg: 2 g single dose, then 0.5 g/day for 6 days >34 kg: one dose, 4.5 g/1 day, then 2 g/day for 6 days
Taeniasis saginata (***Taenia saginata,*** **Beef tapeworm**)			
Drug of Choice:	Praziquantel	1 dose, 5–10 mg/kg	> 4 yrs: 1 dose, 5–10 mg/kg
Taeniasis solium (***Taenia solium,*** **Beef tapeworm**)			
Drug of Choice:	Praziquantel	1 dose, 5–10 mg/kg	> 4 yrs: 1 dose, 5–10 mg/kg
Tapeworms (Larval or Tissue Stage)			
Cysticercosis (***Taenia solium*** **cysticercus**)			
Drug of Choice:	Praziquantel	Total of 50 mg/kg daily in 3 divided doses for 14 days. Corticosteroid (prednisolone) administered for 2–3 days before and throughout treatment	Total of 50 mg/kg daily in 3 divided doses for 14 days. Corticosteroid (prednisolone) administered for 2–3 days before and throughout treatment
Alternative:	Albendazole	15 mg/kg/daily for 30 days	15 mg/kg/daily for 30 days
Dermal Cysticercosis (***Taenia solium*** **cysticercus**)			
Drug of Choice:	Praziquantel	Total 60 mg/kg daily in 3 divided doses for 6 days	Total 60 mg/kg daily in 3 divided doses for 6 days
Echinococcosis (***Echinococcus granulosus,*** **Hydatid Cyst**)			
Drug of Choice:	Albendazole	400 mg/28 days, repeated as necessary	15 mg/kg/day for 28 days, repeated as necessary

Infection	Drug	Adult Dosage	Pediatric Dosage
Echinococcosis (*Echinococcis mutilocularis*)			
Surgery appears to be the only treatment, although albendazole or mebendazole have been suggested as alternative treatment.			
Toxocariasis (See Visceral Larval Migrans)			
Toxoplasmosis (*Toxoplasma gondii*)			
Drugs of Choice:	Pyrimethamine* and Sulfaiazine	Pregnant women: 25 mg/day for 3–4 wks but not before 2nd trimester Chorioretinitis in adults: 75 mg/day for 3 days	Neonates with no overt disease born to mothers infected during pregnancy: 1 mg/kg/day for 4 wks Neonates with overt disease: 1 mg/kg/day for 6 mos
*Because pyrimethamine has teratogenic potential, it cannot be used during the 1st trimester of pregnancy. Spiramycin, which is less effective, is substituted.			
Trematodes			
Clonorchiasis (*Clonorchis sinensis*)			
Drug of Choice:	Praziquantel	1 dose, 25 mg/kg 3 times/day/2 days	> 4 yrs: 1 dose, 25 mg/kg 3 times/day/2 days
Fascioliasis (*Fasciola hepatica*)			
Drug of Choice:	Praziquantel	25 mg/kg 3 times/day/1 day	25 mg/kg 3 times/1 day
Alternative:	Bithionol	30–50 mg/kg on alternate days, total of 10–15 doses	30–50 mg/kg on alternate days, total of 10–15 doses
Fasciolopsiasis (*Fasciolopsis buski*)			
Drug of Choice:	Praziquantel	25 mg/kg 3 times day/2 days	> 4 yrs: 25 mg/kg 3 times day/2 days
Heterophyidiasis (*Heterophyes heterophyes*)			
Drug of Choice:	Praziquantel	25 mg/kg 3 times day/2 days	> 4 yrs: 25 mg/kg 3 times/2 days
Alternative:	Tetrachoroethylene	0.1–0.12 ml/kg (max. 5 ml)	0.1 ml/kg (max. 5 ml)
Echinostomiasis (*Echinostoma* spp.)			
Drug of Choice:	Praziquantel	25 mg/kg 3 times day/2 days	> 4 yrs: 25 mg/kg 3 times day/2 days
Metagonimiasis (*Metagonimus yokogawai*)			
Drug of Choice:	Praziquantel	25 mg/kg 3 times day/2 days	> 4 yrs: 25 mg/kg 3 times day/2 days
Opisthorchiasis (*Opisthorchis felineus, O. viverrini*)			
Drug of Choice:	Praziquantel	25 mg/kg 3 times day/2 days	> 4 yrs: 25 mg/kg 3 times day/2 days
Paragonimiasis (*Paragonimus* spp.)			
Drug of Choice:	Praziquantel	25 mg/kg 3 times day/2 days	> 4 yrs: 25 mg/kg 3 times day/2 days
Trichomoniasis (*Trichomonas vaginalis*)			
Drug of Choice:	Metronidazole	1 dose, 2 g orally (sexual contacts should be treated at same time)	1 dose, orally, 2 g
Trichuriasis (*Trichuris trichiura*)			
Drugs of Choice:	Albendazole	Mild to moderate infections: 1 dose 400 mg	> 2 yrs: 1 dose 400 mg

	or Mebendazole	Mild to moderate infections: 1 dose 500 mg	> 2 yrs: 1 dose 500 mg
	Albendazole	Heavy infections: 400 mg/day/3 days	
	or Mebendazole	Heavy infections: 500 mg/day/3 days	
	or Flubendazole	Heavy infections: 500 mg/day/3 days	
Trypanosomiasis gambiense (*Trypanosoma brucei gambiense*, West African Sleeping Sickness)			
Drug of Choice:	Pentamidine	Early disease: 4 mg/kg in each of 7–10 intramuscular injections/daily or every other day	
		Late disease:	
		Day 1: Pentamidine, 4 mg/kg intramuscularly	
		Day 2: Pentamidine, 4 mg/kg intramuscularly	
		Day 4: Melarsopol, 1.2 mg/kg	
		Day 5: Melarsopol, 2.4 mg/kg	
		Day 6: Melarsopol, 3.6 mg/kg	
		Day 17: Melarsopol, 1.2 mg/kg	
		Day 18: Melarsopol, 2.4 mg/kg	
		Day 19: Melarsopol, 3.6 mg/kg	
		Day 20: Melarsopol, 3.6 mg/kg	
		Day 30: Melarsopol, 1.2 mg/kg	
		Day 31: Melarsopol, 2.4 mg/kg	
		Days 32–33: Melarsopol, 3.6 mg/kg/day	
Trypanosomiasis rhodesiense (*Trypanosoma brucei rhodesiense*, East African Sleeping Sickness)			
Drug of Choice:	Suramin Sodium	Day 1: Suramin sodium, 5 mg/kg Melarsopol, 5 mg/kg	Same as for adult
		Day 3: Suramin sodium, 10 mg/kg Melarsopol, 10 mg/kg	
		Day 5: Suramin sodium, 20 mg/kg Melarsopol, 20 mg/kg	
		Day 11: Suramin sodium, 20 mg/kg Melarsopol, 20 mg/kg	
		Day 17: Suramin sodium, 20 mg/kg Melarsopol, 20 mg/kg	
		Day 23: Suramin sodium, 20 mg/kg Melarsopol, 20 mg/kg	
		Day 30: Suramin sodium, 20 mg/kg Melarsopol, 20 mg/kg	
Visceral Larval Migrans (*Toxocaris canis, T. cati*)			
Drug of Choice:	Diethylcarbamazine	1 mg/kg/2 times daily raised progressively to 3 mg/kg/2 times/day for total of 20 days	1 mg/kg/2 times daily raised progressively to 3 mg/kg/2 times/day for total of 20 days

Appendix C

ADVERSE EFFECTS OF ANTIPARASITIC DRUGS

Albendazole (*Zentel*)
Occasional: diarrhea; abdominal distress; migration of *Ascaris* through nose and mouth.
Rare: leukopenia; alopecia; increased serum transaminase.

Benznidazole (*Rochagan*)
Frequent: allergic rash; dose-dependent polyneuropathy; GI disturbances; psychic disturbances.

Bithionol (*Bithin*)
Frequent: photosensitivity skin reactions; vomiting; diarrhea; abdominal pain; urticaria.

Chloroquine (*Aralen*; and others)
Occasional: pruritus; vomiting; headache; confusion; depigmentation of hair; skin eruptions; corneal opacity; irreversible retinal injury (especially when total dosage exceeds 100 g); weight loss; partial alopecia; extraocular muscle palsies; exacerbation of psoriasis; eczema and other exfoliative dermatoses; myalgias.
Rare: discoloration of nails and mucous membranes of mouth; nerve-type deafness; blood discrasias; photophobia.

Crotamiton (*Eurax*; *Crotan*)
Occasional: skin rash; conjunctivitis.

Dehydroemetine
Similar to emetine hydrochloride, but possibly less severe.

Diethylcarbamazine Citrate USP (*Hetrazan*)
Frequent: severe allergic or febrile reactions due to filarial infection; GI disturbances.
Rare: encephalopathy; loss of vision.

Diiodohydroxyquin (*Iodoquinol*)
Occasional: rash; acne; slight enlargement of thyroid gland; nausea; diarrhea; cramps; anal pruritis.
Rare: optic atrophy and loss of vision after prolonged use in high dosage (for months); iodine sensitivity.

Diloxanide Furoate (*Furamide*)
Frequent: flatulence.
Occasional: nausea; vomiting; diarrhea; urticaria; pruritis.

Emetine Hydrochloride USP
Frequent: cardiac arrhythmias; precordial pain; muscle weakness; cellulitis at site of injection.
Occasional: diarrhea; vomiting; peripheral neuropathy; heart failure.

Flubendazole (similar to Mebendazole)

Furazolidone (*Furoxone*)
Frequent: nausea; vomiting.
Occasional: allergic reactions, including pulmonary infiltration; headache; orthostatic hypotension; hypoglycemia; polyneuritis; MAO inhibitor interactions.
Rare: hemolytic anemia in G6PD deficiency in infants less than one month old.

Halofantrine (*Halfan*)
Occasional: diarrhea; abdominal distress; pruritis.

Iodoquinol (*Yodoxin*) (same as diiodohydroxyquin)

Ivermectin (*Mectizan*)
Occasional: Mazzotti-type reaction seen in onchocerciasis, including fever, pruritis, tender lymph nodes, headache, and joint and bone pain.
Rare: hypotension.

Lindane (*Kwell*; *Gamene*)
Occasional: eczematous skin rash; conjunctivitis.
Rare: convulsions; aplastic anemia.

Mebendazole (*Vermox*)
Occasional: diarrhea; abdominal pain.
Rare: leukopenia.

Mefloquine (*Lariam*)
Frequent: vertigo; nausea; other GI disturbances; nightmares; visual disturbances; headache.
Occasional: confusion.
Rare: psychosis; hypotension; convulsions; coma; paresthesia.

Melarsoprol (*Mel B*; *Arsobal*)
Frequent: myocardial damage; albuminuria; hypertension; colic; Herxheimer-type reaction; encephalopathy; vomiting; peripheral neuropathy.
Rare: shock.

Metrifonate (*Bilarcil*)
Occasional: nausea; vomiting; bronchospasm; weakness; diarrhea; abdominal pain.

Metronidazole (*Flagyl*)
Frequent: nausea, especially with single high dose; headache; dry mouth; metallic taste.
Occasional: vomiting; diarrhea; insomnia; weakness; stomatitis; vertigo; paresthesia; rash; urethral burning; phlebitis at injection site.
Rare: ataxia; encephalopathy; pseudomembranous colitis; neutropenia.

Niclosamide (*Nicloside*)
Occasional: nausea; abdominal pain.

Nifurtimox (*Bayer* 2502; *Lampit*)
Frequent: anorexia; vomiting; weight loss; loss of memory; sleep disorders; tremors; paresthesia; weakness; polyneuritis.
Rare: convulsions.

Niridazole (*Ambilhar*)
Frequent: immunosuppression; vomiting; cramps; dizziness; headache.
Occasional: diarrhea; slight ECG changes; rash; insomnia; paresthesia.
Rare: psychosis; hemolytic anemia in G6PD deficiency; convulsions.

Ornidazole (*Tiberal*)
Occasional: dizziness; headache; GI disturbances.
Rare: reversible peripheral neuropathy.

Oxamniquine (*Vansil*)
Occasional: headache; fever; dizziness; somnolence; nausea; diarrhea; rash; insomnia; hepatic enzyme changes; ECG changes.
Rare: convulsions.

Paromycin (*Sulfate Humatin*)
Frequent: GI disturbances.
Rare: eighth nerve damage (mainly auditory); renal damage.

Pentamidine Isethionate (*Pentam* 300*; Lomidine*)
Frequent: hypotension; hypoglycemia; vomiting; blood discrasia; renal damage; pain at injection site.
Occasional: may aggravate diabetes; shock; liver damage.
Rare: Herxheimer-type reaction; acute pancreatitis.

Piperazine Citrate USP (*Antepar*; others)
Occasional: dizziness; urticaria; GI disturbances.
Rare: exacerbation of epilepsy; visual disturbances; ataxia; hypotonia.

Praziquantel (*Biltricide*)
Frequent: sedation; abdominal discomfort; fever; sweating; nausea; eosinophilia.
Occasional: headache; dizziness.

Primaqine Phosphate USP
Frequent: hemolytic anemia in G6PD deficiency.
Occasional: neutropenia; GI disturbances; methemoglobinemia in G6PD deficiency.
Rare: CNS symptoms; hypertension; arrhythmia.

Pyrantel Pamoate (*Antiminth*)
Occasional: GI disturbances; headache; dizziness; rash; fever.

Pyrimethamine USP (*Daraprim*)
Occasional: blood dyscrasias; folic acid deficiency.
Rare: rash; vomiting; convulsions; shock.

Pyrvinium Pamoate USP (*Povan*)
Frequent: red stool.
Occasional: vomiting; diarrhea.
Rare: photosensitivity skin reactions.

Quinicrine Hydrochloride USP (*Atabrine*)
Frequent: dizziness; headache; vomiting; diarrhea; yellow staining of skin.
Occasional: toxic psychosis; insomnia; bizarre dreams; blood dyscrasias; urticaria; blue and black nail pigmentation; psoriasis-like rash.
Rare: acute hepatic necrosis; convulsions; severe exfoliative dermatitis; ocular effects similar to those caused by chloroquine.

Quinine Dihydrochloride and **Quinine Sulfate**
Frequent: cinchonism (tinnitus, headache, nausea, abdominal pain, visual disturbance)
Occasional: hemolytic anemia; other blood dyscrasias; photosensitivity reactions.
Rare: blindness; sudden death if injected too rapidly.

Sodium Stibogluconate (*Pentostam*)
Frequent: muscle pain and joint stiffness; bradycardia.
Occasional: colic; diarrhea; rash; pruritis; myocardial damage.
Rare: liver damage; hemolytic anemia; renal damage; shock; sudden death.

Spiramycin (*Rovamucin*)
Occasional: GI disturbances.
Rare: allergic reactions.

Suramin Sodium (*Germanin*)
Frequent: vomiting; pruritis; urticaria; paresthesia; hyperesthesia of hands and feet; photophobia; peripheral neuropathy.
Occasional: kidney damage; blood dyscrasias; shock; optic atrophy.

Tetrachloroethylene (*Nema Worm Capsules*; *Vet*)
Frequent: epigastric burning; dizziness; headache.
Occasional: drowsiness; Antabuse-like effect with alcohol.
Rare: hepatic necrosis.

Thiabendazole (*Mintezol*)
Frequent: nausea; vomiting; vertigo.
Occasional: leukopenia; cryustalluria; rash; hallucinations; olfactory disturbances; Stevens–Johnson syndrome.
Rare: shock; tinnitus.

Tinidazole *(Fasigyn)*
Occasional: metallic taste; nausea; vomiting; rash.

Tryparsamide
Frequent: nausea; vomiting.
Occasional: impaired vision; optic atrophy; fever; exfoliative dermatitis; allergic reactions; tinnitus.

Glossary

Acquired immunity a host's immune response to a previous infection.

Amastigote a form of hemoflagellate that develops intracellularly, characterized by subspherical shape and the presence of a very short flagellum.

Amphid a small depression or pit located anteriorly on the body surface of most nematodes and believed to be a chemoreceptor.

Anthrax a bacterial disease of humans, cattle, and sheep, transmitted by tabanid flies.

Antibody a protein synthesized in response to an antigen or, in varying degrees, to molecules of similar structure; an antibody usually binds with a specific antigen.

Antigen any substance, usually proteinaceous, capable under appropriate conditions of inducing a host to synthesize antibodies.

Apical complex a combination of structures found in the apical region of sporozoites and merozoites of members of the phylum Apicomplexa.

Apolysis the release of gravid, or egg-filled, proglottids from tapeworm strobila.

Arbovirus a virus transmitted from one human to another by an arthropod.

Autoinfection reinfection by a parasitic organism without its leaving the host.

Axoneme a microtubular element usually extending the length of a flagellum or cilium.

Axostyle a tube-shaped sheath of microtubules observed in many flagellates, that usually extends from a basal body to the posterior end.

B cell a specialized lymphocyte that produces humoral, or circulatory, antibodies.

Basal body an organelle, morphologically identical to a centriole, from which the flagellum or cilium originates.

Biological vector an arthropod used by a disease-producing organism for transmission and as a vehicle for reproduction and/or development.

Blackwater fever massive lysis of vertebrate erythrocytes that, at times, accompanies falciparum malaria.

Blepharophast See *Basal body.*

Bothrium a groove on the scolex of some tapeworms.

Bradyzoite a stage in the life cycle of various coccidia, such as *Toxoplasma*. Similar to a merozoite, it is found in pseudocysts in the tissues of nonfeline hosts.

Breakbone fever an arbovirus-caused disease. See *Dengue.*

Calabar swelling a transient, subcutaneous swelling caused by the nematode *Loa loa.*

Capitulum a small, anterior projection of acarines that bears the mouthparts.

Cell-mediated reaction the effect produced by specialized cells, e.g., T lymphocytes, mobilized to arrest and, in most cases, eventually destroy a parasite.

Cellular reaction See *Cell-mediated reaction.*

Cercocystis a modified cysticercoid larva of *Hymenolepis nana* found in the intestinal villus of the definitive host.

Cercomer the posterior extension of procercoid and cysticercoid larvae, usually retaining the oncospheral hooks.

Chagas' disease a disease, also known as American trypanosomiasis, caused by *Trypanosoma cruzi.*

Chemokine one of a variety of usually glycoprotein molecules of relatively low molecular weight released by or a part of a cell, which have effects on other cells. See *Cytokine.*

Chigger a mite of the family Trombiculidae.

Chromatoidal bar a structure considered by many to be deposits of nucleic acids in members of the genus *Entamoeba.*

Cirrus the penis or ejaculatory duct of a flatworm.

Coenurus a larval tapeworm of certain cyclophyllideans in which numerous scolices bud from an internal germinal epithelium.

Commensalism a symbiotic relationship between two species in which neither species is physiologically dependent upon the other.

Conoid a truncated cone of spirally arranged, fibrillar structures in the apical complex of certain members of the suborder Eimeriina, e.g., *Toxoplasma gondii.*

Coracidium an oncosphere surrounded by a ciliated embryophore.

Corrion's disease a severe, often fatal, bacterial infection found among inhabitants of parts of South America and transmitted by sandflies.

Costa a striated rod, associated with the basal bodies of many flagellates, that courses along the base of an undulating membrane.

Creeping eruption the irritation and rash caused by hookworm larvae in an unnatural host.

Cutaneous larval migrans a condition caused by the migration of nematode larvae in the skin of an unnatural host. See *Creeping eruption.*

Cysticercoid the tapeworm larva, featuring a cercomer and a fully developed scolex enclosed within a multilayered cyst wall, that develops from the oncosphere of some cyclophyllideans.

Cysticercosis infection with cysticercus larvae.

Cysticercus a tapeworm larva, developing from the oncosphere of some cyclophyllideans, that is characterized by a fully developed scolex invaginated into a fluid-filled vesicle, or bladder; also called bladderworm.

Cystogenous glands in some cercariae of digenetic trematodes, secretory cells that give rise to metacercarial cysts.

Cytokine any of several soluble chemical mediators that are secreted by cells and react with other cells.

Definitive host See *Host, definitive.*

Delayed hypersensitivity increased reactivity to a specific antigen, mediated by cells rather than antibodies, usually requiring up to 24 hours to reach maximum intensity. See *T lymphocyte.*

Dengue a disease caused by a mosquito-transmitted virus; also known as blackwater fever.

Ectoparasite a parasite that lives on the exterior surface of the host.

Ectopic site abnormal or unexpected site of infection.

Edema fluid accumulation in intercellular spaces, resulting in localized swelling.

Endoparasite a parasite that lives inside the host.

Epidemiology the study of the occurrence of a particular disease, including ecological factors, transmission, prevalence, and incidence.

Epimastigote a form of hemoflagellate, equipped with a short undulating membrane, in which the kinetoplast lies near but anterior to the nucleus.

Espundia a disease caused by *Leishmania braziliensis*, also known as mucocutaneous leishmaniasis, uta, pian bois, and chiclero ulcer.

Facultative parasite an organism that, given the opportunity, can assume a parasitic existence.

Flagellar pocket a depression in flagellates from which the flagellum emerges.

Flame cell excretory system a protonephridial excretory system with a current-producing mechanism at the closed end.

Gastrodermis the tissue lining the digestive tract, as found in digenetic trematodes.

Genital atrium a circumscribed area in the body wall of flatworms into which male and female genital ducts open; also known as common genital pore.

Germ cell cycle asexual reproduction in digenea during which progeny arise through differentiation of germinal cells passed from one generation to the next.

Glycocalyx the carbohydrate-containing outer coat found on the free surface of most cells.

Glycosome a membrane-bound, microbody-like organelle, peculiar to the hemoflagellates, that contains enzymes essential for glycolysis.

Gonotyl the muscular sucker or specialized structure surrounding the genital pore of some digeneans.

Ground itch a localized irritation and rash caused by penetrating larvae of hookworms and accompanying bacteria.

Gynaecophoric canal the ventral fold or groove in male schistosomes in which female worms are held *in copula.*

Halzoun the disease resulting from nasopharyngeal blockage due to the attachment of worms, such as pentastomids or young digenea, to buccal or pharyngeal membranes.

Hemocoel the major body cavity of arthropods, typically containing hemolymph.

Hemozoin granules, seen in erythrocytes infected with *Plasmodium malariae*, that may represent residues from incomplete hemoglobin digestion.

Heterogonic describing a life cycle in which free-living generations may alternate periodically with parasitic generations.

Homogonic describing a lifestyle that is consistently either parasitic or free living.

Host, definitive the host in which a parasite attains sexual maturity.

Host, intermediate the host in which a parasite undergoes developmental changes but does not yet reach sexual maturity.

Host, paratenic the host in which a parasite resides without further development; a transfer host.

Host, reservoir a host, usually nonhuman, in which a parasite lives and remains a source of infection but usually produces no symptoms.

Host specificity the extent to which a parasite can exist in more than one host species.

Humoral reaction the effect produced when specialized molecules of the circulatory system interact with a parasite, usually immobilizing or destroying it.

Hydatid a larval tapeworm, of the cyclophyllidean genus *Echinococcus*, in which numerous scolices bud from secondary cysts.

Hydrogenosome a membrane-bound organelle in the cytoplasm of some flagellates (e.g., trichomonads) that is involved in carbohydrate metabolism, an end-product of which may be molecular hydrogen.

Hypnozoite the dormant stage of *Plasmodium vivax* and *Plasmodium ovale* in hepatocytes of the human host.

Hypobiosis a lag phase at some stage of development in the life cycle of a nematode.

Hypodermis the tissue that secretes the nematode cuticle.

Infraciliature in a ciliophoran, numerous basal bodies interconnected by fibrils.

Interleukin one of a variety of molecules secreted by leukocytes that affect other leukocytes.

K-strategist an organism employing a survival strategy characterized by low reproductive capability, low mortality, long life span, and saturation of an environment.

Kala-azar a disease, also known as visceral leishmaniasis and dumdum fever, caused by *Leishmania donovani.*

Kinetoplast a portion of the mitochodrion of the Kinetoplastidae containing K-DNA. Usually associated with the kinetosome.

Kinetosome See *Basal body.*

Laurer's canal a canal, originating on the surface of the oviduct near the seminal receptacle in some digenetic trematodes, that may represent a vestigial vagina.

Leishmaniasis a disease caused by members of the genus *Leishmania.*

Lysosomotropic agent one of a group of chemical compounds, such as chloroquine, that demonstrate an affinity for lysosomes.

Macrogametocyte the cell that gives rise to a macrogamete.

Macrophage a large phagocytic cell of the mononuclear leukocyte series.

Macrophage-activating factor one of several cytokines, including interferon, released by T cells which make macrophages more efficient in phagocytosis and cytotoxicity.

Malpighian tubule an excretory organ of terrestrial insects and most acarines.

Maurer's dots aggregates in the cytoplasm of erythrocytes infected with *Plasmodium falciparum.*

Mechanical vector a passive carrier of a disease-producing agent.

Mehlis' gland a group of unicellular glands that empty into the ootype region of flatworms.

Merogony See *Schizogony.*

Merozoite one of many cells resulting from schizogony.

Metacercaria the larval stage between cercaria and adult in the life cycle of many digenetic trematodes.

Metacyclic describing a form of parasite infective to its vertebrate host, e.g., metacyclic trypomastigote.

Metacystic trophozoite a small trophozoite of *Entamoeba* spp. that emerges from the cyst in the intestine of the host.

Metraterm the muscular, distal portion of the uterus of digenetic trematodes.

Microfilaria the juvenile, first-stage larva of filarial nematodes.

Microgametocyte the cell that gives rise to microgametes.

Microneme a small, convoluted structure that lies parallel to rhoptries and appears to merge with them at the apices of sporozoites and merozoites.

Microthrix (plural, *microthrices*) a specialized microvillus that projects from the outer, limiting membrane of the tapeworm tegument.

Miracidium the ciliated larva that emerges from the egg of digenetic trematodes.

Molecular mimicry the production of or covering by hostlike molecules, especially on the body surface of a parasite.

Mutualism a symbiotic relationship in which each partner is physiologically dependent on the other.

Nagana a disease of domestic ruminants, caused by *Trypanosoma brucei brucei, T. congolense*, and *T. vivax*.

Natural immunity the type of immunity conferred by the presence in an organism of certain naturally occurring proteins that exhibit structural properties of antibodies to specific antigens even in the absence of previous exposure to those antigens.

Oncosphere the hexacanth embryo of a tapeworm.

Oocyst a rounded cyst containing sporoblasts.

Ookinete the motile, elongated zygote of many apicomplexans.

Ootype a specialized region of the flatworm oviduct that is surrounded by Mehlis' gland.

Open circulatory system the system, characteristic of arthropods and most molluscs, in which blood flows slowly through large sinuses (the hemocoel) back to a dorsal, tubular heart.

Operculum a lidlike structure at one end of the eggshell of many digenetic trematodes and some cestodes.

Oriental sore a disease, also known as cutaneous leishmaniasis, caused by *Leishmania tropica.*

Parabasal body the Golgi complex of protozoans.

Parabasal filament a fibril running from the cisternae of the Golgi complex to one or more basal bodies.

Parasitism a symbiotic relationship in which only one of the organisms, the parasite, is physiologically dependent upon the other, the host.

Parasitophorus vacuole within a cell, a vacuole containing a parasite (e.g., an amastigote).

Paratenic host See *Host, paratenic.*

Parenchyma in flatworms, mesodermal tissue filling all available body spaces.

Parthenogenesis development of an unfertilized egg into a new individual.

Phasmid a small, sensory pit, believed to be a chemoreceptor, located posteriorly on the body surface of members of the nematode class Secernentea.

Phoresis a nonobligatory form of commensalism in which one organism is mechanically carried by the other.

Plasma cell an effector B cell that secretes into the circulation large numbers of antibodies of the same specificity as its cell surface receptors.

Plerocercoid the larval form that develops from the procercoid, as in *Diphyllobothrium latum.*

Polar rings electron-dense structures, circling the apical region, that constitute part of the apical complex of sporozoites and merozoites of apicomplexans such as *Plasmodium* spp.

Polyembryony the formation of multiple embryos from a single zygote with no intervening gamete stage.

Premunition a form of acquired immunity dependent upon retention of the infective agent.

Procercoid the larval form that develops from the coracidium.

Proglottid one segment in a tapeworm strobila complete with a full complement of reproductive organs.

Promastigote a hemoflagellate form bearing an anterior flagellum and a kinetoplast well anterior to the nucleus.

Protandrogony initial maturation of male organs which subsequently disappear, followed by maturation of female organs in hermaphroditic organisms. Also termed *Protandry*.

Protoscolex the immature scolex found in coenurus and hydatid larvae.

Pseudocyst a cluster of amastigotes of *Trypanosoma cruzi* in a muscle fiber.

r-strategist an organism employing a survival strategy characterized by high reproductive rates, high mortality, and short life span.

Receptor cell a functionally specialized lymphocyte that produces a specific antibody.

Recrudescence a sudden increase in a previously persistent, low-level parasite population (e.g., *Plasmodium malariae*).

Redia a larval form that arises asexually from within a sporocyst or a primary redia of a digenetic trematode.

Renette a large, unicellular gland that empties to the exterior through a pore and serves as the basic component of the nematode excretory system.

Reservoir host See *Host, reservoir.*

Resistance the ability of an organism to withstand infection.

Retroinfection reinfection by nematode larvae (e.g., *Enterobius vermicularis*) that hatch on skin and reenter the host's body.

Rhoptry part of the apical complex of the sporozoites and merozoites of apicomplexans, composed of electron-dense bodies extending posteriorly from the apex.

Romano's sign early symptoms of Chagas' disease, consisting of unilateral, periorbital edema and conjunctivitis.

Rostellum the small, rounded projection, sometimes bearing hooks, on the apex of the scolex of some tapeworms.

Schüffner's dots fine granules distributed throughout erythrocytes infected with *Plasmodium vivax.*

Schistosomule in a blood fluke, the juvenile stage that develops following cercarial penetration of the definitive host. Sometimes called a schistosomulum.

Schizogony a form of asexual reproduction characterized by rapid organellar and nuclear divisions, followed by cytoplasmic divisions, resulting simultaneously in many daughter cells (e.g., merozoites).

Schizont a multinucleated cell undergoing schizogony, prior to cytoplasmic division.

Scolex the holdfast organ of tapeworms.

Scrub typhus rickettsial disease transmitted by chigger mites.

Shell–yolk gland a cluster of cells that synthesizes globules essential to eggshell formation in many flatworms.

Sleeping sickness a disease caused by *Trypanosoma brucei rhodesiense* and *T. b. gambiense* in Africa.

Sparganosis infection with plerocercoid larvae.

Sporoblast in the oocyst of apicomplexans, a cell that divides into sporozoites while still enclosed by the sporoblast membrane.

Sporocyst the larval stage of a digenetic trematode into which the miracidium metamorphoses, usually in a mollusc.

Sporogony multiple divisions of a zygote.

Stichocyte one of a series of unicellular glands surrounding the capillary-like esophagus of many adenophorean nematodes, e.g., *Trichuris trichiura.*

Strobila in tapeworms, a chain of segments formed by budding.

Strobilization the formation of a strobila by a tapeworm.

Sylvatic animal an animal that lives in the wild.

Syngamy the union of gametes.

T lymphocyte a specialized lymphocyte, processed through the thymus, that elicits cell-mediated reactions.

Tachyzoite a form of merozoite in *Toxoplasma*, found in parasitophorous vacuoles of vertebrate hosts.

Tegument the syncytium that covers the surface of trematodes and cestodes.

Trophozoite the motile, feeding stage of protozoans.

Trypomastigote a hemoflagellate form with an elongated undulating membrane and kinetoplast located posterior to the nucleus.

Tularemia a bacterial disease of humans transmitted by tabanid flies and for which rabbits often serve as sylvatic reservoir hosts.

Undulating membrane that portion of the plasma membrane or cytoplasm of a flagellate that is drawn away from the cell during the beating of a recurrent flagellum.

Vagina in tapeworms, a tubular organ that joins the oviduct and carries sperm from the genital atrium to the oviduct.

Variant antigenic type one of a set of divergent surface antigens that arise as the result of the ability of trypomastigote populations circulating in the bloodstream to change the chemical composition of their glycocalyces.

Vector any agent, most commonly an arthropod, that actively transmits a disease-producing organism.

Vermicle the infective stage, analogous to a sporozoite, of *Babesia* spp. transmitted by ticks.

Visceral larval migrans migration of second-stage larvae of nematodes in the internal organs of unnatural hosts.

Vitellaria See *Shell–yolk gland.*

Winterbottom's sign symptom of African sleeping sickness characterized by enlarged, sensitive cervical lymph nodes.

Xenodiagnosis diagnostic technique in which researchers identify a disease by infecting a laboratory animal and assessing its symptoms.

Yaws a fly-transmitted disease that is caused by the spirochete *Treponema.*

Yellow fever a viral disease transmitted by the mosquito *Aedes aegypti.*

Zoonosis any disease of animals that can be transmitted to humans.

Photo and Illustration Credits

Chapter 1

Fig. 1-1 From Thomas Cheng, 1986, *General Parasitology,* 2nd ed. Adapted with permission of Academic Press. **Fig. 1-2** Adapted with permission of Bobbs-Merrill Co., an imprint of Macmillan Publishing Company, from *Symbiosis: Organisms Living Together* by Thomas C. Cheng. Copyright © 1986 by Macmillan Publishing Company.

Chapter 2

Fig. 2-2 Adapted from E. B. Sandborn, 1972, *Light and Electron Microscopy of Cells and Tissues,* with permission of Academic Press, Orlando, FL.

Chapter 3

Fig. 3-2 Reproduced from I. R. Gibbons and A. V. Grimstone in *Journal of Biophysical/Biochemical Cytology*, 1960, 7, by copyright permission of The Rockefeller University Press. **Fig. 3-3** THE CELL 5/E. by SWANSON/WEBSTER, © 1985, p. 215. Reprinted by permission of Prentice-Hall, Inc., Upper Saddle River, NJ. **Fig. 3-4** From Cleveland P. Hickman, Jr., Larry S. Roberts, and Frances M. Hickman, 1988, *Integrated Principles of Zoology,* 8th ed., St. Louis: © 1988 Times Mirror/Mosby College Publishing. Reproduced with permission of The McGraw-Hill Companies. Original artwork by William C. Ober, M.D. **Fig. 3-5** Photo courtesy of Dr. Keith Vickerman, University of Glasgow. **Fig. 3-6** THE CELL 5/E. by SWANSON/WEBSTER, © 1985, p. 216. Reprinted by permission of Prentice-Hall, Inc., Upper Saddle River, NJ. **Fig. 3-7** From *Cells and Organelles,* 2nd ed., by Alex B. Novikoff and Eric Holtzman, copyright © 1976 by Holt, Rinehart and Winston, Inc., reproduced by permission of the publisher. **Fig. 3-9** © Don Fawcett/Photo Researchers, Inc. **Fig. 3-10** © Don Fawcett/Photo Researchers, Inc. **Fig. 3-11** Photos courtesy of Dr. M. Aikawa, Case Western Reserve University, School of Medicine, reproduced from M. Aikawa, P. K. Hepler, C. G. Huff, and H. Sprintz, *The Journal of Cell Biology,* 1966, 28,362, by copyright permission of The Rockefeller University Press.

Chapter 4

Fig. 4-3 Armed Forces Institute of Pathology, Negative No. 74-2981. **Fig. 4-4** © Institut Pasteur/Phototake, NYC. **Fig. 4-9a,b,c** Adapted from *Introduction to Animal Parasitology,* 1994, 3rd ed., by J. D. Smyth, Cambridge University Press, Cambridge and New York. **Fig. 4-9d** Photo courtesy, Dr. Lawrence Ash, University of California, Los Angeles, School of Public Health. **Fig. 4-10a,b,c** Adapted from *Introduction to Animal Parasitology,* 1994, 3rd ed., by J. D. Smyth, Cambridge University Press, Cambridge and New York. **Fig. 4-10d** © Phototake, NYC. **Fig. 4-11** From Thomas Cheng, 1986, *General Parasitology,* 2nd ed. Adapted with permission of Academic Press.

Chapter 5

Fig. 5-2a, b Photos courtesy of Dennis E. Feeley, University of Nebraska Medical Center, Lincoln, and Stanley L. Erlandsen, University of Minnesota, School of Medicine. Reprinted from *Parasitology Today,* 4(3), W. J. Bemrick and S. L. Erlandsen, "Giardiasis: Is it really zoonosis?" pp. 69–71. Copyright 1988 with permission of Elsevier Science. **Fig. 5-2c** Photo courtesy of Dr. Robert L. Owen, University of California, San Francisco, Veterans Administration Medical Center, reprinted from *Journal of Infectious Diseases,* **140**:222–228, by P. C. Nemanic, R. L. Owen, D. P. Stevens, and J. C. Mueller, by permission of The University of Chicago Press, © 1979 The University of Chicago. **Fig. 5-7** Reprinted with permission from D. R. Pitelka, *Electron Microscope Structure of Protozoa,* copyright © 1963, Pergamon Press PLC.

Chapter 6

Fig. 6-2 Adapted from *Introduction to Animal Parasitology,* 1994, 3rd ed., by J. D. Smyth, Cambridge University Press, Cambridge and New York. **Fig. 6-3** Adapted from *Introduction to Animal Parasitology,* 1994, 3rd ed., by J. D. Smyth, Cambridge University Press, Cambridge and New York. **Fig. 6-4** From A. M. Fallis (ed.), 1971, *Ecology and Physiology of Parasites,* p. 75. Adapted by permission of the University of Toronto Press. **Fig. 6-5** Adapted by permission of Dr. Keith Vickerman, University of Glasgow. **Fig. 6-6** From Keith Vickerman, 1971, "Morphological and physiological considerations of extra-cellular blood protozoa," in A. M. Fallis (ed.), 1971, *Ecology and Physiology of Parasites,* Fig. 13, p. 75. Adapted by permission of the University of Toronto Press and the author. **Fig. 6-8** Adapted from *Introduction to Animal Parasitology,* 1994, 3rd ed., by J. D. Smyth, Cambridge University Press, Cambridge and New York. **Fig. 6-9** © James Webb/Phototake, NYC. **Fig. 6-10** © Institut Pasteur/ Phototake, NYC. **Fig 6-11** Adapted from *Rockefeller Foundation Illustrated,* 4(1), April 1978, by permission of The Rockefeller Foundation. **Fig. 6-12** Reprinted with the permission of Carolina Biological Supply Company, Burlington, NC 27215. **Fig. 6-13** Adapted from *Rockefeller Foundation Illustrated,* 4(1), April 1978, by permission of The Rockefeller Foundation. **Fig. 6-14** From K. Vickerman and J. D. Barry, 1982,"African trypanosomiasis," in S. Conen and K. S. Warren (eds.), *Immunology of Parasitic Infections,* 2nd ed., p. 210, Oxford: Blackwell Scientific Publications. Courtesy of K. Vickerman. **Fig. 6-15** After E. J. A. Brumpt, 1910, *Precis de Parasitologie.* Adapted with permission of MASSON, Paris. **Fig. 6-17** Courtesy, Dr. Julius P. Kreier, Department of Microbiology, Ohio State University.

Chapter 7

Fig. 7-2 Photos courtesy of M. Aikawa. Reproduced from *The Journal of Cell Biology,* 1981, **91**, p. 56, by copyright permission of The Rockefeller Uinversity Press. **Fig. 7-3** Photos courtesy of Dr. M. Aikawa, Case Western Reserve University, School of Medicine, reproduced from M. Aikawa et al., "Erythrocyte entry by malarial parasites: A moving juncture between erythrocyte and parasite," *The Journal of Cell Biology,* 1978, **77**:75, by copyright permission of The Rockefeller University Press. **Fig. 7-4** Photos courtesy of Dr. M. Aikawa, Case Western Reserve University, School of Medicine, from M. Aikawa et al., 1966, "Comparative feeding mechanisms of avian and primate malarial parasites," in Research in Malaria: An International Panel Workshop, Contribution #95, from Army Research Program on Malaria, *Military Medicine: The Official Journal of AMSUS.* **131**(9):969–983, Supplement September 1966. **Fig. 7-5** From "Epidemiological assessment of malaria and chloroquine resistance, 1986," *World Health Statistics Quarterly,* 1988, **41**(2):69–71. Adapted with permission of the World Health Organization. **Fig. 7-7** Photo courtesy of Dr. M. Aikawa, Case Western Reserve University, School of Medicine, from M. Aikawa *et al.* (1983), *J. Parasitol.* **69**(2), 435–437, with permission.

Chapter 8

Fig. 8-3 From E. Scholtyseck, 1979, *Fine Structure of Parasitic Protozoa: An Atlas of Micrographs, Drawings and Diagrams,* Springer-Verlag, New York. Adapted with permission of the publisher. **Fig. 8-4** Adapted from Y. Matsumoto and Y. Yoshida, *Parasitology Today,* **2**(5), "Advances in *Pneumocystis* biology," pp. 137–142, Copyright 1986, with permission of Elsevier Science Publishers. **Fig. 8-5** From M. P. Goheen et al. 1991. The effect of primaquine on the ultrastructural morphology of *Pneumocystis carinii, Journal of Protozoology* **38**:164S. Copied with permission of the *Journal of Protozoology.* **Fig. 8-6** From M. P. Goheen et al. 1991. The effect of primaquine on the ultrastructural morphology of *Pneumocystis carinii, Journal of Protozoology* **38**:1645. Copied with permission of the *Journal of Protozoology.* **Fig. 8-7** From E. Dei-Cas et al. 1991. Ultrastructural observations on the attachment of *Pneumocystis carinii* in vitro. *Journal of Protozoology* **38**:205S. Copied with permission of the *Journal of Protozoology.* **Fig. 8-9** From T. Aji et al. 1991. Ultrastructural study of asexual development of *Cryptosporidium parvum* in a human intestinal cell line. *Journal of Protozoology* **38**:83S. Copied with permission of the *Journal of Protozoology.* **Fig. 8-10** From T. Aji et al. 1991. Ultrastructural study of asexual development of *Cryptosporidium parvum* in a human intestinal cell line. *Journal of Protozoology* **38**:83S. Copied with permission of the *Journal of Protozoology.*

Chapter 9

Fig. 9-2 Courtesy, Dr. Burton J. Bogitsh. **Fig. 9-4** Courtesy, Dr. Burton J. Bogitsh. **Fig. 9-5** Courtesy, Dr. Burton J. Bogitsh. **Fig. 9-6** From Thomas Cheng, 1986, *General Parasitology,* 2nd ed. Adapted with permission of Academic Press. **Fig. 9-7** Courtesy, Dr. Burton J. Bogitsh. **Fig. 9-8** From Asa C. Chandler and Clark P. Read, 1961, *Introduction to Parasitology,* 10th ed. Copyright © 1930, 1936, 1940, 1944, 1949 by Asa C. Chandler. Copyright © 1955, 1961 by John Wiley & Sons, Inc. All rights reserved. **Fig. 9-9** From Thomas Cheng, 1986, *General Parasitology,* 2nd ed. Adapted with permission of Academic Press. **Fig. 9-10** From Thomas Cheng, 1986, *General Parasitology,* 2nd ed. Adapted with permission of Academic Press. **Fig. 9-13** Courtesy, Dr. Burton J. Bogitsh. **Fig. 9-14** Courtesy, Dr. Burton J. Bogitsh. **Fig. 9-15a** From Thomas Cheng, 1986, *General Parasitology,* 2nd ed. Adapted with permission of Academic Press. **Fig. 9-15b** Courtesy, Dr. Burton J. Bogitsh. **Fig. 9-16a, b, c, e** © Phototake, NYC. **Fig. 9-16d** © Camera M. D. Studios, 1989. All rights reserved. **Fig. 9-16f** © John Durham/Science Photo Library/Photo Researchers, Inc. **Fig. 9-18** D. L. Belding, *Textbook of Parasitology,* 3rd ed., copyright © 1965. Reprinted by permission of Appleton-Century-Crofts, Norwalk, CT. **Fig. 9-21** Redrawn after T. C. Cheng and H. A. James, 1960, *Transactions of the American Microscopical Society.* Adapted with permission of the American Microscopical Society. **Fig. 9-23** Courtesy, Dr. Burton J. Bogitsh. **Fig. 9-24** From E. A. Meuleman et al, 1978,"Ultrastructural changes in the body wall of *Schistosoma mansoni* during the transformation of the mother sporocyst in the snail host, *Biophalaria pfeifferi,*" *Parasitology Research,* **56**:227–242. Copyright © 1978, Springer-Verlag, New York. Adapted by permission of the publisher.

Chapter 10

Fig. 10-1a Supplied by Carolina Biological Supply Company. **Fig. 10-1b** Courtesy, Dr. Lawrence Ash, University of California, Los Angeles, School of Public Health. **Fig. 10-2** Reprinted with permission of Macmillan Publishing Company from *Principles of Parasitology* by W. C. Marquardt and R. S. Demaree. Copyright © 1986 by William C. Marquardt and Richard S. Demaree. **Fig. 10-3** From H. Yoshimura, 1965, "The life cycle of *Clonorchis sinensis:* A comment on the presentation in the Seventh Edition of Craig and Faust's *Clinical Parasitology,*" *Journal of Parasitology,* **51**:961–966. **Fig. 10-4** Supplied by Carolina Biological Supply Company. **Fig. 10-5** Reprinted with permission of Macmillan Publishing Company from *Principles of Parasitology* by W. C. Marquardt and R. S. Demaree. Copyright © 1986 by William C. Marquardt and Richard S. Demaree. **Fig. 10-7** Redrawn after Monnig, 1934, *Veterinary Helminthology and Entomology,* as adapted in Thomas Cheng, 1986, *General Parasitology,* 2nd ed. Adapted with permission of Academic Press. **Fig. 10-8a** From Thomas Cheng, 1986, *General Parasitology,* 2nd ed. Adapted with permission of Academic Press. **Fig. 10-8b** After R. T. Leiper, 1913, *Transactions of the Royal Society of Tropical Medicine & Hygiene,* London. Adapted by permission of the Royal Society of Tropical Medicine & Hygiene. **Fig. 10-11a** © Bruce Iverson. **Fig. 10-11b** From Thomas Cheng, 1986, *General Parasitology,* 2nd ed. Reproduced with permission of Academic Press.

Chapter 11

Fig. 11-1 From *The Control of Schistosomiasis: Second Report of the WHO Expert Committee,* Geneva, World Health Organization, 1993, WHO Technical Report Series, No. 830. **Fig. 11-3** Courtesy, Dr. Ming Ming Wong, University of California, San Francisco, School of Medicine. **Fig. 11-5** © Bruce Iverson. **Fig. 11-6** H. W. Brown and F. A. Neva, *Basic Clinical Parasitology,* 5th ed., copyright © 1983. Reprinted by permission of Appleton-Century-Crofts, Norwalk, CT. **Fig. 11-7** Courtesy, Dr. Burton J. Bogitsh. **Fig. 11-8a** H. W. Brown and F. A. Neva, *Basic Clinical Parasitology,* 5th ed., copyright © 1983. Reprinted by permission of Appleton-Century-Crofts, Norwalk, CT. **Fig. 11-8b** From Thomas Cheng, 1986, *General Parasitology,* 2nd ed. Adapted with permission of Academic Press. **Fig. 11-10** H. W. Brown and F. A. Neva, *Basic Clinical Parasitology,* 5th ed., copyright © 1983. Reprinted by permission of Appleton-Century-

Crofts, Norwalk CT. **Fig. 11-11** © Camera M. D. Studios, 1989. All rights reserved.

Chapter 12

Fig. 12-2 © Bruce Iverson. **Fig. 12-3a** From E. Loser, 1965, "Die Eibildug bei Cestoden," *Zeischrift fur Parasitenkunde,* **25**:556–80. Copyright © 1985, Springer-Verlag, Heidelberg. Adapted with permission of the publisher. **Fig. 12-6** From Thomas Cheng, 1986, *General Parasitology,* 2nd ed. Adapted with permission of Academic Press. **Fig. 12-11** From E. Loser, 1965, "Die Eibildug bei Cestoden," *Zeitschrift fur Parasitenkunde,* **25**:556–580. Copyright © 1985, Springer-Verlag, Heidelberg. Adapted with permission of the publisher. **Fig. 12-13** © Bruce Iverson.

Chapter 13

Fig. 13-8 From Asa C. Chandler and Clark P. Read, 1961, *Introduction to Parasitology,* 10th ed. Copyright © 1930, 1936, 1940, 1944, 1949 by Asa C. Chandler. Copyright © 1955, 1961 by John Wiley & Sons, Inc. All rights reserved.

Chapter 14

Fig. 14-1 Photo courtesy, Formosan Medical Association, Taiwan, Republic of China, from Wang and Cross, 1974, *Journal of the Formosan Medical Association,* 73:173–77. **Fig. 14-2** © Bruce Iverson. **Fig. 14-3a** Photo by Dr. Warren Buss, provided courtesy of Dr. Gerald D. Schmidt, University of Northern Colorado, from Gerald D. Schmidt and Larry S. Roberts, 1985, *Foundations of Parasitology,* 3rd ed., St. Louis, copyright © 1985, Times Mirror/Mosby College Publishing. Reproduced with permission of The McGraw-Hill Companies. **Fig. 14-3b** Photo courtesy, Dr. A. Flissner, Ciudad Universitaria, Instituto de Investigaciones Biomedicas, from chapter by Dr. Genaro Horacio-Zenteno-Alanis in A. Flissner (ed.), 1982, *Cysticercosis: Present State of Knowledge and Perspectives.* Reproduced with permission of Academic Press. **Fig. 14-4** Adapted from Frank A. Brown (ed.), 1950, *Selected Invertebrate Types,* copyright © 1950 by John Wiley & Sons, Inc. All rights reserved. **Fig. 14-5** Adapted from *Parasitology Today,* **2**(6), D. P. McManus and J. D. Smyth, "Hydatidosis: Changing concepts in epidemiology and speciation," pp. 163–168, Copyright 1986, with permission of Elsevier Science. **Fig. 14-6** Adapted from Frank A. Brown (ed.), 1950, *Selected Invertebrate Types,* copyright © 1950 by John Wiley & Sons, Inc. All rights reserved. **Fig. 14-7** Adapted from *Parasitology Today,* **2**(6), D. P. McManus and J. D. Smyth, "Hydatidosis: Changing concepts in epidemiology and speciation," pp. 163–168, Copyright 1986, with permission of Elsevier Science. **Fig. 14-8** Photos by Dr. Calum McPherson, provided courtesy of Dr. D. P. McManus, Imperial College of Science and Technology, London. Adapted from *Parasitology Today,* **2**(6), D. P. McManus and J. D. Smyth, "Hydatidosis: Changing concepts in epidemiology and speciation," pp. 163–168, Copyright 1986, with permission of Elsevier Science.

Chapter 15

Fig. 15-1 Reprinted with permission of Macmillan Publishing Company from *Introduction to Parasitology* by W. C. Marquardt and R. S. Demaree. Copyright © 1986 by William C. Marquardt and Richard S. Semaree. **Fig. 15-2** Photo courtesy, Dr. Don L. Lee, University of Leeds, UK, from Don L. Lee, 1977, *Comparative Biology of Skin,* Zoological Society of London Symposia, Vol. **39**:150. **Fig. 15-3** From Thomas Cheng, 1986, *General Parasitology,* 2nd ed. Adapted with permission of Academic Press. **Fig. 15-4** From Thomas Cheng, 1986, *General Parasitology,* 2nd ed. Adapted with permission of Academic Press. **Fig. 15-6** Reproduced from J. Rosenbluth, *The Journal of Cell Biology,* 1965, **26**:580, by copyright permission of The Rockefeller University Press. **Fig. 15-7** Adapted from *Introduction to Animal Parasitology,* 1994, 3rd ed., by J. D. Smyth, Cambridge University Press, Cambridge and New York. **Fig. 15-8a,b** From H. D. Crofton, 1966, *Nematodes,* Hutchinson University Library, published by Unwin Hyman, Ltd., London. Adapted by permission of the publisher. **Fig. 15-8c** From Thomas Cheng, 1986, *General Parasitology,* 2nd ed. Adapted by permissin of Academic Press. **Fig. 15-9** From F. G. W. Jones, 1959, *Plant Pathology: Problems and Progress 1908–1958,* © 1959 University of Wisconsin Press. Adapted with permission of the publisher. **Fig. 15-10** Adapted from *Introduction to Animal Parasitology,* 1994, 3rd ed., by J. D. Smyth, Cambridge University Press, Cambridge and New York. **Fig. 15-11a** After S. Vottenlogel, 1902, *Zoologische Jahrbeucher Abteilung Anat.* Adapted with permission of VEB Gustav Fischer Verlag, DDR. **Fig. 15-11b, c** After J. G. de Man, 1907, *Memoires de la Société Zoologique de France.* Adapted with permission of the Société Zoologique de France. **Fig. 15-13a, b, e** © Bruce Iverson. **Fig. 15-13c** © Martin Rotker/Phototake, NYC. **15-13d** Courtesy, Dr. Lawrence Ash, University of California, Los Angeles, School of Public Health. **Fig. 15-13f** ©

ames Webb/Phototake, NYC. ʼig. **15-14** From Don L. Lee, 1965, *The Physiology of Nematodes.* \dapted with permission of Oliver and Boyd, Publishers, London. ʼig. **15-15** From Thomas Cheng, 1986, *General Parasitology,* 2nd ed. \dapted with permission of \cademic Press.

ʒhapter 16

ʼig. **16-1** H. W. Brown and F. A. Neva, *Basic Clinical Parasitology,* 5th ed., copyright © 1983. Reprinted by permission of \ppleton-Century-Crofts, Norwalk, CT. **Fig. 16-3** Adapted from *ntroduction to Parasitology,* 1994, 3rd ed., by J. D. Smyth, Cambridge Jniversity Press, Cambridge and New York. **Fig. 16-5a** © Dickson Despommier/Photo Researchers, nc. **Fig. 16-5b** From Thomas Cheng, 1986, *General Parasitology,* 2nd ed. Adapted with permission of \cademic Press. **Fig. 16-6** After E. W. Faust, 1949, *Human Helminthology: A Manual for Physicians, Sanitarians and Medical Zoologists.* Adapted with permission from Kimpton Medical Publications, London. **Fig. 16-11** © James Webb/Phototake, NYC. **Fig. 16-12** Adapted from *Introduction to Parasitology,* 1994 3rd ed., by J. D. Smyth, Cambridge University Press, Cambridge and New York. **Fig. 16-14** Courtesy, Dr. Burton J. Bogitsh. **Fig. 16-15** © Camera M. D. Studios. All rights reserved. **Fig. 16-16** Reprinted with permission of Macmillan Publishing Company from *Invertebrate Zoology Laboratory Workbook,* 3rd ed., by D. E. Beck And L. F. Braithwaite. Copyright © 1968 by Macmillan Publishing Company. **Fig. 16-17** Reprinted with permission of Macmillan Publishing Company from *Introduction to Parasitology* by W. C. Marquardt and R. S. Demaree. Copyright © 1986 by William C. Marquardt and Richard S. Demaree. **Fig. 16-18** © Phtotake, NYC.

Chapter 17

Fig. 17-2 © Institut Pasteur/ Phototake, NYC. **Fig. 17-3** Reprinted with permission of Macmillan Publishing Company from *Introduction to Parasitology* by W. C. Marquardt and R. S. Demaree. Copyright © 1986 by William C. Marquardt and Richard S. Demaree. **Fig. 17-4a** © Bruce Iverson. **Fig. 17-4b** Armed Forces Institute of Pathology, Negative No. 68–7638–3. **Fig. 17-5** Armed Forces Institute of Pathology, Negative No. 67–5368–1. **Fig. 17-6** © Phototake, NYC.

Chapter 18

Fig. 18-1 (top) Courtesy, National Center for Communicable Diseases, U.S. Public Health Service, Atlanta, GA. **Fig. 18-1** (bottom) From Thomas Cheng, 1986, *General Parasitology,* 2nd ed. Adapted with permission of Academic Press. **Fig. 18-4b** From Thomas Cheng, 1986, *General Parasitology,* 2nd ed. Adapted with permission of Academic Press. **Fig. 18-4c** Adapted from C. L. Metcalf and W. P. Flint, 1962, *Destructive and Useful Insects,* with permission of The McGraw-Hill Companies, New York. **Fig. 18-5** After R. E. Snodgrass, *Smithsonian Miscellaneous Collection 110,* Number 10, Fig. 2.7. Reprinted by permission of the Smithsonian Institution Press. **Fig. 18-6** From Thomas Cheng, 1986, *General Parasitology,* 2nd ed. Adapted with permission of Academic Press. **Fig. 18-7** From Thomas Cheng, 1986, *General Parasitology,* 2nd ed. Adapted with permission of Academic Press. **Fig. 18-8** Courtesy, National Center for Communicable Diseases, U.S. Public Health Service, Atlanta, GA. **Fig. 18-9** © 1986 L. West/Photo Researchers Inc. **Fig. 18-10a, d** From Thomas Cheng, 1986, *General Parasitology,* 2nd ed. Adapted with permission of Academic Press. **Fig. 18-10** From W. Byam and R. G. Archibald, 1921–23, *The Practice of Medicine in the Tropics,* Hodder & Stoughton, N. Pomfret, VT. **Fig. 18-11a** Adapted from Robert Matheson, 1950, *Medical Entomology,* 2nd ed. Copyright © 1950 by Comstock Publishing Company, Inc. Used by permission of the publisher, Cornell University Press. **Fig. 18-11b, c** From Thomas Cheng, 1986, *General Parasitology,* 2nd ed. Adapted with permission of Academic Press. **Fig. 18-12** Armed Forces Institute of Pathology, Negative No. 75–5783. **Fig. 18-13a** Adapted from E. Francis, 1919, *Public Health Reports,* U.S. Department of Health and Human Services. **Fig. 18-13b** From Thomas Cheng, 1986, *General Parasitology,* 2nd ed. Adapted with permission of Academic Press. **Fig. 18-14a, c** From Thomas Cheng, 1986, *General Parasitology,* 2nd ed. Adapted with permission of Academic Press. **Fig. 18-14b** After E. A. Brumpt, 1910, *Precis de Parasitologie,* adapted with permission of MASSON, Paris. **Fig. 18-15** Armed Forces Institute of Pathology, Negative No. 65–5015. **Fig. 18-16** Courtesy, National Center for Communicable Diseases, U.S. Public Health Service, Atlanta, GA. **Fig. 18-17** Adapted from G. T. Strickland, *Hunter's Tropical Medicine,* 6th ed., copyright © 1984 by Saunders College Publishing, a division of Holt, Rinehart and Winston, Inc., reproduced by permission of the publisher. **Fig. 18-18** From A. W. Bacot and C. S. Martin, 1914, *Journal of Hygiene, Epidemiology, Microbiology and Immunology.* Adapted with permission of Karger Libri AG, Basel, Switzerland. **Fig. 18-19** Armed Forces Insititute of Pathology, Negative No. 219900–7B. **Fig. 18-20** © Institut Pasteur/Phototake, NYC. **Fig. 18-21a, b** From D. Keilin and G. H. F. Nuttall, 1930, *Parasitology.* Adapted with permission of Cambridge University Press, Cambridge, U.K. **Fig. 18-21c** From Thomas Cheng, 1986, *General Parasitology,* 2nd ed. Adapted with permission of Academic Press. **Fig. 18-22** From James R. Busvine, 1975, *Arthropod Vectors of Disease,* Studies in Biology, No. 55, Edward Arnold Publishers, London. Adapted with permission of the author. **Fig. 18-23** © Alfred Pasieka/Bruce Coleman, Inc. **Fig. 18-24** From James R. Busvine, 1975, *Arthropod Vectors of Disease,* Studies in Biology, No. 55, Edward Arnold Publishers, London. Adapted with permission of the author.

Color Section

Reproduced by permission of WHO, from *Bench Aids for the Diagnosis of Malaria,* Geneva, World Health Organization, 1988.

Index

References to photographs and illustrations are printed in boldface type.

D

E

Q

R